ILLUSTRATED VETERINARY PATHOLOGY
(General & Systemic Pathology)

A widely preferred text book of Veterinary Pathology for second year
BVSc & AH students under Veterinary Council of India (VCI) Syllabus

Prof. R.S. Chauhan

M.V.Sc., Ph.D. (Path.), FNAVS, FSIIP, FIAVP
Joint Director (CADRAD)
Centre for Animal Disease Research and Diagnosis
Indian Veterinary Research Institute
Izatnagar - 243 122 Bareilly, U.P. India
E-mail : rs_chauhan123@rediffmail.com

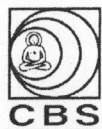

CBS

CBS Publishers & Distributors Pvt. Ltd.

New Delhi • Bengaluru • Chennai • Kochi • Kolkata • Mumbai
Hyderabad • Nagpur • Patna • Pune • Vijayawada

Illustrated Veterinary Pathology
(General & Systemic Pathology)

ISBN: 978-93-85915-88-8

First CBS Reprint: 2016

Published by:
Satish Kumar Jain for CBS Publishers & Distributors Pvt. Ltd.,
4819/XI Prahlad Street, 24 Ansari Road, Daryaganj, New Delhi - 110002
delhi@cbspd.com, cbspubs@airtelmail.in • www.cbspd.com
Ph.: 23289259, 23266861, 23266867 • Fax: 011-23243014

Corporate Office: 204 FIE, Industrial Area, Patparganj, Delhi - 110 092
Ph: 49344934 • Fax: 011-49344935
E-mail: publishing@cbspd.com • publicity@cbspd.com

Branches:
- *Bengaluru:* 2975, 17th Cross, K.R. Road, Bansankari 2nd Stage, Bengaluru - 70 • Ph: +91-80-26771678/79 • Fax: +91-80-26771680 E-mail: cbsbng@gmail.com, bangalore@cbspd.com
- *Chennai:* No. 7, Subbaraya Street, Shenoy Nagar, Chennai - 600030 Ph: +91-44-26681266, 26680620 • Fax: +91-44-42032115 E-mail: chennai@cbspd.com
- *Kochi:* Ashana House, 39/1904, A.M. Thomas Road, Valanjambalam, Ernakulum, Kochi • Ph: +91-484-4059061-65 Fax: +91-484-4059065 • E-mail: cochin@cbspd.com
- *Kolkata:* 6-B, Ground Floor, Rameshwar Shaw Road, Kolkata - 700014 Ph: +91-33-22891126/7/8 • E-mail: kolkata@cbspd.com
- *Mumbai:* 83-C, Dr. E. Moses Road, Worli, Mumbai - 400018 Ph: +91-9833017933, 022-24902340/41 • E-mail: mumbai@cbspd.com

Representatives:

- Hyderabad: 0-9885175004
- Patna: 0-9334159340
- Vijayawada: 0-9000660880
- Nagpur: 0-9021734563
- Pune: 0-9623451994

Printed at:
India Binding House, Noida (UP)

FOREWORD TO THE FIRST EDITION

The past few decades have seen a tremendous change in concepts of livestock and poultry diseases, many new diseases being added up. The large quantity of information unearthed, most coming in small analytical bits, undigested and unrelated, needed to be properly categorized, and incorporated in books in updated form.

The book, "Illustrated Veterinary Pathology" written by Dr. R.S. Chauhan, National Fellow/Professor, Department of Pathology, College of Veterinary Sciences, G.B. Pant University of Agriculture and Technology, Pantnagar, is an appropriate attempt to fill the gap in the study of Veterinary Pathology. The syllabi of Veterinary Sciences has been changed as per modern requirements and has been in vogue in almost all the Veterinary Colleges of the country. The book prepared as per the requirement of the new syllabus of Veterinary Council of India, has been divided into two sections.

The General Pathology section covers topics including introductory part, historical milestones, general concepts of pathology such as degenerative and vascular changes, healing, concretions, calcification, growth disturbances and inflammation and their etiological factors. Each pathological condition has been described with relevant photographs and diagrams to make it more understandable. Similarly, section two has been divided in ten chapters covering systemic pathology of animals and poultry. Pathology of each organ and system has been nicely presented with macroscopic and microscopic features supported by photographs and diagrams. The practical aspect has been covered in appendices containing post-mortem techniques, viscera examination, collection and preservation of material, necropsy of veterolegal cases and dispatch of material to forensic laboratory for diagnosis. Steps of post-mortem examination are suitably presented with photographs and diagrams. In the end of each chapter, model questions are given for self assessment of the students and is one of the unique feature of the book.

I am sure the book will prove of immense value to the students, teachers and veterinarians for better understanding of Veterinary Pathology and disease processes.

N.P. Singh
Former Prof. Path. and Dean
Faculty of Veterinary Sciences, Pantnagar
International Consultant IICA,
Fed. Mini. Agri. (Nigeria)/World Bank

PREFACE TO THE SECOND EDITION

Since the first edition of this book "Illustrated Veterinary Pathology" exhausted, I received messages in the form of letters, phones, SMSs, etc. from the students of BVSc&AH, from different parts of the country to bring out its second edition and make it available to the students. During last 4 years various suggestions and appreciations were also received about the book. Illustrated Veterinary Pathology book has been revised as per the need of its readers. Differential features of various Pathological conditions are given to present in an easily understandable form. Various chapters are updated with some new photographs. The latest classification of viruses has been incorporated in the chapter 'Etiology'. Students of Veterinary Pathology will find it suitable for their study and to prepare for competitive examinations like ICAR, NET, ASRB, etc. Feedback received from the readers is given due care while preparing second edition of the book and most of the suggestions are incorporated.

In my opinion, it will become were useful to not only the students but also to the teachers, field veterinarians and diagnosticians. I must extend thanks to all those who helped me in this meticulous task.

RS Chauhan

Centre for Animal Disease Research and Diagnosis (CADRAD),
Indian Veterinary Research Institute, Izatnagar–243 122, Bareilly (UP) India
Email: rs_chauhan123@rediffmail.com

PREFACE TO THE FIRST EDITION

Ever since the VCI course curriculum was implemented, need of suitable literature for students was felt at many fora. In the busy curriculum of veterinary sciences, the subject of pathology forms a vital link between basic subjects of anatomy, biochemistry and physiology on one hand, and the clinical subjects of surgery, gynaecology and medicine, on the other. The students face difficulty in understanding pathology since they are confronted with the dilemma of choosing between exhaustive and voluminous books of Veterinary Pathology, most of them without photographs/illustrations. Majority of available textbooks on Veterinary Pathology are written by western authors and English being a foreign language in this country, most of our students find it hard to understand and reproduce the highly technical subject from these books. Most of the available textbooks were written a decade or more than that back,and are out dated in present scenario. Needless to say that some of the books written by Indian authors are also too exhaustive and without illustrations, thus, creating confusion in the mind of students.

In preparing this textbook, I have kept these problems in mind and recalled the difficulties I faced as a student. How far have I succeeded in my endeavour is for the students and my professional colleagues to judge.

The very purpose of the **Illustrated Veterinary Pathology** is to provide the undergraduate Veterinary students a textbook with diagrams and photographs to make the text comprehensive. To broaden the scope further, laboratory methods, including post-mortem examination, histopathological procedures and clinicopathological procedures are also included in the appendices.

Physically, the book is of the standard textbook size, each chapter being well illustrated and provided with salient features of macroscopic and microscopic observations. The book is divided into two sections of General Pathology and Systemic Pathology. The text provides a complete, uptodate and concise coverage of the traditionally difficult subject in simple, lucid and clear language. Wherever new terms/unfamiliar words appear in the text, they are first defined and explained. The material has been organized meticulously in such a way that the student can easily understand, retain and reproduce it. Various levels of headings, sub-headings, bold type set and italics given in the text are meant to aid the student for quick revision of the subject. Another major point of this book is inclusion of original and high standard questions including fill in the gaps, true/false, definitions, short notes and multiple choice questions (MCQ), which are not only helpful in their self-assessment but also in preparation for competitive examinations like ICAR junior research fellowship (JRF) etc.

In a work of this magnitude, it is natural for the sole author of a book to solicit help and cooperation from others. The most overwhelming enthusiasm, good will, love and affection have generously come from my students for which I shall remain always indebted to them. I wish to express gratitude to the Vice-Chancellor, Dr. J.B. Chowdhary, who always encouraged me to produce such a useful textbook for undergraduate students. The support and encouragement from Dr. Harpal Singh, Dean, PGS & former Dean, V.Sc., Dr. Amresh Kumar, Dean, V.Sc. and Dr. S.P. Singh, Head, Pathology in accomplishing this academic work is thankfully acknowledged. I wish to thank my colleagues who helped me a lot during preparation of the text book, including Dr. G.K. Singh, Prof . & Head, Anatomy, Dr. D.K. Agrawal, Assoc. Prof., Pathology and Dr. Avadhesh Kumar, SMS. The valuable suggestions and criticism from Dr. Lokesh Kumar, Dr. B.P. Singh, Dr. Rajesh Kumar and Dr. Sumeet Bagga is thankfully acknowledged. My teacher, Dr. Nagendra P. Singh, Ex-professor Pathology and Dean, Veterinary Sciences, has been a source of constant inspiration and encouragement to me for successful completion of this work. Some of the illustrations provided by Dr. Ramesh Somvanshi, IVRI, Dr. Arup Das, Dr. Stayendra Kumar, Dr. Avadhesh Kumar, Dr. R. Sharma, Dr. G.K. Singh and others are duly acknowledged. I am thankful to Agricultural Research Service, United States, Department of Agriculture (ARS/USDA) for the photographs of various unusual and rare disease conditions and consent to produce them in this text book for the benefit of students. The meticulous type setting and photograph setting by Sri. Navin Joshi and Tasabber Khan are thankfully acknowledged.

Finally, I would be failing in my duties, if I fail to mention the contributions of my family. The cooperation and help provided by my wife, Mrs. Vandana, and the children, Ms. Mahima and Master Yatishwar cannot be overlooked because it was their time that I used to spend in preparation of this book.

Lastly, in spite of my best efforts at perfection, element of human error is still likely to creep in which the readers are welcome to point out since that would help me in improving the text book further.

College of Veterinary Sciences
G.B. Pant University of Agri. & Tech.
Pantnagar- 263145. Uttaranchal, INDIA
E mail: rs_chauhan123@rediffmail.com
August, 2001

R.S. CHAUHAN
M.V.Sc. Ph.D. FNAVS
National Fellow
Department of Pathology

CONTENTS

Part A
General Veterinary Pathology

1
INTRODUCTION

- **Definitions**

- **Historical Milestones**

- **Model Questions**

DEFINITIONS

Pathology

Pathology is the study of the anatomical, chemical and physiological alterations from normal as a result of disease in animals. It is a key subject because it forms a vital bridge between preclinical sciences (Anatomy, Physiology, Biochemistry) and clinical branches of medicine and surgery. Pathology is derived from the Greek word *pathos* = disease, *logos* = study. It has many branches, which are defined as under:

General Pathology

General Pathology concerns with basic alterations of tissues as a result of disease. *e.g.* fatty changes, thrombosis, amyloidosis, embolism, necrosis (Fig. 1.1).

Systemic Pathology

Systemic Pathology deals with alterations in tissues/organs of a particular system. *e.g.* respiratory system, genital system etc. (Fig. 1.2).

Specific Pathology

Specific Pathology is the application of the basic alterations learned in general pathology to various specific diseases. It involves whole body or a part of body. *e.g.* tuberculosis, rinderpest.

Experimental Pathology

Experimental Pathology concerns with the production of lesion through experimental methods. *e.g. Rotavirus* → calves → enteritis/ diarrhoea in calves (Fig. 1.3).

Clinical Pathology

Clinical Pathology includes certain laboratory methods which help in making the diagnosis using animal excretions/secretions/blood/skin scrapings/ biopsy etc. *e.g.* urine examination, blood examination (Fig. 1.4).

Post-mortem Pathology

Post-mortem Pathology is examination of an animal after death. Also known as *Necropsy* or *Autopsy*. It forms the base for study of pathology (Fig. 1.5).

Microscopic Pathology

Microscopic Pathology deals with examination of cells/tissues/organs using microscope. It is also known as histopathology/cellular pathology. *e.g.* microscopy, electronmicroscopy (Figs. 1.6 & 1.7).

Humoral Pathology

Humoral Pathology is the study of alterations in fluids like antibodies in serum (Fig. 1.8).

Chemical Pathology

Chemical Pathology is the study of chemical alterations of body fluids/tissues. *e.g.* enzymes in tissue.

Physiological Pathology

Physiological Pathology deals with alteration in the functions of organ/system. It is also known as Pathophysiology. *e.g.* indigestion, diarrhoea, miscarriage (Fig. 1.9).

Nutritional Pathology

Nutritional Pathology is the study of diseases due to deficiency or excess of nutrients. *e.g.* Vit.-A deficiency induced nutritional roup, rickets due to calcium deficiency (Fig. 1.10).

Comparative Pathology

Comparative Pathology is the study of diseases of animals with a comparative study in human beings and other animals. *e.g.* zoonotic diseases such as tuberculosis (Fig. 1.11).

Oncology

Oncology is the study of cancer/tumor/neoplasms.

Immunopathology

Immunopathology deals with the study of diseases mediated by immune reactions. It includes Immunodeficiency diseases, autoimmunity and hypersensitivity reactions (Fig. 1.12).

Cytopathology

Cytopathology is the study of cells shed off from the lesions for diagnosis.

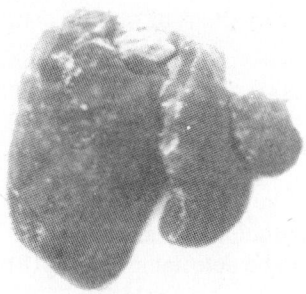

Fig. 1.1 Necrosis in liver

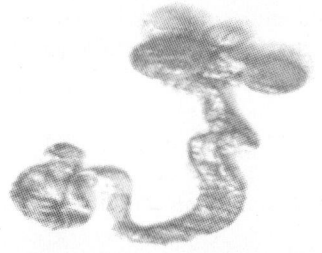

Fig.1.2. Female genital system of poultry

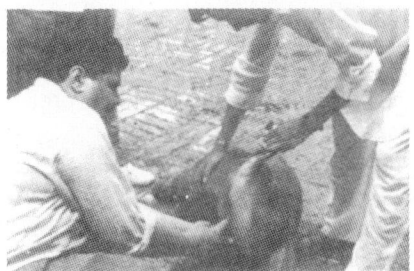

Fig.1.3. Experimental Pathology

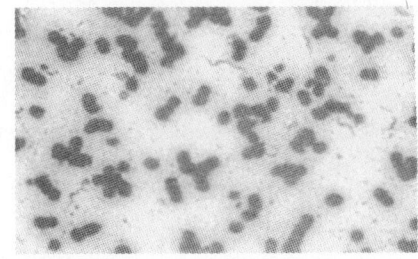

Fig.1.4. Examination of blood for protozoan parasites

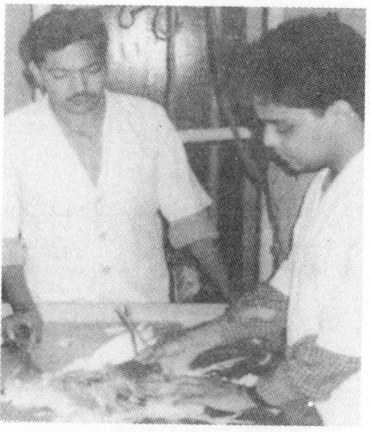

Fig. 1.5. Post-mortem examination of poultry

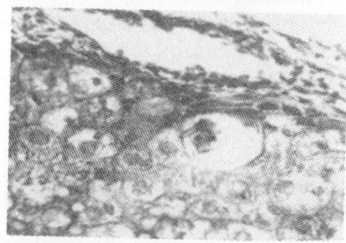

Fig. 1.6. Histopathological examination of skin section showing inclusions of poxvirus infection.

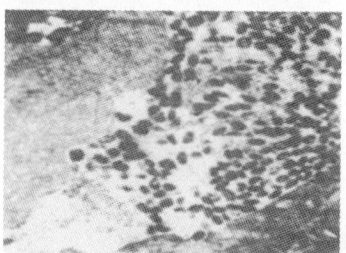

Fig. 1.7. Electronmicrophotograph showing poxvirus in cytoplasm of a cell

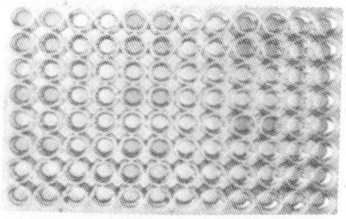

Fig.1.8. Detection of antibodies in serum using ELISA

Health

Health is a state of an individual living in complete harmony with his environment/surroundings (Fig. 1.13).

Disease

Disease is a condition in which an individual shows an anatomical, chemical or physiological deviation from the normal. (Discomfort with environment & body) (Fig. 1.14).

Illness

Illness is the reaction of an individual to disease in the form of illness.

Forensic Pathology

Forensic Pathology includes careful examination and recording of pathological lesions in case of veterolegal cases.

Homeostasis

Homeostasis is the mechanism by which body keeps equilibrium between health and disease. *e.g.* Adaptation to an altered environment.

Toxopathology

Toxopathology or Toxic Pathology deals with the study of tissue/organ alterations due to toxins/poisons (Fig.1.15).

Etiology

Etiology is the study of causation of disease (Fig. 1.16).

Diagnosis

Diagnosis is an art of precisely knowing the cause of a particular disease (*Dia*= thorough, *gnosis*= knowledge) (Fig 1.17).

Symptoms

Any subjective evidence of disease of animal characterized by an indication of altered bodily or mental state as told by owner (complaints of the patients).

Signs

Indication of the existence of something, any objective evidence of disease, perceptible to veterinarian (observations of the clinicians).

Syndrome

A combination of symptoms caused by altered physiological process.

Lesion

Lesion is a pathological alteration in structure/ function that can be detectable (Fig. 1.18).

Pathogenesis

Pathogenesis is the progressive development of a disease process. It starts with the entry of causal agent in body and ends either with recovery or death. It is the mechanism by which the lesions are produced in body.

Incubation period

Incubation period is the time that elapses between the action of a cause and manifestation of disease.

Course of disease

Course of disease is the duration for which the disease process remains till fate either in the form of recovery or death.

Prognosis

Prognosis is an estimate by a clinician of probable severity/outcome of disease.

Morbidity rate

Morbidity rate is the percentage/proportion of affected animals out of total population in a particular disease outbreak. *e.g.* out of 100 animals 20 are suffering from diarrhoea, the morbidity rate of diarrhoea will be 20%.

Mortality rate

Mortality rate is the percentage/proportion of animals out of total population died due to disease in a particular disease outbreak. *e.g.* if in a population of 100 animals, 20 fall sick and 5 died, the mortality rate will be 5%.

Case fatality rate

Case fatality rate is the percentage/proportions of

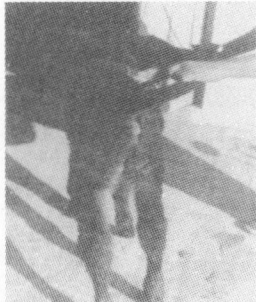

Fig.1.9. A calf showing diarrhoea

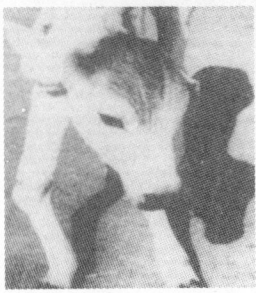

Fig. 1.10. Calcium deficiency causing rickets in calf.

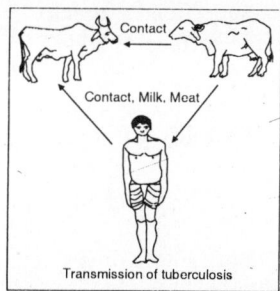

Fig. 1.11. Transmission of disease from animals to man.

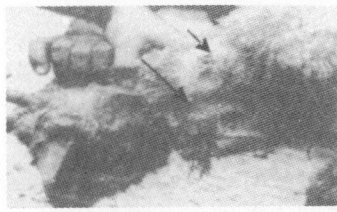

Fig.1.12. Lamb showing DTH reaction on neck

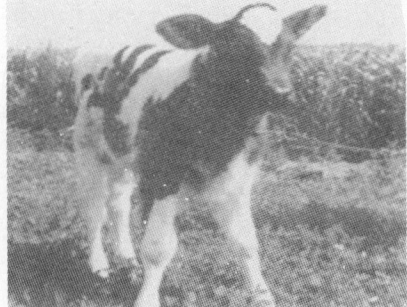

Fig. 1.13. A healthy calf

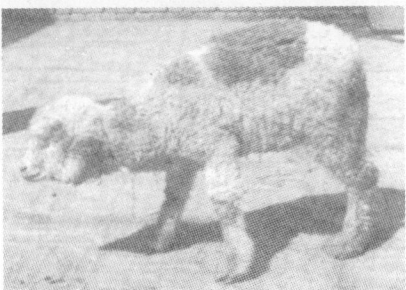

Fig. 1.14. Lamb suffering from pneumonia

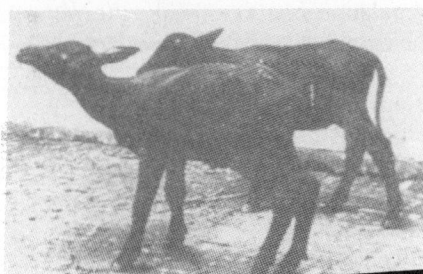

Fig. 1.15. Strychnine poisoning in calf

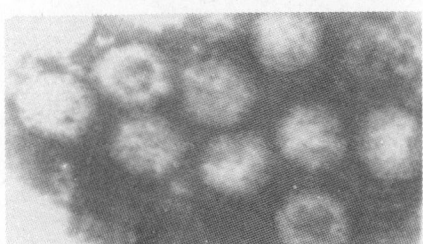

Fig. 1.16. Rotavirus – A cause of diarrhoea

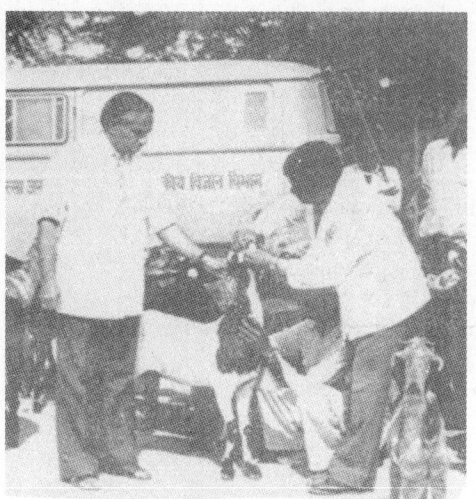

Fig. 1.17. *Diagnosis of diseases in animals.*

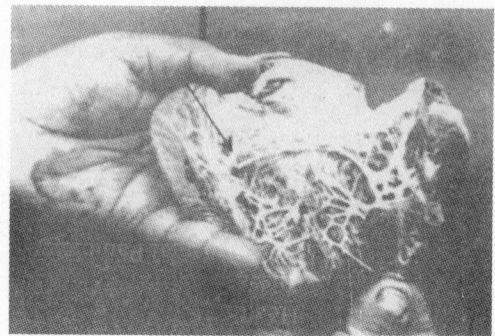

Fig. 1.18. *Haemorrhagic lesion in heart*

animals died among the affected animals. If in a population of 100 animals, 20 fall sick and 5 die,. the case fatality rate will be 25%.

Biopsy

Biopsy is the examination of tissues received from living animals.

Infection

Infection is the invasion of the tissues of the body by pathogenic organisms resulting in the development of a disease process.

Infestation

Infestation is the superficial attack of any parasite/organism on the surface of body.

Pathogenicity

Pathogenicity is the capability of an organism for producing a disease.

Virulence

Virulence is the degree of invasiveness of pathogenic organism.

HISTORICAL MILESTONES

2500-1500 BC	Shalihotra (Indian)	• First known veterinarian of the world • Wrote *Haya Ayurved/ Ashwa- Ayurved* in Sanskrit, 8 volumes on equine medicine with diagnosis, treatment, effect of planetary forces and evils on health
	Muni Palkapya (Indian)	• Wrote a treatise on elephants — *Gaj Ayurved*
2100 BC	Hammurabi	Conduct of Veterinary Practitioners, "Laws of Hammurabi"

1000 BC	Krishna (Indian)	• Mathura is known for best cattle production/milk production
	Nakul (4th Pandav) (Indian)	• Wrote *Ashwa- Chikitsa*, a book on equine medicine. • He is considered as an expert of equine management
	Sahdev (5th Pandav) (Indian)	• Expert in cattle rearing and disease management.
800 BC	Charak (Indian)	• Wrote *Charak Sanhita* with details of cause of diseases and impact of environment.
500 BC	Jeevak (Indian)	• Described the pathology of brain.
460-375 BC	Hippocrates (Greece)	• Physician, studied malaria, pneumonia , also known as "Father of Medicine"
384-323 BC	Aristotle (Greece)	• Humoral theory of disease • Father of Zoology • Originator of Modern Anatomy & Physiology
300 BC	Chandra Gupta Maurya period	• In Kautilya, Arthshashtra description on "Animal Husbandry and Veterinary Sciences", rules on animal ethics and jurisprudence
	Samrat Ashok	• First Veterinary Hospital established for treatment of animal diseases • Prevention of cruelty on animals advertised through writings on walls.
53 BC-37 AD	Cornelius Celsus (Rome)	• Wrote 8 volumes of pathology (1st special pathology) Cardinal signs of inflammation (redness, swelling, heat and pain)
131-206 AD	Claudius Galen (Rome)	• Meat inspection • 5th cardinal sign of inflammation "Loss of function"
450-500 AD	Renatus Vegetius (Rome)	• Father of Veterinary Medicine • Disregard divine pleasure • Disease of animals' influence on man
600 AD	Madhav	• Described pathology of diarrhoea, dysentery, icterus, tuberculosis and various toxic conditions.

980-1037 AD	Avicenna	• Cause of disease are minute organism • Spreads through air, food, water.
1497 AD-1558 AD	Jean Fernel	• Compiled the information of his time *First to attempt to codify the knowledge of Pathology.*
1564 AD-1642 AD	Galileo Galilei	• Developed single microscope
1578-1657 AD	William Harvey	• Blood vascular system and its impact on pathology
1617 AD-1619 AD	Drebbel	• Developed double lens microscope
1617-1680 AD	Solleysel (French)	• Book on *Le Parfact Marechal*
1632 AD-1723 AD	Antony van Leeuwen-hoek	• Saw microbes first • Book — *Little animals*
1682-1771 AD	G.B. Morgagni (Italian)	• Conducted 700 autopsies • Began modern pathology • Book *The seats and causes of disease*
1712-1779 AD	Bourgelat, C (French)	• New knowledge of equine medicine
1728- 1793 AD	John Hunter (English)	• First experimental pathologist
1753-1793 AD	Saint Bel (French)	• Teacher at Alfort established Vet School in England 1791 and in 1793 died due to glanders.
1762 AD	Bourgelat, C (French)	• 1st Veterinary school established — Ecole Veterinaire Nationale'd Alfort
1771-1802 AD	Bichat (French)	• Father of pathological anatomy • Foundation for the study of histology • Father of histology
1801-1858 AD	Mueller. J. (German)	• Cellular pathologist, known for his work "The fine structure and form of morbid tumors"
1804-1878 AD	Carl Rokitan-Skey (German)	• Supreme descriptive pathologist
1818-1865 AD	Semmelwiss (Hungarian)	• Surgery/autopsy • Started hospital sanitation

1821-1902 AD	R. Virchow (German)	• Journal *Virchow's Archives* • Great work on cellular pathology, "Father of modern Pathology"
1822-1895 AD	Louis Pasteur (French)	• Bacteria cause of disease
1839-1884 AD	J. Cohnheim (German)	• Originator of modern experimental pathology • Detected leucocytes at the site of inflammation • His work forms the basis for the pathology of inflammation • Introduced frozen sections
1843-1890 AD	R. Koch (German)	• Koch's postulates • Identified Tuberculosis, Staphylococcus and Vibrio as cause of disease
1850-1934 AD	W.H. Welch (U.S.A)	• Professor Pathology • Started pathology in USA.
1869 AD	Bruck Muller (USA)	• Textbook of pathological anatomy of domestic and zoo animals.
1883-1962 AD	G.N. Papanicolaou	• Father of exfoliative cytology
1884 AD	E. Metchnikoff	• Phagocytosis (microphages/macrophages)
1884-1955 AD	Robert Feulgen (German)	• Founder of Histochemistry
1885-1979 AD	William Boyd (Canadian)	• Author of Textbook of Pathology
1889 AD		• Establishment of Imperial Bacteriological Laboratory at Mukteshwar (Now IVRI)
1905-1993 AD	L. Ackerman (American)	• Authority on interpretation of frozen sections.
1913 AD	India	• Imperial Bacteriological Laboratory (now IVRI) established at new campus at Izatnagar- Bareilly
1924 AD	India	• The Publication of Indian Veterinary Journal started
1926 AD	E. Joest	• Wrote 5 volumes of Veterinary Pathology
1931 AD	India	• The publication of Indian Journal of Veterinary Sciences and Animal Husbandry (Presently Indian Journal of Animal Sciences) started

1933 AD	Ruska and Lorries	• First developed electronmicroscope.
1936 AD	Bittner	• Milk transmission of cancer
1938 AD	R.A. Runnels	• Wrote book on "Animal Pathology".
1953 AD	Watson and Crick	• Structure of DNA
1968 AD	G.A. Sastry (India)	• Author of *Veterinary Pathology* textbook.
1973 AD		• The Publication of Indian Veterinary Medical Journal started from Lucknow
1976 AD		• The publication of Indian Journal of Veterinary Pathology started from Izatnagar
1983 AD		• Indian Association of Veterinary Pathologist established.
1989 AD		• Veterinary Council of India established • Dr. C.M. Singh became 1st President of VCI • 1st Veterinary and Animal Sciences University established in Madras (now Chennai).
1998 AD		• Establishment of " Society for Immunology and Immunopathology" at Pantnagar. • Publication of "Journal of Immunology and Immunopathology" started from Pantnagar

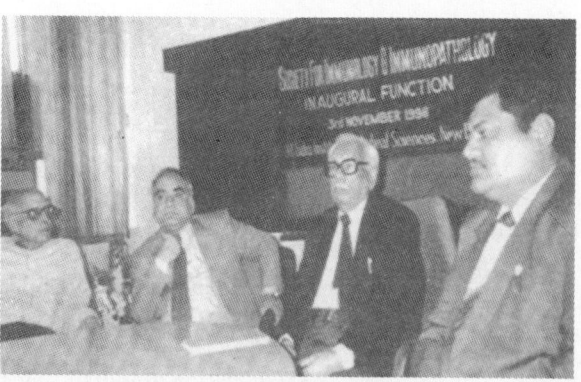

From left to right: Dr. Ramesh Kumar, professor. Microbiology, AIIMS;
Dr. N.K. Ganguly, Director General Indian Council of Medical Research;
Dr. C.M. Singh, Former Director, IVRI and President VCI; Dr. R.S. Chauhan, National Fellow,
at inaugural function of Society for Immunology and Immunopathology.

MODEL QUESTIONS

Q. 1. In a dairy farm a total of 1000 cows are kept for milk purpose. On 3.1.2001, 80 animals were found sick and were suffering from nasal discharge, fever and diarrhoea. Out of these 30 animals died till 18.1.2001 and rest recovered. The blood and serum samples were collected from affected animals for laboratory examination. The dead animals were necropsied and their tissue samples were also collected for microscopic examination. Based on this describe the followings:
1. Morbidity rate
2. Mortality rate
3. Case fatality rate
4. Course of disease
5. State the branch of pathology under which following activity falls:
   (a) Examination of blood ....
   (b) Examination of dead animals ....
   (c) Examination of serum for Ca, P, enzymes ....
   (d) Microscopic examination of tissues ....
   (e) Examination of serum for antibodies ....
   (f) Examination of urine and faeces of affected animals. ....

Q. 2. *Fill in the blanks with suitable word(s).*
1. ....is the father of Veterinary Medicine.
2. ....gave 4 cardinal signs of inflammation which included ...., ..., ... and .... while the fifth cardinal sign .... was given by ....
3. ....deals with study of diseases of animals and man.
4. Immunopathology deals with the study of diseases mediated by ...... and it includes ...., ... and ....
5. Symptoms are any .... evidence of disease of animals while signs are the existence of any .... evidence that is the observations of the clinicians.
6. ....is the progressive development of a disease process; it starts with the .... of causal agent in body and ends either with .... or ....
7. .... is the examination of tissues received from living animals.

Q. 3. *Define the following.*

1.	Health	6.	Diagnosis
2.	Disease	7.	Syndrome
3.	Experimental Pathology	8.	Prognosis
4.	Oncology	9.	Lesion
5.	Homeostasis	10.	Infection

Q. 4. *Justify the statement "Pathology is a key subject in Veterinary Sciences, which is quite helpful in prevention and control of diseases in animals".*

Q. 5. *Select most appropriate word(s) from the four options given with each question.*
1. The process of phagocytosis by macrophages was first described by...............
   (a) B. Muller   (b) E. Metchnikoff   (c) Bittner   (d) Bichat

2. First Veterinary School was established in the year ....
   (a) 1762   (b) 1884   (c) 1889   (d) 1773

3. The originator of modern Experimental Pathology is ....
   (a) R. Koch   (b) J. Cohnheim   (c) John Hunter   (d) R. Virchow

4. Study of tumors is known as ....
   (a) Cytopathology   (b) Clinical Pathology   (c) Chemical Pathology   (d) Oncology

5. Study of zoonotic diseases fall under the branch of .... Pathology.
   (a) Nutritional   (b) Comparative   (c) Experimental   (d) Systemic

6. Humoral Pathology is the study of alterations in..............in animals.
   (a) Antibodies   (b) Fibrin   (c) Urine   (d) Faeces

7. Immunodeficiency disorders of animals fall under the branch of ....
   (a) Cytopathology   (b) Humoral Pathology   (c) Microscopic Pathology
   (d) Immunopathology

8. General Pathology does not include one of the following activity
   (a) Fatty changes   (b) Embolism   (c) Inflammation (d) Digestive system
   disorders.

9. Examination of dead animals is known as ....
   (a) Necropsy   (b) Autopsy   (c) Lethopsy   (d) Microscopy

10. Nutritional roup is an example of ....Pathology.
    (a) Chemical   (b) Nutritional   (c) Humoral   (d) Post-mortem

2
ETIOLOGY

- **Intrinsic Causes**
- **Extrinsic Causes**
  - **Physical Causes**
  - **Biological Causes**
  - **Chemical Causes**
  - **Nutritional Causes**
- **Model Questions**

ETIOLOGY

Etiology is the study of cause of disease. It gives precise causal diagnosis of any disease. Broadly, the cause of diseases can be divided into two:

    a. Intrinsic causes.
    b. Extrinsic causes.

INTRINSIC CAUSES

Those causes which determine the type of disease present within an individual over which he has no control. These causes are further divided into following subgroups:

Genus

Specific diseases occur in a particular genus or species of animals. *e.g.* Hog cholera in pigs, Canine distemper in dogs

Breed/Race

Diseases do occur in particular breed of animals such as: dairy cattle are more prone for mastitis. Brain tumors are common in Bull dog/ Boxer.

Family

Genetic relationship plays a role in occurrence of diseases in animals. *e.g.* some chickens have resistance to leucosis; hernia in pigs due to weak abdominal wall.

Age

Age of animal may also influence the occurrence of diseases such as:

- At young age diarrhoea/pneumonia (Fig. 2.1).
- Old age tumor
- Canine distemper – Young dogs
- Strangles – Young horse
- Prostatic hyperplasia – Old dogs
- Coccidiosis – Young chickens

Sex

Reproductive disorders are more common in females

- Milk fever, mastitis and metritis in females.

- Nephritis is more common in male dogs than female, but Bovine nephritis is more common in females.

Colour

Colour may also play role in occurrence of diseases. *e.g. s*quamous cell carcinoma in white coat colour cattle, melanosarcoma in grey and white horses

Idiosyncracy

An unusual reaction of body to some substances such as:

- Drug reaction: Small dose of drug may produce reaction.
- Individual variations.

EXTRINSIC CAUSES

Some etiological factors which are present in the outside environment may cause/influence the occurrence of disease. These are also known as exciting cause/acquired cause. Majority of causes of diseases fall under this group which are further classified as physical, chemical, biological and nutritional causes.

PHYSICAL CAUSES
TRAUMA

Traumatic injury occurs due to any force or energy applied on body of animal *e.g.* during control / restraining, shipping or transport of animal.

Contusions/Bruises

Contusions or bruises arise from rupture of blood vessel with disintegration of extravassated blood (Fig. 2.2).

Abrasions

Abrasions are circumscribed areas where epithelium has been removed by injury and it may indicate the direction of force (Fig. 2.3).

Erosions

Partial loss of surface epithelium on skin or mucosal surface is termed as erosion (Fig. 2.4).

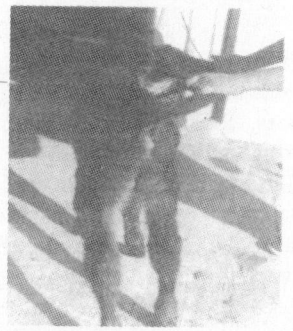

Fig. 2.1. Rotaviral diarrhoea in young calf

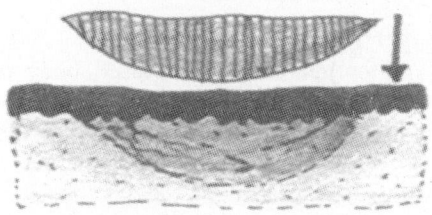

Fig. 2.2. Diagram showing contusion

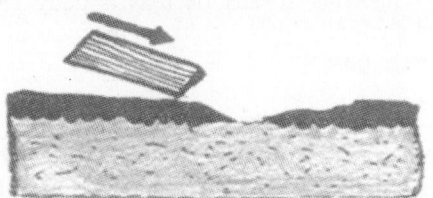

Fig. 2.3. Diagram showing abrasion

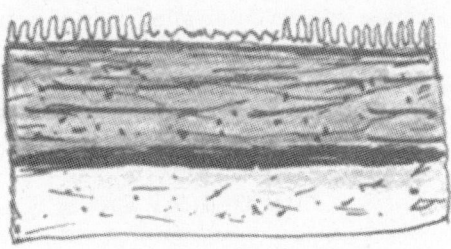

Fig. 2.4. Diagram showing erosion

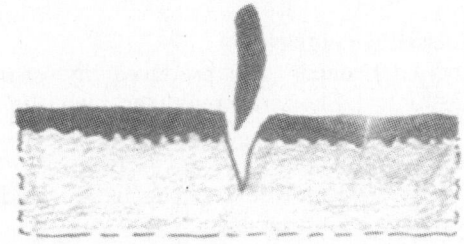

Fig. 2.5. Diagram showing incised wound

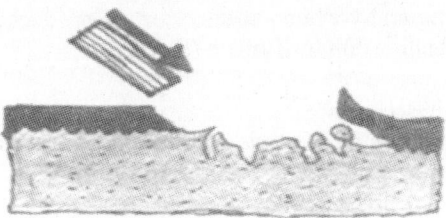

Fig. 2.6. Diagram showing laceration

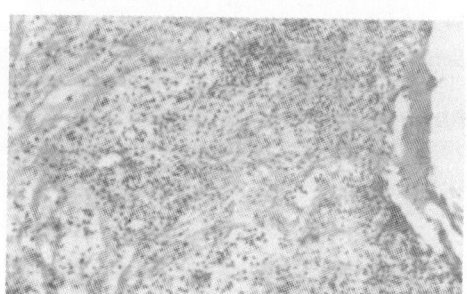

Fig. 2.7. Photomicrograph of third degree burn in skin

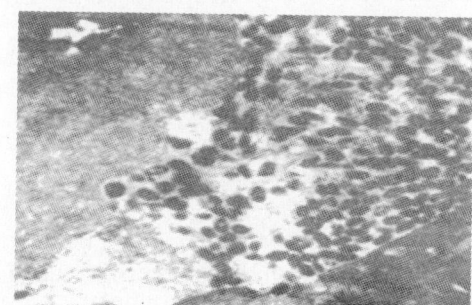

Fig. 2.8. Electronmicrophotograph of poxvirus in CAM

Incised wounds/cuts

Incised wounds are produced by sharp-edged instrument. They are longer than deep (Fig. 2.5).

Stab wound

Stab wounds are deeper than longer produced by sharp edged instrument.

Laceration

Severance of tissue by excessive stretching and is common over bony surfaces or are produced by cut through a dull instrument (Fig. 2.6).

Compression

Compression injury is produced as a result of force applied slowly *e.g.* during parturition.

Blast injury

Force of compression waves against surfaces followed by a wave of reduced pressure. It can rupture muscles/viscera.

Bullet wound

Hitting at 90° by firearms to produce uniform margins of abrasion. Exit wounds are irregular and lacerated.

ELECTRICAL INJURY

High voltage current induces tetanic spasms of respiratory muscles and hits the respiratory centre of brain. It also produces flash burns. Lightning causes cyanotic carcass, post-mortem bloat, congestion of viscera, tiny haemorrhage and skin damage.

TEMPERATURE

Burns

I degree burns

There is only congestion and injury to the superficial layers of epidermis *e.g.* sun burn on hairless parts or white skinned animal.

II degree burns

Epidermis is destroyed; hair follicles remain intact and provide a nidus for healing of epithelium.

III degree burns

Epidermis and dermis both are destroyed leading to fluid loss, local tissue destruction, laryngeal and pulmonary oedema, renal failure, shock and sepsis. Till 20 hrs of burn, the burn surface remains sterile then bacterial contamination occurs. After 72 hrs millions of bacteria enter in the affected tissue. Bacteria such as Staphylococci, Streptococci and *Pseudomonas aeruginosa* invade the deeper layers of skin and cause sepsis. There is a state of immunosuppression in severe burns leading to impaired phagocytosis by neutrophils (Fig. 2.7).

Hyperthermia

Hyperthermia means increased body temperature due to high environmental temperature *e.g.* pets in hot environment without water. Hyperthermia leads to increased respiration (hyperpnoea), rapid heart beat (tachycardia), and degeneration in myocardium, renal tubules and brain.

Hypothermia

Hypothermia means decreased body temperature and includes freeze induced necrosis of tissues at extremities

RADIATION INJURY

Radiation as a result of exposure to X-rays, Gamma rays or ultra violet (UV) rays leads to cell swelling, vacuolation of endoplasmic reticulum, swelling of mitochondria, nuclear swelling and chromosomal damage resulting in mutation. The impact of radiation is more on dividing cells of ovary, sperm, lymphocytes, bone marrow tissue and intestinal epithelium. It is characterized by vomiting, leucopenia, bone marrow atrophy, anemia, oedema, lymphoid tissue and epithelial necrosis.

BIOLOGICAL CAUSES

Virus

Viruses are smallest organisms, which have only one type of nucleic acid DNA or RNA in their core covered by protein capsid.

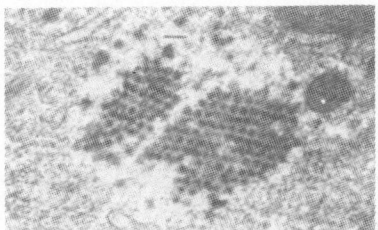

Fig. 2.9. *Electron microphotograph of reovirus in CAM*

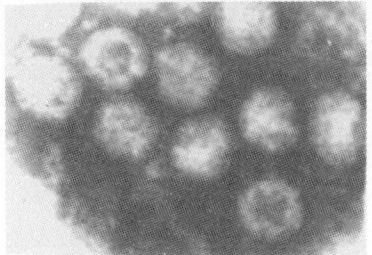

Fig. 2.10. *Electronmicrophotograph of rotavirus*

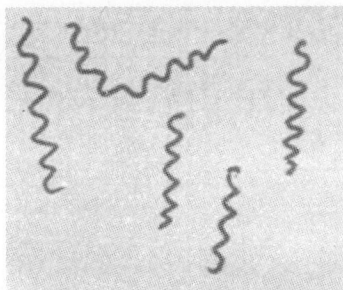

Fig. 2.11. *Diagram of Leptospira.*

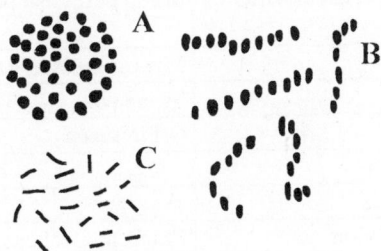

Fig. 2.12. *Diagram of bacteria (a) Staphylococci, (b) Streptococci (c) Bacilli*

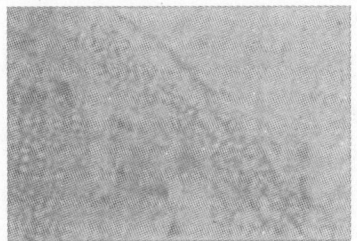

Fig. 2.13. *Photomicrograph of Trichophyton sp. a cause of ringworm*

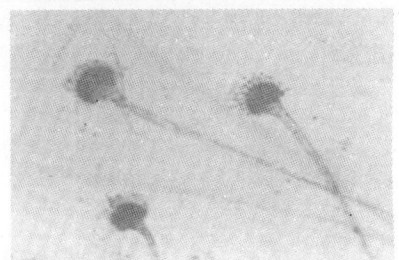

Fig. 2.14. *Photomicrograph of Aspergillus flavus*

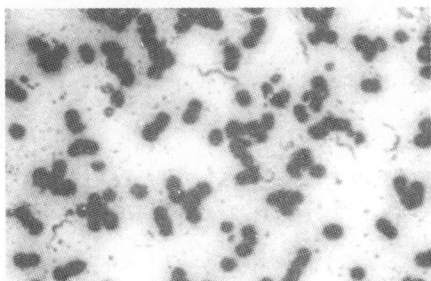

Fig. 2.15. *Photomicrograph of Trypanosoma evansi infection*

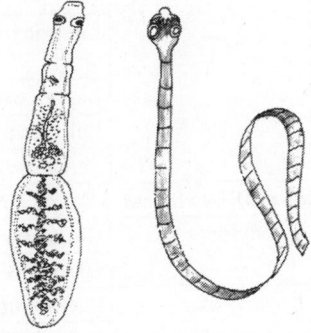

Fig. 2.16. *Diagram of Echinococcus and Taenia spp.*

17

Viruses of Veterinary Importance with their classification
(International Committee on taxonomy of viruses, 2005)

DNA Viruses (Fig. 2.8)

S.No.	Family	Genus	Virus species	Disease
Group I - ds DNA viruses (Double stranded DNA virus)				
1.	Adenoviridae	Aviadenovirus Atadenovirus Mastadenovirus	Fowl adenovirus Ovine adenovirus A Canine adenovirus 1	IBH, EDS, HPS in birds Pneumonia in Sheep ICH in Dog
2.	Herpesviridae	Alphaherpes virus	Herpes suis	Pseudorabies in pigs
			Bovine herpes virus – 1 (BHV-1)	IBR, IPV in cattle
			Equine herpes virus – 1 (EHV-1)	Equine viral abortion
			Equine herpes virus – 4 (EHV-4)	Rhinopneumonitis in equines
			Equine herpes virus – 3 (EHV-3)	Coital exanthema
			Avian herpes virus type-1 (AHV-1)	ILT in birds
		Betaherpes virus	Porcine cytomegalo virus	Inclusion body rhinitis in pigs
		Gammaherpes virus	Malignant catarrhal fever virus	MCF in cattle
			Marek's disease virus	Marek's disease in birds
3.	Papillomaviridae	Papillomavirus	Bovine papillomavirus	Cutaneous papilloma in cattle Oral papilloma in dogs
			Canine oral papillomavirus Rabbit papillomavirus	Cutaneous papilloma in rabbits
4.	Poxviridae	Orthopox virus	Vaccinia virus, Cowpox virus, Buffalopox virus, Monkeypox virus, Rabbitpox virus Camelpox virus	Pox in animals
		Avipox virus	Fowlpox virus, Pigeonpox virus, Turkeypox virus, Canarypox virus	Fowl pox, Pigeon pox, Turkeypox, Canarypox
		Capripox virus	Sheeppox virus, Goatpox virus	Sheep pox, Goat pox
		Leporipox virus	Myxoma virus	Myxomatosis in Rabbits
		Suipox virus	Swinepox virus	Swine pox
		Parapox virus	Orfpox virus	Orf in sheep
Group II - ss DNA viruses (Single stranded DNA virus)				
1.	Circoviridae	Circovirus	Porcine circovirus	-
		Gyrovirus	Chicken anemia virus	Chicken infectious anemia
2.	Parvoviridae	Parvovirus	Murine minute virus	
		Bocavirus	Bovine parvovirus	Diarrhoea in cattle
			Canine parvovirus	Enteritis, myocarditis in dogs
			Porcine parvovirus	Infertility, fetal death in pigs

RNA Viruses (Figs. 2.9 & 2.10)

S.No.	Family	Genus	Virus species	Disease
Group III - ds RNA virus (Double stranded RNA virus)				
1.	Birnaviridae	Avibirnavirus	IBD virus	IBD in birds
		Aquabirnavirus	Infectious pancreatic necrotic virus	Infectious pancreatic necrosis
2.	Reoviridae	Orthoreovirus	Mammalian orthoreo virus	Pneumoenteritis in calves
		Orbivirus	Blue tongue virus	Blue tongue in sheep
		Rotavirus	Rotavirus	Diarrhoea in neonates
Group IV - (+ve) ss RNA virus (Positive single stranded RNA or M RNA like)				
1.	Arteriviridae	Arterivirus	Equine arteritis virus	Equine viral arteritis
2.	Coronaviridae	Coronavirus	Infectious bronchitis virus	Infectious bronchitis in birds
			Bovine coronavirus	Diarrhoea in calves
3.	Astroviridae	Avastrovirus	Turkey astrovirus	-
4.	Calciviridae	Vesivirus	Swine vesicular exanthema virus	Vesicular exanthema in pigs
		Lagovirus	Rabbit haemorrhagic disease virus	Haemmorhagic disease in rabbit
		Norovirus	Norwalk virus	-
5.	Flaviviridae	Flavirus	Yellow fever virus	Yellow fever in man
		Hepacivirus	Hepatitis C virus	Hepatitis in man
		Pestivirus	BVD virus, CSF virus	BVD, CSF
6.	Picornaviridae	Enterovirus	Poliovirus	Polio in man
		Rhinovirus	Rhinovirus	Rhinitis
		Hepatovirus	Hepatitis A virus	Hepatitis
		Cardiovirus	Encephalomyocarditis virus	Encephalomyocarditis
		Aphthovirus	FMD virus	FMD
		Erbovirus	Equine rhinitis B virus	Respiratory disease in equines
7.	Togaviridae	Alphavirus	Equine Encephalomyelitis virus	Equine encephalomyelitis
		Rubivirus	Rubellavirus	
Group V – (-ve) ss RNA virus (Negative single stranded RNA)				
1.	Paramyxoviridae	Paramyxovirus	Parainfluenza virus 1 (PI-1)- Pigs,	Respiratory diseases in pigs
			Parainfluenza virus 2 (PI-2)- Dogs,	Kennel cough in dogs
			Parainfluenza virus 3 (PI-3)- Cattle	Respiratory disease in cattle
		Avulavirus	Ranikhet disease virus	Ranikhet disease in birds
		Morbillivirus	Canine Distemper virus Rinderpest virus PPR virus	CD in dogs RP- in animals PPR – sheep, goat

19

S.No.	Family	Genus	Virus species	Disease
2.	Bornaviridae	Borna disease virus	Borna disease virus	Borna disease in sheep
3.	Filoviridae	Ebolavirus	-	-
		Filovirus	-	-
4.	Rhabdoviridae	Vesiculovirus	Vesicular stomatitis virus	Vesicular stomatitis in bovines
		Lyssavirus	Rabies virus	Rabies
		Ephemerovirus	Ephemeral fever virus	Ephemeral fever in animals
5.	Bunyaviridae	Hantavirus	Hantaanvirus	Hantavirus pulmonary syndrome, Korean haemorragic fever
		Phlebovirus	Nairobi sheep disease virus, Rift valley fever virus, Akabana disease virus	Nairobi Sheep disease, RVF Akabana disease
6.	Orthomyxoviridae	Influenza virus A Influenza virus B Influenza virus C	Influenza virus A Influenza virus B Influenza virus C	Influenza in animals
Group VI ss RNA-RT virus (Single stranded RNA virus with reverse transcriptase)				
1.	Retroviridae	Alpharetrovirus	Avian leucosis virus	ALC in birds
		Betaretrovirus	Mouse mammary tumour virus	Cancer in mice
		Gammaretrovirus	Murine leukemia virus	Leukemia in mice
			Feline leukemia virus	Leukemia in cats
		Deltaretrovirus	Bovine leukemia virus	Bovine leukemia
		Lentivirus	Bovine immunodeficiency virus	Bovine immunodeficiency syndrome
			Feline immunodeficiency virus	Feline immunodeficien(syndrome
Group VII ds DNA-RT virus (Double stranded DNA virus with reverse transcriptase)				
1.	Hepadnaviridae	Orthohepadnavirus	Hepatitis B virus	Hepatitis
		Avihepadna virus	Duck hepatitis B virus	Duck hepatitis

20

Subviral agents

- Prion proteins are infectious proteins without any nucleic acid. *e.g.* Bovine spongiform encephalopathy.

- Viroids have only nucleic acid without proteins. They do not cause any disease in animals. However, They are associated with plant diseases.

Rickettsia

Coxiella burnetti causes Q-fever

Mycoplasma

Mycoplasma mycoides is responsible for pneumonia, joint ailments and genital disorders

Chlamydia

Chlamydia trachomatis, C. psittaci cause abortions, pneumonia, and eye ailments.

Spirochaete

Leptospira sp. causes abortion, icterus.

Borrelia ansernia causes fowl spirochetosis in chickens (Fig. 2.11).

Bacteria

Bacteria are classified as Gram positive and Gram negative on the basis of Gram's staining. Gram positive bacteria include Staphylococci, Streptococci, Corynebacterium, Listeria, Bacillus Clostridia. Gram negative bacteria are *Escherichia coli*, Salmonella, Proteus, Klebsiella, Pasteurella, Pseudomonas, Brucella, Yersinia, Campylobactor etc. Besides, there are certain organisms stained with Zeihl Neelson stain and are known as acid fast bacilli *e.g.Mycobacterium tuberculosis* and *M. paratuberculosis* (Fig. 2.12).

Fungi

Fungi pathogenic for animals mostly belong to fungi imperfecti. *e.g.* Histoplasmosis.

Fungi cause three type of disease – Mycosis *e.g.* Actinomycosis; Allergic disease *e.g.* Ringworm; Mycotoxicosis *e.g.* Aflatoxicosis (Figs. 2.13, 2.14).

Parasites

Parasites are classified mainly in 3 groups:

Protozoan parasites

Trypanosoma evansi, Theileria annulata, Babesia bigemina, Toxoplasma gondii, Eimeria Spp. (Fig. 2.15).

Helminths

Nematodes – Roundworms *e.g.* Ascaris.

Trematod – Flat worms *e.g.* Liverfluke.

Cestodes – Tapeworms *e.g* Taenia spp. (Fig. 2.16).

Arthropods

Ticks, Mites, Flies, Lice (Figs. 2.17, 2.18, 2.19, 2.20).

TRANSMISSION

Biological agents are transmitted from one animal to another through horizontal or vertical transmission.

Horizontal Transmission

Horizontal transmission of biological causes occurs through direct contact or indirectly via animal or inanimate (fomites) objects. It is also known as lateral transmission as it occurs in a population from one to another. Various methods of horizontal transmission are as under:

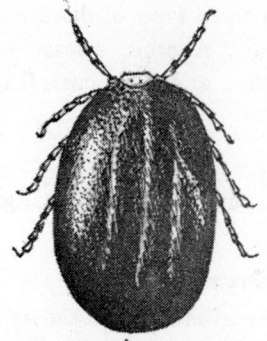

Fig. 2.17. Diagram of a tick

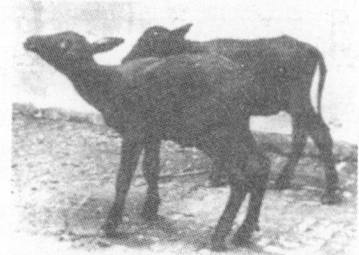

Fig. 2.21. Photograph of calves with strychnine poisoning

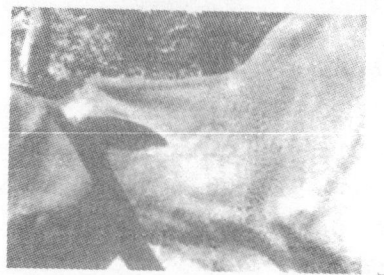

Fig. 2.18. Photograph of bullock with tick infestation

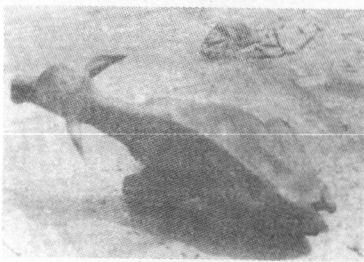

Fig. 2.22. Photograph of calves with strychnine poisoning

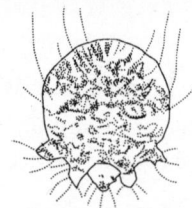

Fig. 2.19. Diagram of a Mite

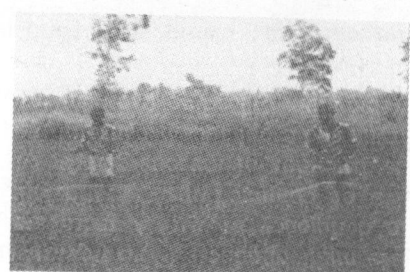

Fig. 2.23. Pesticide spray in crops

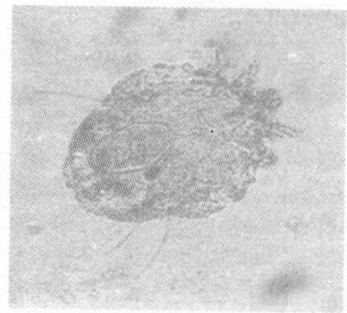

Fig. 2.20. Photomicrograph of Sarcoptes scabei

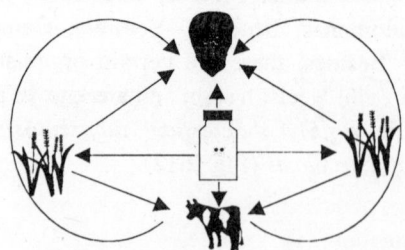

Fig. 2.24. Pesticide cycle in environment

Ingestion
Food, water, faecal-oral route *e.g.* Salmonellosis, Johne's disease, Rotavirus infection.

Inhalation
Air-borne infections, droplet infection *e.g.* R.P., FMD, Tuberculosis.

Contact
Fungal infection, Bacterial dermatitis, Flu, Brucellosis, Rabies through bite.

Inoculation
Introduction of infection in body through puncture either mechanically through needles or by arthropods such as by ticks. Ticks transmit diseases through transovarian (one generation to next generation) or transstadial (through developmental stages) transmission.

Iatrogenic
Transmission of infection during surgical procedures or caused by doctor, through dirty instrument and contaminated preparations.

Coitus
Through sexual contact of animals, biological agents spread from one to another animals. *e.g.* Campylobacteriosis, Trichomonosis.

Vertical Transmission
Vertical transmission occurs from one generation to another generation *in ovo/in utero* or through milk. These include:

Hereditary
Infection/disease carried in the genome of either parent *e.g.* Retrovirus

Congenital
Diseases acquired either *in utero/in ovo*
- Infection in ovary/ ovum (Germinative transmission) *e.g.* ALC in chickens, lymphoid leukemia in mice, Salmonellosis in poultry.
- Infection through placenta. *e.g.* Feline panleukopenia virus (Transmission to embryo)

- Ascending infection from lower genital canal to amnion / placenta *e.g.* Staphylococci.
- Infection at parturition: Infection from lower genital tract during birth. *e.g.* Herpex simplex virus.

MAINTENANCE OF INFECTION
Biological agents face difficulty of survival at both places – in environment and in host. Two types of hazards which create problem to agent are:
Internal hazards e.g. Host's immune system
External hazards e.g. Desiccation, UV light
Agents try to maintain themselves by adopting following maintenance strategies:
- Avoidance of a stage in the external environment.
- Resistant forms *e.g.* Anthrax spores.
- Rapidly in-rapidly out strategy *e.g.* Viruses of respiratory tract.
- Persistence within the host *e.g. Mycobacterium tuberculosis*, Slow viral diseases.
- Extension of host range.
- Infection in more than one host *e.g.* Foot and mouth disease.

CHEMICAL CAUSES
Biological Toxins
Snake venom
Snake venom has phospholipase A_2 which causes lytic action on membranes of RBC and platelets.
The presence of hyaluronidase, phosphodiesterase and peptidase in snake venom are responsible for oedema, erythema, haemolytic anemia, swelling of facial/laryngeal tissues, haemoglobinurea, cardiac irregularities, fall in blood pressure, shock and neurotoxicity.

Microbial toxins
Microbial toxins are those toxins/poisons that are produced by microbial agents particularly by bacteria and fungi.

Bacterial toxins
Bacterial toxins include structural proteins (endotoxins) and soluble peptides/ secretary toxins (exotoxins). Endotoxins are present in cell wall of

Gram-negative bacteria and are found to be responsible for septicemia and shock. Exotoxins are secreted by bacteria outside their cell wall and are responsible for protein lysis and damage to cell membrane. *e.g.* Clostridium toxins suppress metabolism of cell. Most potent clostridial toxins are botulinum and tetanus, which are the cause of hemolysis and are powerful neurotoxin. Besides, *Clostridium chauvei* toxins are responsible for black leg disease in cattle.

Fungal Toxins (Mycotoxins)

There are several fungi known for production of toxins. Such toxins are known as mycotoxins and they are mostly found in food/ feed items, which cause disease in animals through ingestion.

Aflatoxins

Aflatoxins are produced by several species of fungi including mainly *Aspergillus flavus, A. parasiticus* and *Penicillium puberlum*. These aflatoxins are classified as B_1, B_2, G_1, G_2, M_1, M_2, B_2a, G_2a and aspertoxin. Aflatoxins are produced in moist environment in grounded animal/poultry feed on optimum temperature and are more common in tropical countries where storage conditions are poor and provide suitable environment for the growth of fungi. These toxins are known to cause immunosuppression, formation of malignant neoplasms and hepatopathy.

Ergot

Ergot is produced by *Claviceps purpura* in grains which causes blackish discoloration. It produces gangrene by chronic vasoconstriction, ischemia and capillary endothelium degeneration. It is also associated with summer syndrome in cattle characterized by gangrene of extremities.

Fusarium toxins

Fusarium toxins are produced by *Fusarium tricinctum* in paddy straw, which are found to cause gangrene in extremities. Zearalenone toxin is the cause of ovarian abnormality in sow.

Ochratoxins

Ochratoxins are produced by *Aspergillus ochraceous* and *A. viridicatum* fungi in grounded feed on optimum temperature and moisture and are found to cause renal tubular necrosis in chickens and pigs.

Plant toxins

Over 700 plants are known to produce toxin. *e.g.* Braken fern which causes haematuria and encephalomalacia. Strychnine from *Strychnos nuxvomica* is highly toxic and causes death in animals with nervous signs. It is used for dog killing in public health operations to control rabies (Figs. 2.21 & 2.22). HCN is found in sorghum which is known to cause clonic convulsions and death in animals characterized by haemorrhage in mucous membranes.

Drug toxicity

- *Antibiotics:* Cause direct toxicity by destroying gut microflora. Oxytetracyline, sulfonamides are nephrotoxic. Neomycin and Lincomycin cause Malabsorption diarrhoea and immunosuppression.
- *Anti-inflammatory drugs,* like acetaminophen causes hepatic necrosis, icterus and hemolytic anemia.
- *Anticoccidiostate drug:* Monensin is responsible for necrosis of cardiac and skeletal muscles.
- *Trace elements:* There are various trace elements, excess of which may cause poisoning in animals. *e.g.* Selenium poisoning "Blind staggers" or "Alkali Disease" in cattle characterized by chronic debilitating disease. It also causes encephalomalacia in pigs.

Environmental pollutants

Environment is polluted due to presence of unwanted materials in food, water, air and surroundings of animals, particularly by agrochemicals including pesticides and fertilizers. The environmental pollutants exert their direct or indirect effect on the animal health and production. The main pollutants are:

- Heavy metals such as mercury, lead, cadmium are found in industrial waste, automobile and generator smoke, soil, water and also as contaminants of pesticides and fertilizers. They are responsible for damage in kidneys, immune system and neuropathy. They are also associated with immune complex mediated glomerulonephritis.
- Sulphur dioxide is produced by automobiles, industries and generators. It is responsible for loss of cilia in bronchiolar epithelium.
- Hydrogen sulphide is produced by animal's decay and in various industries. It inhibits mitochondrial cytochrome oxidase leading to death.
- Pesticides are agrochemicals used in various agricultural, animal husbandry and public health operations. They are classified as insecticides, herbicides, weedicides and rodenticides. Chemically, insecticides are grouped mainly as organochlorine organophosphates, carbamates and synthetic pyrethroids. Acute poisoning of pesticides causes death in animals after nervous clinical signs of short duration. Chronic toxicity is characterized by immunosuppression, nephropathy, neuropathy, hypersensitivity and autoimmunity in animals (Figs. 2.23 & 2.24).

NUTRITIONAL CAUSES

Malnutrition causes disease in animals either due to deficiency or excess of nutrients. It is very difficult to diagnose the nutritional causes and sometimes it is not possible to find a precise cause as in case of infectious disease because functions of one nutrient can be compensated by another in cell metabolism. Experimental production of nutritional deficiency is not identical to natural disease. When tissue concentration of nutrient falls down to the critical level, it leads to abnormal metabolism and the abnormal metabolites present in tissues can be detected in urine and faeces. First changes of nutritional deficiency are recorded in rapidly metabolizing tissues *e.g.* skeletal muscle, myocardium and brain. Immature animals are more

susceptible to nutritional disease. *e.g.* calves, chicks, piglets etc.

Types of deficiency
- Acute/chronic *e.g.* thiamine deficiency in pigs.
- Multiple deficiencies: *e.g.* poor quality food.
- Nutritional imbalance: *e.g.* imbalance in calcium: phosphorus (2:1) ratio.
- Protein malnutrition: *e.g.* malabsorption.
- Calorie deficiency: *e.g.* Loss of fat/ muscle wasting.

Factors responsible for nutritional deficiency
- Interference with intake *e.g.* anorexia, G.I. tract disorders.
- Interference with absorption *e.g.* intestinal hypermotility, Insoluble complexes in food (Fat/Calcium)
- Interference with storage *e.g.* hepatic disease leads to deficiency of vit. A.
- Increased excretion *e.g.* polyuria, sweating and lactation
- Increased requirement *e.g.* fever, hyperthyroidism and pregnancy
- Natural inhibitors *e.g.* presence of thiaminases in feed, leads to thiamine deficiency.

Calorie deficiency
Calorie deficiency in animals occurs due to food deprivation or starvation.

Food deprivation
Dietary deficiency of food in terms of quantity/quality leads to emaciation, loss of musculature, atrophy of fat, subcutaneous oedema, cardiac muscle degeneration and atrophy of viscera including liver and pancreas. The volume of hepatocytes reduced by 50% and mitochondrial total volume also reduced by 50%.

Starvation
Starvation is the long continued deprivation of food. It is characterized by fatty degeneration of liver, anemia and skin diseases. Young and very old animals are more susceptible to starvation while in pregnant animals it causes retarded growth

of foetus. In animals, following changes can be seen due to starvation.

Intestinal involution
Absorptive surface is reduced with shrunken cells and pyknotic nuclei. Villi become shorter and show atrophy.

Atrophy of muscles
There is decrease in muscle mass.

Lipolysis
Increased cortisol leads to increased lipolysis resulting in formation of fatty acids in liver which in turn converts into ketones used by brain.

Gluconeogenesis
In early fasting blood glucose level drops down. The insulin level becomes low while glucagon goes high in starvation. The glucose comes from skeletal muscle, adipose tissue and lymphoid tissue during starvation. Twenty-four hours of food deprivation causes reduction in liver glycogen and blood glucose. Fatty acid from adipose tissue forms glucose and in mitochondria after oxidation it forms acetoacetate, hydroxybutyrate and acetone. These are also known as **ketone bodies** and are present in blood stream during starvation. This state is also known as ketosis *e.g.* ketosis/acetonemia in bovines. Lack of glucose in blood leads to oxidation of fatty acids which form ketone bodies as an alternate source of energy. They are normal/ physiological at certain level but may become pathological when their level is high.

Clinically it is characterized by anorexia, depression, coma, sweet smell in urine. Concentration of acetone increases in milk, blood and urine along with hyperlipimia and acidosis. A similar condition also occurs in sheep known as pregnancy toxaemia which is characterized by depression, coma and paralysis. This situation occurs when many foetus are present in uterus. There are fatty changes in liver, kidneys, and heart, with subepicardial petechiae or echymosis.

Protein deficiency
Generally, protein deficiency does not occur. However, the deficiency of essential amino acids has been reported in animals when certain ingredients are deficient in certain amino acids. *e.g.* maize is deficient in lysine and tryptophan that leads to slow growth; peanuts and soybean are deficient in methioine. Protein deficiency is characterized by hypoproteinemia, anemia, poor growth, delayed healing, decreased or cesation of cell proliferation, failure of collagen formation, atrophy of testicles and ovary, atrophy of thymus and lymphoid tissue.

Deficiency of Lipids
Generally, there is no deficiency of fat in animals. However, essential fatty acids, including linolenic acid, linoleic acid and arachdonic acid, deficiency may occur which causes dermatoses in animals. Fat has high calorie value and it is required in body because there are certain vitamins soluble in fat only.

Deficiency of Water
Deficiency of water may lead to dehydration and slight wrinkling in skin. Deficiency may occur due to fever, vomiting, diarrhoea, haemorrhage and polyuria, which can be corrected through adequate oral water supply or through intravenous fluid therapy.

Deficiency of Vitamins
Vitamin deficiency may occur due to starvation. There are two types of vitamins viz., fat soluble and water soluble. Fat soluble vitamins are vit. A, D, E and K and water soluble are vit B complex and C.

Vitamin A
It is also known as retinol. It is derived from its precursor carotene. It is found in abndance in plants having yellow pigment, animal fat, liver, cod liver oil, shark liver oil. β-carotene is cleaved in gut mucosa into two molecules of retinol (Vit. A aldehyde) which, after absorption, is stored in liver. Bile salts and pancreatic juice are responsible for

absorption of vit. A from gut. Deficiency of vit. A occurs due to damage in liver.

Vit. A deficiency may lead to following disease conditions:

Squamous metaplasia of epithelial surfaces in esophagus, pancreas, bladder and parotid duct, which is considered pathognomonic in calves. Destruction of epithelium/ goblet cell in respiratory mucosa is generally replaced by keratin synthesizing squamous cells in vit. A deficient animals. There are ***abnormal teeth*** in animals due to hypoplasia of enamel and its poor mineralization. Vitamin A deficiency is also associated with ***still birth*** and ***miscarriages*** in pigs. It causes night blindness (***Nyctalopia***) in animals. Due to deficiency of Vit. A there are recurrent episodes of conjunctivitis/ keratitis. In poultry, there is distention of mucous glands, which opens in pharynx and esophagus because of metaplasia of duct epithelium leading to enlargement of esophageal glands due to accumulation of its secretions. The glands become spherical, 1-2 mm dia. over mucosa. It is considered pathognomonic for hypovitaminosis A. and is known as ***Nutritional roup*** (Fig. 2.25a&b). Inflammation of upper respiratory tract lead to coryza. Urinary tract of cattle, sheep and goat suffers due to formation of calculi, which may cause obstruction in sigmoid flexure of urethra in males. Such calculi are made up of desquamated epithelial cells and salts and the condition is known as ***urolithiasis***. Deficiency of vit. A may also lead to in abnormal growth of cranial bones and there may be failure of foramen ovale to grow leading to constriction of optic nerves which results in blindness in calves, increased CSF pressure, blindness at birth and foetal malformations. In sows, piglets are born without eyes (***Anophthalmos***) or with smaller eyes- (***Microphthalmos***).

Vitamin D

Vitamin D occurs in three forms viz. vitamin D_2 or calciferol, Vit. D_3 or cholecaliciferol and Vit D_1 or impure mixture of sterols. About 80% Vit. D is synthesized in body skin through UV rays on 7-hydrocholesterol. In diet containing egg, butter, it is found in abundant quantity in milk, plants, grains etc. Active forms of vit. D are 25-hydroxy vit. D and 1, 25 dihydroxy vit D. (Calcitriol) which is 5 to 10 times more potent than former. Vit D is stored in adipose tissue in body. The main functions of vit D are absorption of Ca and P from intestines and kidneys, mineralization of bones, maintenance of blood levels of Ca and P and immune regulation as it activates lymphocytes and macrophages.

- The deficiency of vitamin D is associated with rickets in young animals (Fig. 2.26), osteomalacia in adult animals and hypocalcemic tetany.
- Excess of vitamin D leads to the formation of renal calculi, metastatic calcification and osteoporosis in animals.

Vitamin E (α- tocopherol)

Source of vitamin E is grains, oils, nuts, vegetables, and in body it is stored in adipose tissue, liver and muscles. It has antioxidant activity and prevents oxidative degradation of cell membrane.

- Deficiency of vit E causes degeneration of neurons in peripheral nerves. There is denervation of muscles leading to muscle dystrophy e.g. ***White muscle disease*** in cattle and ***Stiff lamb disease*** in sheep and ***Myoglobinuria*** in horses. Deficiency of vit. E causes degeneration of pigments in retina and reduces life span of RBC, leading to anemia and sterility in animals. Crazy chick disease (***Encephalomalacia***) is also caused by vit E deficiency; the chicks become sleepy with twisting of head and neck. There is muscular dystrophy in chickens due to vit. E deficiency (Fig. 2.27).

Vitamin K

Vit. K occurs in two forms namely vit. K_1 or phylloquinone found in green leaf and vegetables and Vit- K_2 or menadione which is produced by gut microflora. Its main function is coagulation of blood. Deficiency of vit K may leads to hypoprothrombinemia and haemorrhages.

(a)

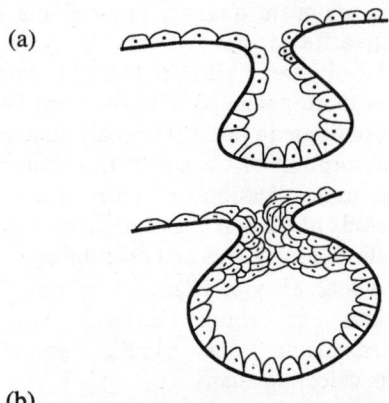

(b)

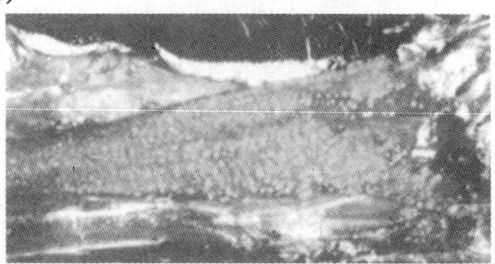

Fig. 2.25.(a) Diagram of squamous metaplasia in esophageal glands due to vitamin A deficiency (b) Photograph of eosophagus of poultry showing nutritional roup.

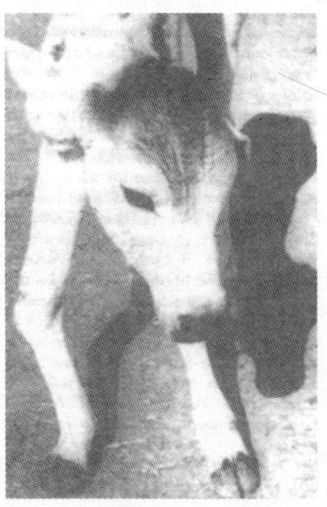

Fig. 2.26. Photograph of a calf showing rickets

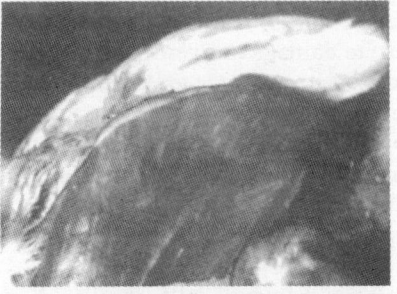

Fig 2.27. Muscular dystrophy due to vitamin E deficiency

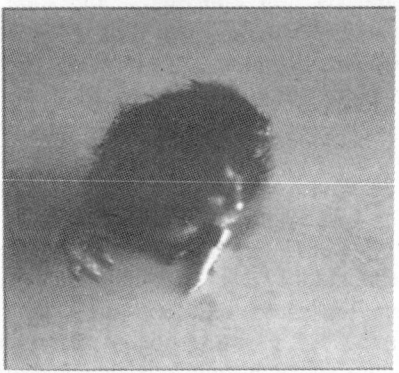

Fig. 2.28. Curled toe paralysis in a chick due to Riboflavin deficiency

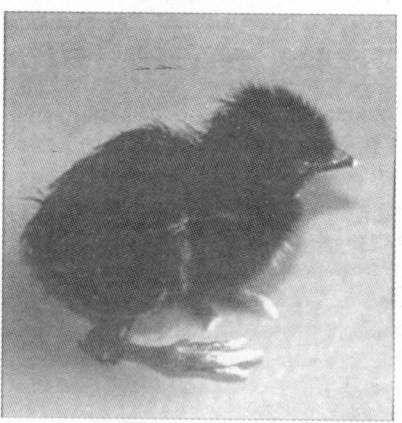

Fig. 2.29. Slipped tendon or perosis in chicks

Vitamin B

Vitamin B is a water soluble vitamin which has at least 9 sub types including B_1 or thiamine, B_2 or riboflavin, B_6 or pyridoxine, B_{12} or cyanocobalamin, niacin or nicotinic acid, folate or folic acid, choline, biotine and pantothenic acid.

Thiamine

In ruminants, synthesis of thiamine occurs in rumen. Sources of vit. B are pea, beans, pulses, green vegetables, roots, fruits, rice, wheat bran etc. Strong tea, coffee have antithiamine action. It is stored in muscles, liver, heart, kidneys and bones of animals. Thiamine plays active role in carbohydrate metabolism

- Deficiency of thiamine may lead to *Beriberi disease* characterized by Ataxia and neural/lesions. *Chastek paralysis* in cats, fox and mink and *stargazing* attitude of chicks due to thiaminase (thiamine deficiency) in meal may be observed. Bracken fern poisoning in cattle and horses may cause deficiency of thiamine due to presence of thiaminase enzyme in bracken fern. Toxicity of thiamine splitting drugs like amprolium, a coccidiostate, may cause polioencephalomalcia in cattle and sheep. Cardiac dialation in pigs has also been observed due to vit. B_1 deficiency.

Riboflavin

Riboflavin is a component of several enzymes and is found in plants, meat, eggs and vegetables.

- Deficiency of riboflavin may cause *Curled Toe Paralysis* in chicks and swelling of sciatic and brachial nerves (Fig. 2.28).

Niacin

Role of niacin (NAD/NADP, nicotinamide adenine dinucleotide) is in electron transport in mitochondria of cells. It is found in grains, cereals, meat, liver, kidneys, vegetables and plants.

- Deficiency of niacin is associated with skin disorders in man *Pellegra*; anorexia, diarrhoea, anemia in pigs and mucous hyperplasia, haemorrhage in gastrointestinal tract and black tongue in dogs which is also known as *Canine pellegra*.

Pyridoxine

It is found in egg, green vegetables, meat, liver etc.

- Deficiency of pyridoxine causes uremia, convulsions, dermatitis and glossitis

Pantothenic acid

- Pantothenic acid deficiency is associated with stunted growth of chicks.

Folate

- Folic acid is required in formation of erythrocytes and hence its deficiency leads to anemia.

Cyanocobalamin

Deficiency of cyanocobalamin may also lead to anemia, as it is also needed in RBC formation.

Biotin

Biotin deficiency causes paralysis of hind legs in calves and perosis in chicks.

Choline

Choline deficiency is associated with fatty changes in liver and perosis.

Vitamin C (Ascorbic acid)

It is found in green plants and citrus fruits.
Deficiency of vit. C may cause retardation of fibroplasia, scurvy in G. pigs, haemorrhage, swelling, ulcers and delayed wound healing in animals.

MINERALS

Various minerals are also necessary for survival of animals. Deficiency of any one of them or in combination may cause serious disease in animals. Some of the important minerals are:

- Sodium chloride
- Calcium
- Phosphorus
- Magnesium
- Iodine
- Iron
- Copper
- Cobalt
- Manganese
- Potassium
- Fluorine
- Sulphur
- Selenium
- Zinc

Sodium chloride

Sodium chloride is an essential salt which maintains osmotic pressure in blood, interstitial tissue and the cells because 65% of osmotic pressure is due to sodium chloride. Chloride ions of hydrochloric acid present in stomach also come from sodium chloride.

- The excess of sodium chloride causes gastroenteritis in cattle, gastroenteritis and eosinophilic meningoencephalitis in pigs and ascites in poultry.
- Deficiency of sodium chloride is characterized by anorexia, constipation, loss of weight in sows and pica, weight loss, decreased milk production and polyurea in cattle. Deficiency of salt occurs due to diarrhoea, dehydration and vomiting.

Calcium

Normal range of calcium is 10-11 mg/100 ml blood in body of animals. If it increases above 12 mg/100 ml blood, metastatic calcification occurs, while its level less than 8 mg/100 ml blood may show signs of deficiency characterized by tetany.

Absorption of calcium from gut is facilitated by vit. D. Paratharmone stimulates to raise blood Ca level from bones while calcitonin from thyroid stimulates its deposition in bones and thus reduces blood Ca levels.

- In pregnant cows, calcium deficiency occurs just after parturition. During gestation calcium goes to foetus from skeleton of cows, resulting in weak skeleton of dam. If calcium is not provided in diet, it may cause disease in dam characterized by locomotor disturbances, abnormal curvature of back, distortion of pelvis, tetany, incoordination, muscle spasms, unconsciousness and death. Such symptoms occur in animals when their blood calcium level falls below 6 mg/100 ml of blood and if it is less than 3 mg/100ml blood, death occurs instantly.
- Milk fever is a disease of cattle that occurs due to deficiency of calcium just after parturition. Cow suddenly becomes recumbent and sits on sternum with head bending towards flank and is unable of get up. No gross/ microscopic lesion is reported in this disorder. The calcium therapy recovers the animal immediately.
- The excess of calcium may cause metastatic calcification leading to its deposition in soft tissue of kidney, lungs and stomach.

Magnesium

It acts as activator of many enzymes *e.g.* alkaline phosphatase. It is required for activation of membrane transport synthesis of protein, fat and nucleic acid and for generation/ transmission of nerve impulses. The normal blood levels are 2 mg/100 ml of blood.

- Dietary deficiency leads to hypomagnesaemia and a level below 0.7 mg/100 ml causes symptoms in calves characterized by nervous hyperirritability, tonic and clonic convulsions, depression, coma and death.
- The post-mortem lesions of magnesium deficiency includes haemorrhage in heart, intestines, mesentery and congestion of viscera.
- Microscopic lesions include calcification of intimal layer of heart blood vessels (metastatic) muscles and kidneys. *Grass tetany and Grass staggers* occurs due to hypomagnesaemia and are characterized by hyperirritability, abnormal gait, coma and death.

Phosphorus

Normal level of phosphorus is 4-8 mg/100 ml of blood. In bones, it is in the form of calcium phosphate. Deficiency of phosphorus may lead to hypophosphatemia and is characterized by pica, rheumatism and hemoglobinurea.

- Pica is licking/eating of objects other than food. It mainly occurs in cattle, buffaloes and camels, who eat bones, mud and other earthern materials. Such animals have heavy parasitic load in their gut.
- Rheumatism like syndrome is characterized by lameness in hind legs particularly in camels and buffaloes.
- Hemoglobinurea is characterized by the presence of coffee colour urine of animal due to extensive intravascular hemolysis Hemo-

globin urea is thus known as postparturient hemoglobin urea.

Selenium

Deficiency of selenium causes hemolysis as it protects cell membrane of RBC and thus its deficiency leads to anemia. Blind Staggers occurs due to excess of selenium.

Iron

Deficiency of iron leads to anemia, which is hypochromic and microcytic but rarely occurs in animals.

Copper

Deficiency of copper results in anemia and steel wool disease in sheep, which is characterized by loss of crimp in wool. Enzootic ataxia with incoordination of posterior limb has been observed in goats.

Cobalt

Vit. B_{12} is synthesized by ruminal bacteria from cobalt in ruminants. Cobalt also stimulates erythropoiesis. Its deficiency may cause wasting disease, cachexia and emaciation in animals. The pathological lesions are comprised of anemia, hemosiderosis in liver, spleen and kidneys.

Manganese

Deficiency of manganese causes slipped tendon in chicken or perosis characterized by shortening of long bones in chickens. It occurs as the epiphyseal cartilage fails to ossify at 12 week of age and epiphysis becomes loose and thus gastrocnemius tendon slips medially. This condition is known as *Slipped Tendon* or *Perosis* (Fig. 2.29).

Zinc

Deficiency of zinc may cause parakeratosis in pigs at 10-20 weeks' age. Calcium in diet with phytate or phosphate forms a complex with zinc making it unavailable for absorption leading to its deficiency, which is characterized by rough skin of abdomen, medial surface of thigh, which becomes horny. It also causes fascial eczema in cattle, thymic hypoplasia in calves and immunodeficiency in animals.

Iodine

Deficiency of iodine causes goiter in newborn pigs characterized by absence of hair on their skin. Other signs of iodine deficiencies include abnormal spermatozoa, decreased spermatogenesis, loss of libido, reduced fertility, suboestrus, anoestrus, miscarriages, dystocia and hydrocephalus. Excess of iodine may lead to lacrimation and exfoliation of dandruff like epidermal scales from skin.

Fluorine

Excess of fluorine causes mottling in teeth and bones. The teeth become shorter, broader with opaque areas.

MODEL QUESTIONS

Q. 1.   ***Fill in the blanks with suitable word(s) to answer the followings.***
1. .... in severe burns leads to impaired phagocytosis by ....
2. Radiation mainly affects the................cells of body in........., ..., ... and.........
3. Viruses are classified into two major groups viz. .... and .... on the basis of presence of ....
4. Acid fast bacilli causing disease in animals are ...., ... and ....
5. The transmission of infection created by man / doctor is known as ....
6. Snake venom contains ...., ..., ... and .... causing lysis of erythrocytes and platelets leading to .... and............

7. The gangrene on extremities produced by feeding of.............. to the animals and is also known as............... disease.
8. Fungal toxins like............... cause immunosuppression and hepatotoxicity while .... causes renal damage in chickens.
9. Pesticides are classified into four major groups..............., ..., ... and, ... of which a major group is ....
10. Heavy metals such as ...., ... and............... are immunotoxic as well as nephrotoxic in animals.
11. The first changes of nutritional deficiency are recorded in rapidly metabolizing tissues such as ...., ... and ....
12. .... animals are more susceptible to nutritional disorders.
13. Starvation is the .... of food and is characterized by .... , ... and ....
14. Ketone bodies are ...., ... and ....
15. Protein deficiency may lead to failure of collagen formation resulting in atrophy of ....,....................,....................and..................
16. Maize is deficient in................... and ....amino acids.
17. Essential fatty acids are ...., ... and..................
18. The deficiency of Vit. A is the cause of recurrent episodes of .... and .... in animals.
19. Encephalomalacia is caused by deficiency of vitamin ....
20. Perosis is caused by..................., ... and .... deficiency in birds.

Q. 2. **Write true or false against each statement and correct the false statement.**
1. ....Hog cholera occurs only in pigs.
2. ....Beef cattle are more prone to mastitis.
3. ....Nephritis is more common in male in comparison to female bovines.
4. ....Canine distemper occurs in old dogs.
5. ....Burns and surgery may lead to immunosuppression.
6. ....Rabies is caused by lyssavirus which belongs to retroviridae family.
7. ....Pathogenic fungi belong to fungi imperfecti.
8. ....Trypanosomasis may be transmitted through inoculation.
9. ....Ochratoxin causes bile duct hyperplasia and hepatcarcinoma in birds.
10. ....Most of the antibiotics show their deleterious effect on gut microflora, which may lead to gastrointestinal tract problems.
11. ....Newly born piglets are less prone to deficiency diseases.
12. ....Starvation may cause stunted growth of foetus in pregnant animals.
13. ....Presence of ketone bodies in blood should always be suspected for ketosis in cows.
14. ....Soybean is deficient in lysine amino acid.
15. ....Vitamin B complex and C are water-soluble.
16. ....Nyctalopia is caused by vitamin E deficiency.
17. ....Microphthalmos is defined as newborn with smaller eyes.
18. ....Vitamin D regulates the immune system of animals and activates the lymphocytes and macrophages.
19. ....Vitamin K_2 is produced by gastrointestinal flora and is known as phylloquinone.
20. ....Slipped tendon is caused by manganeese deficiency is birds. '

Q. 3. **Define the followings.**

1. Multiple deficiency
2. Lipolysis
3. Dehydration
4. Urolithiasis
5. Anophthalmos
6. Idiosyncracy
7. Burns
8. Mode of transmission
9. Maintenance of infection
10. Aflatoxin
11. Microphthalmos
12. Parakeratosis
13. Perosis
14. Hemoglobinurea
15. Myoglobinurea
16. Drug toxicity
17. Immunotoxicity of environmental pollutants
18. Microbial toxins
19. Electrical injury
20. Radiation injury

Q. 4. **Write short notes on.**

1. Erosions
2. Laceration
3. Latency
4. Septicemia
5. Blind staggers
6. Osteomalacia
7. Gluconeogenesis
8. Ketosis
9. Pregnancy toxemia
10. Nutritional roup
11. Convulsions
12. Neuropathy
13. Exotoxins
14. Hematuria
15. Bacteriostate
16. Factors responsible for nutritional deficiency
17. Milk fever
18. Goiter
19. White muscle disease
20. Salt poisoning

Q. 5. **Select one appropriate word from the four options provided with each question.**

1. Hog cholera occurs in.........................
   (a) Pig   (b) Dog   (c) Horse   (d) Cow
2. Partial loss of epithelium on skin or mucous membrane is known as................
   (a) Abrasion   (b) Erosion   (c) Laceration   (d) Contusion
3. Burn area of skin and tissues remains sterile till..........
   (a) 12 hrs   (b) 16 hrs   (c) 20 hrs   (d) 24 hrs
4. Epidermis and dermis are destroyed leading to shock in ....burn.
   (a) I degree   (b) II degree   (c) III degree   (d) IV degree
5. Radiation affects the dividing cells of.......
   (a) Ovary   (b) Testes   (c) Lymphocytes   (d)All of the above

6. Leptospira is a......... which causes miscarriages in cattle.
   (a) Bacteria   (b) Virus   (c) Chlamydia   (d) Spirochaete
7. *Coxiella burnetti* is a...... which causes Q-fever in animals.
   (a) Mycoplasma   (b) Bacteria   (c) Rickettsia   (d) Chlamydia
8. Ringworm is caused by a.......
   (a) Bacteria   (b) Virus   (c) Fungi   (d) Parasite
9. Transmission of diseases from one generation to another is known as.......
   (a) Vertical   (b) Horizontal   (c) Triangular   (d)All of the above
10. Aflatoxins are produced by..........
    (a) *Aspergillus flavus* (b) *Asperfillus parasiticus* (c) *Penicillium puberlum* (d)All of the above

11. Pesticide includes......
    (a) Insecticide   (b) Rodenticide   (c) Weedicide   (d)All of the above
12. Acetone, β-hydroxybutyrate and acetoacetic acid are known as.......
    (a) Ochratoxins   (b) Ketone bodies   (c) Heinze bodies   (d)Pyknotic bodies
13. Prolonged starvation leads to.................. of muscles
    (a) Hypertrophy   (b) Hyperplasia   (c) Atrophy   (d) Metaplasia
14. Deficiency of vitamin A causes...................
    (a) Nutritional roup   (b) Nyctalopia   (c) Calculi in urethra   (d)All of the above
15. Vitamin D regulates the activity of......................
    (a) Lymphocytes   (b) Macrophages   (c) All of the above   (d) None of the above
16. Star grazing in chicks in caused by .... deficiency
    (a) Vitamin B_1 (b) Vitamin B_2 (c) Vitamin B_6 (d) Vitamin B_{12}
17. Curled toe paralysis is caused by .... deficiency
    (a) Thiamine   (b) Riboflavin   (c) Choline   (d) Biotin
18. Crazy chick disease is caused by .... deficiency
    (a) Vitamin A   (b) Vitamin C   (c) Vitamin D   (d) Vitamin E
19. Perosis is caused by .... deficiency.
    (a) Biotin   (b) Choline   (c) Manganese   (d)All of the above
20. Rheumatism like syndrome is caused by deficiency of ....
    (a) Calcium   (b) Phosphorous   (c) Copper   (d) Zinc

3

GENETIC DISORDERS, DEVELOPMENTAL ANOMALIES AND MONSTERS

- **Genetics**
  - **Chromosomes**
- **Genetic disorders**
  - **Aberrations in chromosomes**
- **Anomalies**
- **Monsters**
- **Model Questions**

GENETICS

Genetics is the branch of science that deals with study of genes, chromosomes and transmittance of characters from one to generation another.

CHROMOSOMES

Chromosomes are thread-like structures present in the form of short pieces in nucleus of a cell. They are in pairs; of which one pair is sex chromosome and others are autosomes.

Table 3.1 Number of chromosomes in different species of animals

Sl. No.	Animal	Chromosomes		Male	Female
		Pairs	Total		
1.	Cattle	30	60	XY	XX
2.	Sheep	27	54	XY	XX
3.	Goat	30	60	XY	XX
4.	Pig	19	38	XY	XX
5.	Dog	39	78	XY	XX
6.	Cat	19	38	XY	XX
7.	Horse	32	64	XY	XX
8.	Poultry	39	78	ZZ	ZW

- Each chromosome is composed of two chromatids connected at centromere.

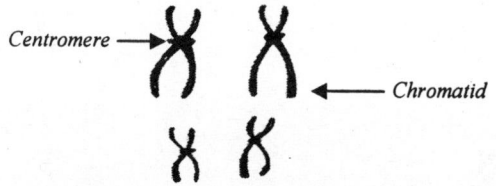

Fig. 3.1 Diagram of Chromosomes

- Chromosomes are grouped together on the basis of their length, location of centromere and this procedure is known as *karyotyping.*
- The study of karyotyping is known as *cytogenetics.*
- Chromosomes are composed of 3 components:
  - DNA - 20%
  - RNA - 10%
  - Nuclear proteins - 70%

Deoxyribo nucleic acid (DNA)

- Double helix structure of polynucleotide chain.
- A nucleotide consists of phosphate, sugar and base of either purine (Adenine, Guanine) or pyrimidine (Thymine, Cytosine).

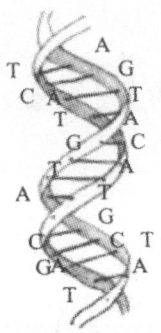

Fig. 3.2. Double helix DNA structure

- A sequence of 3 nucleotide determines the synthesis of an amino acid and is known as *genetic code/codon.*
- During cell division, one half of DNA molecule acts as template for the synthesis of other half by an enzyme DNA polymerase to transmit the genetic information which may also transit some disorders to next progeny.

Gene

- Sequence of nucleotides which controls the synthesis of one specific protein is known as *gene*. It is a unit of function. Study of genes is termed as *Genetics*. In higher animals about 1.0 million genes are present.
- Genes located on X or Y chromosomes are termed as sex linked and all other genes are autosomal genes.
- When the genes at one locus are same from both parents they are termed as *homozygous* but when they are different at one locus they are known as *heterozygous*.
- In heterozygous, characters of one gene are manifested in phenotype and such gene is known as *dominant* while unexpressed gene is called as *recessive.*

Karyotyping

- Karyotyping is the study of chromosomes in cell.
- Collection of blood, separation of lymphocytes using Histopaque-1077 gradient.
- The lymphocytes are cultured with mitogen concanavalin A (ConA) or phytohemagglutinin - M (PHA-M) for 72 hrs.
- Colchicine is used after 72 hrs to arrest the cell division at metaphase stage.
- Hypotonic solution is added to allow cells to swell which causes separation of chromosomes.
- Prepare glass slides and stain with Giemsa or other special stain.
- Identify the chromosomes and photograph them.
- Cut photographs having homologous chromosomes and make pairs.

GENETIC DISORDERS
ABERRATION IN CHROMOSOMES

- A large number of chromosomal aberrations are removed due to death of gamete or zygote which is termed as *"species cleansing effect"*. However, some aberrations persist and are expressed in phenotype leading to illness.

1. **Aberration in number**
- Chromosomes are in pairs (2n). When number of chromosomes are other than (n) or (2n). It is known as *heteroploidy*.

(a) Heteroploidy
- The number of chromosomes are other than (n) or (2n).
- When abnormal number is exact multiplies of the haploid set due to errors in mitosis. The polar body may fail to be extruded from ovum leaving diplod set to be fertilized by sperm (n) i.e. 2n + n = 3n (Triploid zygote).
- When abnormal number is not the exact multiplies of haploid set. It may have specific chromosome in triple number *(trisomy)* or in single number *(monosomy)*.

(b) Duplication and deficiencies
- Duplication or deficiency may occur in a section of chromosome and total number of chromosomes remains same.
- *Translocation* is the rearrangement of a part of chromosome in two non-homologous chromosomes. It may be reciprocal or non-reciprocal. Absence of a piece of chromosome is known as *deletion*.

(c) Mosaicism
- In mosaicism, there is more than one population of cells in body; each population differs in their chromosomes/ genes due to error during development.
- May be due to chromosomal non-disjunction there is, *e.g.* XXY in some cells, XY in other cells.

(d) Chimerism
- In this, one type of cells are acquired *in utero* from a twin *e.g.* Bovine twin, 1 male and 1 female, with joint placenta. The blood cells of male may go in female counterpart. Then the female will have two types of cell population, one of its own and another acquired from twin. Similarly, male may also have XX leucocytes in its blood. Such chimeric bulls are sterile.

2. **Abnormalities in sex chromosomes**
(a) Klinefelters syndrome
- Males have sex chromatin i.e. XXY = 47(2n) in man.
- In some cells, different number of chromosomes i.e. XX, XXY, XXXY, XXYY
- It is recognized in adolscence by small testes, tall body, and low sexual characters, mostly infertile.
- May occur in sheep, cattle and horse.

(b) Tortoiseshell male cat
- Male cat has small testes, lack of libido and absence of spermatozoa in testes with 3n chromosomes (XXY).

(c) Turner's syndrome

- Mare are with XO karyotype having gonadal dysgenesis and such animals are sterile and do not have sex chromatin.
- In mice XO karyotype is normal.

(d) Intersexes

- In this condition ambiguity occurs in genitalia or the secondary sex characters are present for both the sexes including male and female.
- Hermaphrodites have male and female genitalia while pseudohermaphrodites hae external genitalia of one sex and gonads of opposite sex.

(e) Freemartinism

- In bovine twins, one male with (XY) and one female (XX) karyotype but they share placental circulation so cells of embryo establish in other co-twin.

(f) Testicular feminization

- The animal has female genitalia as external and internal organs but in place of ovaries, there are testes. It occurs due to single gene defect and makes tissues unresponsive to androgenic hormones.

3. Abnormalities in autosomal chromosomes
(a) Down's syndrome/ Mongolism

- It occurs as a result of trisomy, number of a particular chromosome increases leaving 2n, as 61 in bovines, 77 in dogs and 47 in man *e.g.* bovine lymphosarcoma occurs in animals with 2n=61. Male dog with 2n= 77 are prone to lymphoma.

(b) Sterility in hybrids

- Donkey has 2n=62 and horse has 2n=64. Their cross mule has 2n=63.
- Cause of sterility in mules is not known, may be due to uneven number of chromosomes.

4. Abnormalities in genes

- Lethal genes are those genes which are responsible for death of zygote.

- Sublethal genes
- X-linked or sex linked: Diseases transmitted by heterozygous carrier females only to male offsprings who are homozygous for X-chromosome.

ANOMALIES

Anomaly is a developmental abnormality that occurs in any organ/tissue. It may be due to genetic disorder and may affect the zygote itself within a few days after fertilization or may occur during any stage of pregnancy. It may be classified as under:

1. Imperfect development
(a) Agenesis

Agenesis is incomplete development of an organ or mostly it is associated with absence of any organ.

- **Acrania** is absence of cranium.
- **Anencephalia** is absence of brain.
- **Hemicrania** is absence of half of head.
- **Agnathia** is absence of lower jaw.
- **Anophthalmia** is absence of one or both eyes.
- **Abrachia** is absence of fore limbs.
- **Abrachiocephalia** is absence of forelimbs and head.
- **Adactylia** is absence of digits.
- **Atresia** is absence of normal opening *e.g. Atresia ani* is absence of anus opening.

(b) Fissures

Fissures are a cleft or narrow opening in an organ on the median line of head, thorax and abdomen.

- **Cranioschisis** is a cleft in skull.
- **Chelioschisis** is a cleft in lips also known as *harelip.*
- **Palatoschisis** is a cleft in palates; also known as *cleft palate.*
- **Rachischisis** is a cleft in spinal column.
- **Schistothorax** is a fissure in thorax.
- **Schistosomus** is a fissure in abdomen.

(c) Fusion

Fusion is joining of paired organs.

- **Cyclopia** is fusion of eyes.

- **Renarcuatus** is fusion of kidneys; also known as *horseshoe kidneys.*

2. Excess of development
- Congenital hypertrophy of any organ.
- Increase in the number of any organ or part /tissue.
    - **Polyotia** is increased number of ears.
    - **Polyodontia** is increased number of teeth.
    - **Polymelia** is increased number of limbs.
    - **Polydactylia** is increased number of digits.
    - **Polymastia** is increased number of mammary gland.
    - **Polythelia** is increased number of teats.

3. Displacement during development
(a) Displacement of organ
- **Dextrocardia** is the transposition of heart into right side instead of left side of thoracic cavity.
- **Ectopia cordis** is the displacement of heart into neck.

(b) Displacement of tissues
- **Teratoma** is a tumor arising due to some embryonic defect and composed of two or more types of tissues. In this at least two tissues should be of origin.
- **Dermoid cyst** is a mass containing skin, hair, feathers or teeth depending on the species and often arranged as cyst. It mostly occurs in the subcutaneous tissues.

MONSTERS
Monster is a disturbance of development in several organs and causes distortion of the foetus *e.g.* Duplication of all or most of the organs (Fig. 3.3).
- Monsters develop from a single ovum; these are the product of incomplete twinning.
- Monsters are classified as under:

1. Separate twins
One twin is well developed while another is malformed and lacks the heart, lungs or trunk, head, limbs.

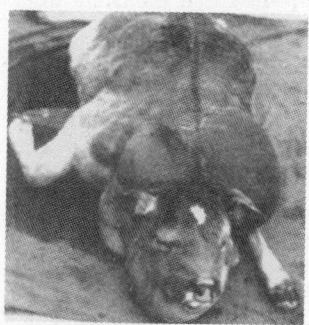

Fig.3.3. Photograph showing monster calf.

2. United twins
These twins are united with symmetrical development and are further classified as:

(a) Anterior twinning
Anterior portion of foetus is having double structures while posterior remains as single.
- **Pyopagus** is a monster twin united in the pelvic region with the bodies side by side.
- **Ischiopagus** is a monster twin united in the pelvic region with the bodies at more than a right angle.
- **Dicephalus** is a monster having two separate heads, neck, thorax, and trunk.
- **Diprosopus** is a monster having double organs in cephalic region without complete separation of heads and with double face.

(b) Posterior twinning
When in monsters, the anterior portion remains single and posterior parts become double.
- **Craniopagus** is a monster having separate brain with separate bodies arranged at an acute angle.
- **Cephalothoracopagus** is the monster having united head and thorax.
- **Dipygus** is the monster having double posterior extremities and posterior parts of body.

(c) Almost complete twining
In some monster, twins have complete development with joining in thorax and abdomen.

- **Thoracopagus** is a monsters united in thorax region.
- **Prosopothoracopagus** is the monster twin united at thorax, head, neck and abdomen.
- **Rachipagus** is the monster in which thoracic and lumber portion of vertebral column are united in twin.

MODEL QUESTIONS

Q. 1.   *Fill in the blanks with suitable word(s).*

1. Chromosomes are grouped together on the basis of ……………. and ……………… and this procedure is known as ………………..

2. ………………. is the rearrangement of a part of chromosome in two non-homologous chromosomes and it may be ………………. or ………………. .

3. Acrania is absence of ………………. while ………………. is absence of forelimbs.

4. …………. is absence of normal opening; for example……………. is absence of anus opening.

5. ………………. is a fissure in lips which is also known as ………………..

6. Palatoschisis is a ………………. in palates and is also known as……………….

7. ………………. is transposition of heart into ………………. of thoracic cavity.

8. Monsters develop from ………………. and are the products of ………………. twinning.

9. ………………. is a monstor united in the pelvic region with the bodies side by side.

10. ………………. is fusion of kidneys and is also known as ………………..

Q. 2.   *Write true or false against each statement. Correct the false statement.*

1. …………Hemicrania is absence of head.
2. …………Polyotia is decreased number of ears.
3. …………Each chromosome contains about 70% DNA.
4. …………Monsters develop from a single ovum.
5. ………….Abrachiocephalia is a absence of forelimbs and head.
6. ………… Chromosomes are thread-like structures, composed to two chromatids connected with a centromere.
7. …………Dipygus is a monster having double anterior extremities and other parts of body.
8. ………….Schistosomus is a fissure in spinal column.
9. …………Dicephalus is a monster having two separate head, neck, thorax and trunk.
10. ………….Prosopothoracopagus is a monster, which is not united at head.

Q. 3.   *Write short notes on the following.*

1. Draw a diagram of DNA structure
2. Karyotyping
3. Freemartinism
4. Anomalies
5. Monsters
6. Dermoid cyst
7. Teratoma
8. Aberration in chromosomes
9. Testicular feminization
10. Mosaicism

Q. 4.   *Define the following with suitable examples.*

1. Cytogenetics
2. Heteroploidy
3. Agnathia
11. Thoracopagus
12. Abrachia
13. Renarcuatus

4. Anophthalmia
5. Cyclopia
6. Polythelia
7. Ischiopagus
8. Ectopia cordis
9. Craniopagus
10. Polymelia

14. Pseudohermaphrodite
15. Rachischisis
16. Hemicrania
17. Chimerism
18. Rachipagus
19. Deletion
20. Cephalothoracopagus

Q. 5. *Each question is provided with four options. Select most appropriate option to fill in or answer the question.*

1. Each chromosome contains the DNA content as..................
   (a) 20%   (b) 10%   (c) 70%   (d) 30%
2. The study of karyotyping of chromosomes falls under ....
   (a) Immunogenetics   (b) Cytogenetics   (c) Moleculer genetics   (d)   Nuclear genetics.
3. In heterozygous, one gene character is manifested in phenotype and such gene is known as...
   (a) Autosomal   (b) Recessive   (c) Dominant   (d) Sex linked
4. In karyotyping, colchicine is added in culture of peripheral blood lymphocytes for arresting the cell division in ....
   (a) Telophase   (b) Meiosis   (c) Anaphase   (d) Metaphase
5. In heteroploidy, the chromosome number will be ....in cells.
   (a) n   (b) 2n   (c) 3n   (d) All of them
6. Intersexes is the condition in animals which occurs due to ambiguity in..............
   (a) Genitalia   (b) Bones   (c) Ears   (d) Eyes
7. In Turner's syndrome, mare have karyotype as....................
   (a) XX   (b) XXX   (c) XXXX   (d) XO
8. Mules have chromosome number as...........
   (a) 61   (b) 62   (c) 63   (d) 64
9. Bovine lymphosarcoma occurs in animals having chromosome number.......
   (a) 60   (b) 61   (c) 62   (d) 64.
10. Dogs with chromosome number......... are more prone to lymphoma
    (a) 76   (b) 78   (c) 77   (d) 75
11. Absence of lower jaw in foetus is known as............
    (a) Acrania   (b) Adactylia   (c) Agnathia   (d) Abrachia
12. Rachischisis is a cleft in ....
    (a) Spinal column (b) Abdomen   (c) Skull   (d) Lips
13. Harelip is due to fissure in lips and is also known as.............
    (a) Palatoschisis (b) Cranioschisis   (c) Schistosomus   (d) Chelioschisis
14. Fusion of eyes occurs in monsters and is known as.................
    (a) Renarcuatus   (b) Columbia   (c) Cyclopia   (d) Anophthalmia
15. Increased number of limbs in monsters is known as ....
    (a) Polythelia   (b) Polymastia   (c) Polymelia   (d) Polydactylia
16. Dextrocardia is transposition of heart in.............
    (a) Right thorax   (b) Left thorax   (c) Neck   (d) Abdomen
17. Tumor arising from embryonic defect and composed of more than two tissue.....
    (a) Dermatoma   (b) Hematoma   (c) Papilloma   (d) Teratoma

18. A monster having two separate brains with bodies separately arranged at an acute angle......
     (a) Cephalothoracopagus (b) Dicephalus   (c) Craniopagus   (d) Cranioschisis
19. A monster united at thorax region and with complete development as twin is known as.........
     (a) Prosopothoracopagus (b) Thoracopagus   (c) Dipygus   (d) Cephalothoracopagus
20. A monster having thorax and lumber portion of vertebral column united in twin is known as.....
     (a) Rachipagus   (b) Craniopagus   (c) Thoracopagus   (d) Dipygus

4

DISTURBANCES IN GROWTH

- **Aplasia**
- **Hypoplasia**
- **Atrophy**
- **Hypertrophy**
- **Hyperplasia**
- **Metaplasia**
- **Anaplasia**
- **Dysplasia**
- **Model Questions**

APLASIA/AGENESIS

Aplasia or agenesis is absence of any organ (Fig. 4.1).

HYPOPLASIA

Hypoplasia is failure of an organ/tissue to attain its full size (Fig. 4.1).

Etiology
- Congenital anomalies *e.g.* hypoplasia of kidneys in calves.
- Inadequate innervation.
- Inadequate blood supply.
- Malnutrition.
- Infections *e.g.* cerebral hypoplasia in bovine viral diarrhoea.

Macroscopic features
- Organ size, weight, volume reduced

Microscopic features
- Reduced size of cells.
- Reduced number of cells.
- Connective tissue and fat is more.

ATROPHY

Atrophy is decrease in size of an organ that has reached its full size (Figs. 4.2 & 4.3).

Etiology
- Physiological *e.g.* senile atrophy.
- Pressure atrophy.
- Disuse atrophy *e.g.* atrophy of immobilized legs.
- Endocrine atrophy *e.g.* atrophy of testicles.
- Environmental pollution *e.g.* atrophy of lymphoid organs.
- Inflammation/ fibrosis.

Macroscopic features
- Size, weight, volume of organ decreased.
- Wrinkles in capsule of organ.

Microscopic features
- Size of cell is smaller.

- Cell number is less.
- Fat and connective tissue cells are more.

HYPERTROPHY

Hypertrophy is increase in size of cells leading to increase in size of organ/ tissue without increase in the number of cells (Fig. 4.4).

Etiology
- Increase in metabolic activity *e.g.* myometrium during pregnancy.
- Compensatory *e.g.* if one kidney is removed, another becomes hypertrophied due to compensatory effect.

Macroscopic features
- Organ becomes large in size.
- Organ weight increases.

Microscopic features
- Size of cells increases.

HYPERPLASIA

Hyperplasia is increase in number of cells leading to increase in size of organ/tissue (Fig. 4.5).

Etiology
- Prolonged irritation *e.g.* fibrosis/nodules in hands, pads.
- Nutritional disorders *e.g.* iodine deficiency
- Infections *e.g.* pox.
- Endocrine disorders *e.g.* prostate hyperplasia.

Macroscopic features
- Increase in size, weight of organ.
- Nodular enlargement of organ.

Microscopic features
- Increased number of cells.
- Displacement of adjacent tissue.
- Lumen of ducts/ tubules obstructed.

METAPLASIA

Metaplasia is defined as transformation of one type of cells to another type of cells (Fig. 4.6 & 4.7).

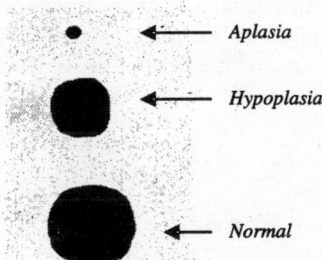

Fig. 4.1. Diagram showing Aplasia and Hypoplasia

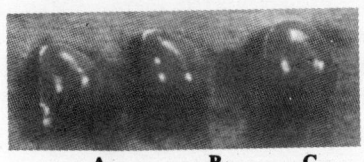

Fig. 4.2. Photograph of spleen showing atrophy (c)

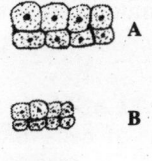

Fig. 4.3. Diagram showing atrophy (a) normal (b) decrease in size and (c) decrease in number of cells

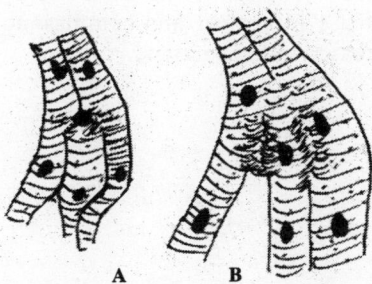

Fig. 4.4. Diagram showing hypertrophy
(a) Normal (b) Hypertrophy

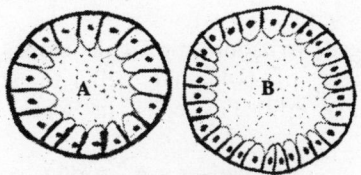

Fig. 4.5. Diagram showing hyperplasia
(a) Normal (b) hyperplasia

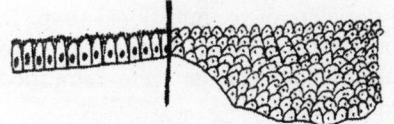

Fig. 4.6. Diagram showing Metaplasia

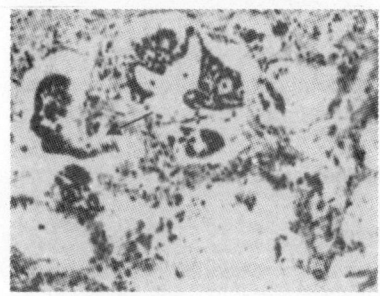

Fig. 4.7. Photograph showing Metaplasia

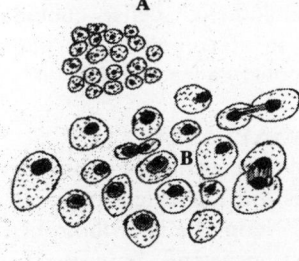

Fig. 4.8. Diagram showing anaplasia (a) Normal (b) Anaplastic cells

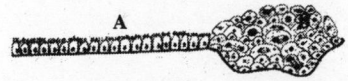

Fig. 4.9. Diagram showing dysplasia
(a). Normal (b) Dysplasia

Etiology

- Prolonged irritation *e.g.* gall stones cause metaplasia of columnar cells to stratified squamous epithelial cells in wall of gall bladder.
- Endocrine disturbances *e.g.* in dog, columnar epithelium of prostate changes into squamous epithelium.
- Nutritional deficiency *e.g.* nutritional roup. In poultry, cuboidal/columnar epithelium of oesophageal glands change into stratified squamous epithelium.
- Infections *e.g.* pulmonary adenomatosis

Macroscopic features

- Mucous membrane becomes dry in squamous metaplasia.
- Presence of nodular glands on oesophageal mucous membrane due to vitamin A deficiency in chickens also known as Nutritional roup.

Microscopic features

- Change of one type of cells to another type.
- In place of columnar cells, there are squamous epithelial cells.
- In place of endothelial cells, cuboidal or columnar cells in alveoli giving it glandular shape. *e.g.* pulmonary adenomatosis.

ANAPLASIA

Anaplasia is defined as reversion of cells to a more embryonic and less differentiated type. It is a feature in neoplasia. Neoplasia is uncontrolled new growth that serves no useful purpose, has no orderly structural arrangement and is undifferentiated or less differentiated in nature with more embryonic characters of the cells (Fig. 4.8).

Etiology

- Chemicals.
- Radiation.
- Viruses *e.g.* oncogenic viruses.

Macroscopic features

- Enlargement of organ/ tissue.
- Nodular growth of tissue, hard to touch.

Microscopic features

- Presence of pleomorphic cells and less or undifferentiated cells.
- Hyperchromasia.
- Size of cells increases.
- Size of nucleus and nucleolus increases.
- Presence of many mitotic figures.
- Seen in neoplastic conditions.

DYSPLASIA

Abnormal development of cells/tissues which are improperly arranged. It is the malformation of tissue during maturation (Fig. 4.9).

1. Spermatozoa head and tailpiece are structurally abnormal or aligned in improper way.
2. Fibrous dysplasia in bones.
3. In gastrointestinal tract, disruption of cellular orientation, variation in size and shape of cells, increase in nuclear and cytoplasmic ratio and increased mitotic activity.

MODEL QUESTIONS

Q. 1. *Fill in the blanks with suitable word(s).*
1. Dysplasia is ....development of cells which are ....arranged during ....
2. In hypoplasia the size of organ is ....and it does not attain its ....
3. The number of cells are ....in atrophy.
4. In atrophied tissue the fat and connective tissues cells are ....
5. Papule in pox is an example of .... growth disturbance.
6. Increase in size of cells in known as.................which occurs as physiological reaction in .... during pregnancy.
7. Metaplasia is defined as .... of one type of cells to another type.
8. In anaplasia, the cells are more .... and less ....
9. Hyperchromasia is a feature of .... growth disturbance.
10. Pulmonary adenomatosis is an example of .... growth disturbance.

Q. 2. *Write True or False against each statement. Correct the false statement.*
1. ....Anaplasia is a feature of neoplasia.
2. ....Metaplasia is increase in size and shape of the cells.
3. ....Dysplasia is malformation in which the cells are arranged in an improper way.
4. ....Hyperplasia is increase in size of cells.
5. ....Atrophy includes the reduction of size of an organ/ tissue.
6. ....Cerebral hypoplasia in calves is caused by an adenovirus.
7. ....In Hypertrophy, the weight of organ does not affect much.
8. ...... Atrophy is reduction in size of cells while hypoplasia is decrease in number of cells.
9. ...... Wrinkles in capsule of spleen are example of atrophy.
10. ....Increased size of nucleus and nucleolus with increase in size of cell occurs in anaplasia.

Q. 3. *Define the followings.*
1. Anaplasia
2. Metaplasia
3. Senile atrophy
4. Hyperplasia
5. Hypertrophy
6. Dysplasia
7. Atrophy
8. Hyperchromasia
9. Neoplasia
10. Hypoplasia

Q. 4. *Write short notes on.*
1. Nutritional roup.
2. Pulmonary adenomatosis.

Q. 5. *Select most appropriate word(s) from the four options given with each statement.*
1. Cerebral hypoplasia in calves is caused by..............
   (a) Adenovirus   (b) Rotavirus   (c) Bovine viral diarrhoea virus   (d) Coronavirus
2. Increase in size of cells leading to increase in size of organ is known as............
   (a) Atrophy   (b) Hyperplasia   (c) Hypertrophy   (d) Metaplasia.
3. Fibrosis may lead to ....
   (a) Atrophy   (b) Hyperplasia   (c) Dysplasia   (d) Hypertrophy

47

4. Transformation of one type of cells to another cell type is known as ....
    (a) Hypoplasia   (b) Dysplasia   (c) Anaplasia   (d) Metaplasia
5. Reversion of cells towards embryonic type is known as........
    (a) Anaplasia   (b) Neoplasia   (c) Metaplasia   (d) Hypoplasia
6. Spermatozoa with defective head and tail piece is an example of ....
    (a) Dysplasia   (b) Anaplasia   (c) Neoplasia   (d) Metaplasia
7. Hyperchromasia in cells with their enlargement is known as ....
    (a) Hyperplasia   (b) Hypertrophy   (c) Metaplasia   (d) Anaplasia
8. Increased number of cells leading to increase in size and weight of organ is known as.........
    (a) Hypertrophy   (b) Anaplasia   (c) Hyperplasia   (d) Metaplasia
9. Environmental pollution may lead to .... of lymphoid organs.
    (a) Atrophy   (b) Aplasia   (c) Agenesis   (d) Hypoplasia
10. Failure of an organ to develop its full size is known as ......
    (a) Hyperplasia   (b) Aplasia   (c) Neoplasia   (d) Hypoplasia

5

DISTURBANCES IN CIRCULATION

- **Congestion / Hyperemia**
- **Haemorrhage**
- **Thrombosis**
- **Embolism**
- **Ischemia**
- **Infarction**
- **Oedema**
- **Shock**
- **Sludged blood**
- **Model Questions**

CONGESTION/ HYPEREMIA

Hyperemia is increased amount of blood in circulatory system. It is of two types, active and passive. In active hyperemia blood accumulates in arteries while in passive hyperemia the amount of blood increases in veins (Figs. 5.1. to 5.4).

Etiology
- As a result of inflammation.
- Obstruction of blood vessels.

Macroscopic features
- Organ becomes dark red/cyanotic.
- Size of organ increases.
- Weight of organ increases.
- Blood vessels become distended due to accumulation of blood.

Microscopic features
- Increased amount of blood in blood vessels.
- Veins/capillaries/arteries are distended due to accumulation of blood.
- Blood vessels become enlarged with blood and their number increases.

HAEMORRHAGE

Escape of all the constituents of blood from blood vessels. It may occur through two processes *i.e. rhexis*- break in wall of blood vessel or through *diapedesis* in which blood leaves through intact wall of blood vessel. It occurs only in living animals (Fig. 5.5).

Etiology
- Mechanical trauma.
- Necrosis of the wall of blood vessels.
- Infections.
- Toxins.
- Neoplasm.

Macroscopic features
- Organ becomes pale due to escape of blood
- As per size, the haemorrhage is classified as under:
  - Pinpoint haemorrhage of about one mm diameter or pinhead size is known as *petechiae* (Fig. 5.6).
  - More than one to 10 mm diameter haemorrhage are known as *ecchymoses* (Fig. 5.6).
  - Irregular, diffuse and flat areas of haemorrhage on mucosal or serosal surfaces are known as *suffusions*.
  - Haemorrhage appear in line in crests or folds on mucous membrane are known as *linear haemorrhage* (Figs. 5.7 & 5.8).
  - *Hematoma* is the accumulation of blood in spherical shaped mass (Fig.5.9).
- According to location, the haemorrhage is classified as:
  - **Hemothorax:** Blood in thoracic cavity.
  - **Hemopericardium:** Blood in pericardial sac. When there is increased amount of blood in pericardial sac, it causes heart failure and is known as *cardiac temponade* (Fig. 5.10).
  - **Hemoperitonium:** Blood in peritoneal cavity.
  - **Hemoptysis:** Blood in sputum.
  - **Hematuria:** Blood in urine.
  - **Epistaxis:** Blood from nose.
  - **Metrorrhagia:** Blood from uterus.
  - **Melena:** Bleeding in faeces.
  - **Hematemesis:** Blood in vomitus.

Microscopic features
- Blood constituents are seen outside the blood vessels.
- Break in blood vessels.
- Presence of red blood cells in tissues outside the blood vessels (Fig. 5.11).

THROMBOSIS

Formation of clot of blood in vascular system in the wall of blood vessel. It occurs due to endothelial injury leading to accumulation of thrombocytes, fibrinogen, erythrocytes and leucocytes (Figs. 5.12 & 5.13).

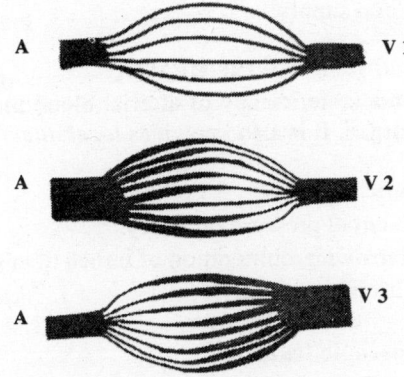

Fig. 5.1. Diagram showing congestion 1. Normal blood vessel A–arterial and V-Venous end, 2. Active congestion and 3. Passive congestion

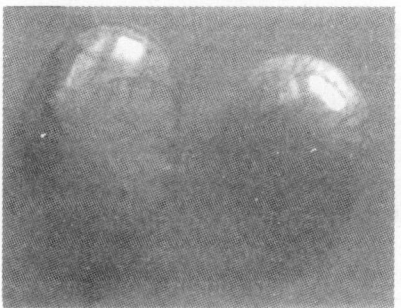

Fig. 5.2. Photograph of testes showing congestion

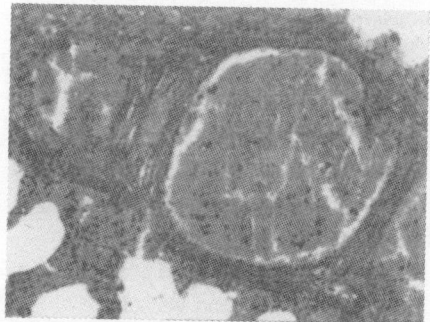

Fig. 5.3. Photomicrograph of lung showing congestion

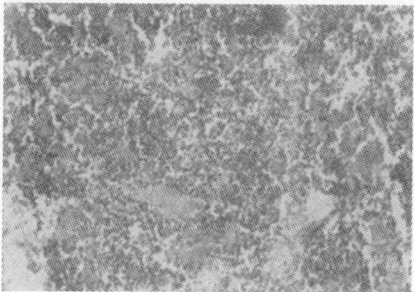

Fig. 5.4. Photomicrograph of lymph node showing congestion

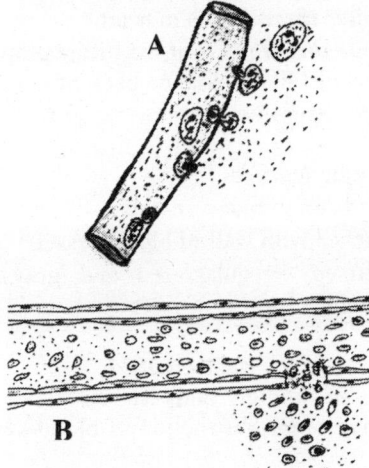

Fig. 5.5. Diagram showing haemorrhage through (A) diapedesis (B) rhexis

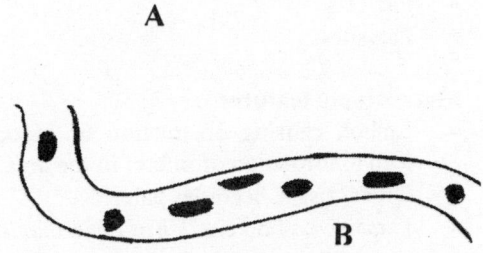

Fig. 5.6. Diagram showing (A) Petechial (B) Ecchymotic haemorrhage

51

Etiology

- Injury in endothelium of blood vessels.
- Alteration in blood flow.
- Alteration in composition of blood.

Macroscopic features

- Blood clot in wall of blood vessels.
- On removal of clot, rough surface exposed.
- Clot may be pale, red or laminated.
- *Occlusive thrombus* totally occlude blood vessels.
- *Mural thrombus* is on the wall of heart.
- *Valvular thrombus* is on valves of heart.
- *Cardiac thrombus* is in heart.
- *Saddle thrombus* is at the bifurcation of blood vessel just like saddle on back of horse.
- *Septic thrombus* contains bacteria.

Microscopic features

- Blood clot in blood vessel.
- Attached with wall of blood vessel.
- Alternate, irregular, red and gray areas in thrombi.

EMBOLISM

Presence of foreign body in circulatory system which may cause obstruction in blood vessel (Fig. 5.14).

Etiology

- Thrombus, Fibrin.
- Bacteria.
- Neoplasm.
- Clumps of normal cells.
- Fat, Gas.
- Parasites.

Macroscopic features

- Emboli causing obstruction of blood vessels lead to formation of infarct in the area.
- Organ/ tissue becomes pale.
- Parasitic emboli *e.g. Dirofilaria immitis*

Microscopic features

- Presence of foreign material in blood.

- Dependent area necrotic due to absence of blood supply.

ISCHEMIA

Ischemia is deficiency of arterial blood in any part of an organ. It is also known as *local anemia*.

Etiology

- External pressure on artery.
- Narrowing/obliteration of lumen of artery.
- Thrombi/emboli.

Macroscopic features

- Necrosis of dependent part.
- Occurrence of infarction.
- Dead tissue replaced by fibrous tissue.

Microscopic features

- Lesions of infarction

INFARCTION

Local area of necrosis resulting from ischemia. Ischemia is the deficiency of blood due to obstruction in artery (Figs. 5.15 & 5.16).

Etiology

- Thrombi.
- Emboli.
- Poisons like Fusarium toxins.

Macroscopic features

- Necrosis in triangular area
- *Red infarct* is observed as red triangle bulky surface.
- *Pale infarct* is grey in colour and seen as triangle depressed surface.

Microscopic features

- Necrosis in cone shaped area.
- Obstruction of blood vessels.

OEDEMA

Accumulation of excessive fluid in intercellular spaces and / or in body cavity (Figs. 5.17 to 5.20).

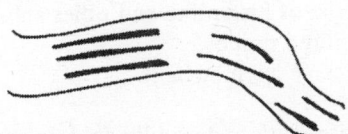

Fig. 5.7. Diagram of linear haemorrhage

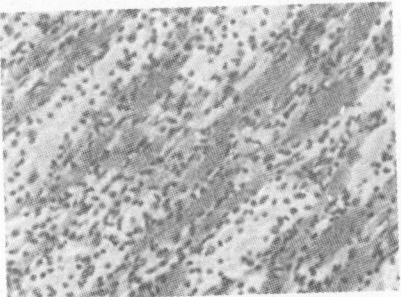

Fig. 5.11. Photomicrograph of kidney showing
haemorrhage

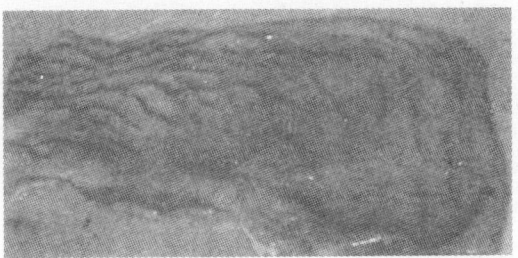

Fig. 5.8. Photograph of Large intestine showing
linear haemorrhage

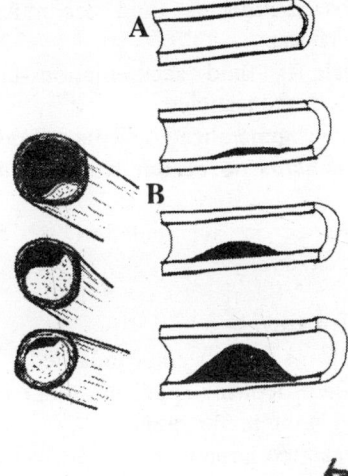

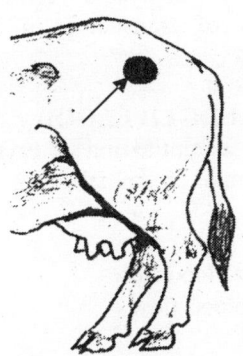

Fig. 5.9. Diagram showing hematoma

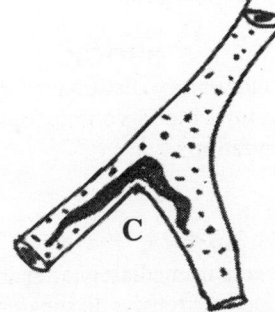

Fig. 5.12. Diagram of thrombi formation in
wall of blood vessel (A) Normal
(B) Thrombi formation (C) Saddle thrombi

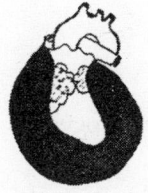

Fig. 5.10. Diagram showing cardiac temponade

Etiology
- Deficiency of protein.
- Passive hyperemia.
- Increased permeability of capillaries.
- Obstruction of lymphatics.

Macroscopic features
- Swelling of tissue / organ / body.
- Weight and size of organ increased.
- Colour becomes light.
- Pitting impressions on pressure.
- *Ascites* is accumulation of fluid in peritoneum. It is also known as *hydroperitonium*.
- *Hydropericardium* is fluid accumulation in pericardial sac.
- *Hydrocele* is fluid accumulation in tunica vaginalis of the testicles.
- *Anasarca* is generalized oedema of body.
- *Hydrocephalus* is accumulation of fluid in brain.
- *Hydrothorax* is accumulation of fluid in thoracic cavity.

Microscopic features
- Intercellular spaces become enlarged.
- Serum/fluid deposits (pink in colour on H&E staining) in intercellular spaces.
- Cells separated farther.

SHOCK
Shock is a circulatory disturbance characterized by reduction in total blood volume, blood flow and by haemconcentration.

Etiology
- *Primary shock*
  - Occurs immediately after injury.
  - Injury / extensive tissue destruction.
  - Emotional crisis.
  - Surgical manipulation.
- *Secondary shock*
  - Crushing injury involving chest and abdomen.
  - Occurs after several hours of incubation.

- Release of histamine and other substances by injured tissue.
- Extensive haemorrhage.
- Burns.
- Predisposing factors like cold, exhaustion, depression.

Macroscopic features
- Acute general passive hyperemia.
- Dilatation of capillaries.
- Cyanosis.
- Numerous petechial haemorrhages.
- Oedema and loose connective tissue.

Microscopic features
- Capillaries and small blood vessels are distended due to accumulation of blood.
- Number of engorged blood vessels increased.
- Focal haemorrhage.
- Oedema, cells separated farther due to accumulation of transudate in intercellular spaces.

SLUDGED BLOOD
Sludged blood is agglutination of erythrocytes in the vascular system of an animal.

Etiology
- Fluctuation in blood flow.
- Slow rate of blood flow.

Macroscopic features
- Oedema.
- Emboli.
- Infarction.
- Necrosis.

Microscopic features
- Clumping of erythrocytes in pulmonary capillaries.
- Infarction, necrosis.
- Oedema.
- Erythrophagocytosis by reticuloendothelial cells.

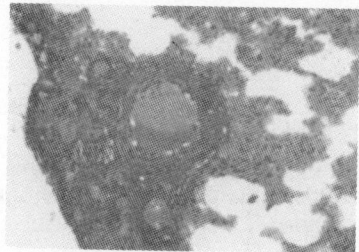

Fig. 5.13. *Photomicrograph of thrombi in blood vessel of lung*

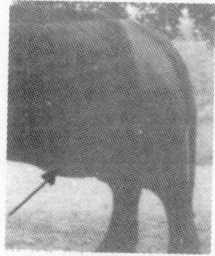

Fig. 5. 17. *Photograph of an elephant showing oedema in s/c region*

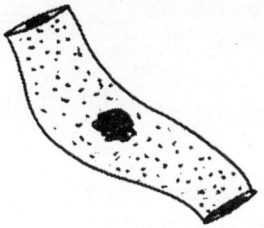

Fig. 5.14. *Diagram of emboli in blood vessel*

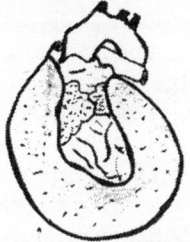

Fig. 5.18. *Diagram showing Hydropericardium*

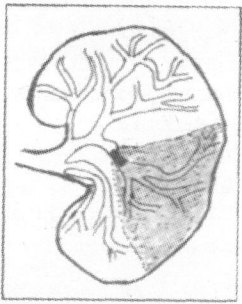

Fig. 5.15. *Diagram of infarction in kidney*

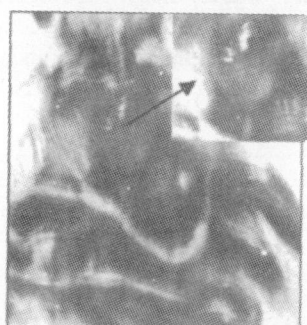

Fig. 5. 19. *Photograph of poultry showing Hydropericardium*

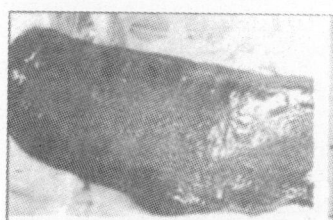

Fig. 5.16. *Photograph of spleen showing infarction*

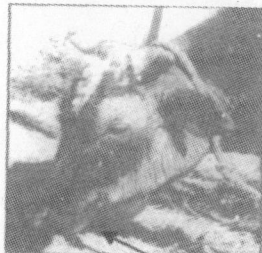

Fig. 5.20. *Photograph of bullock showing oedema in mandibular region*

MODEL QUESTIONS

Q. 1.   *Fill in the blanks with suitable word(s).*
1.   Accumulation of increased amount of blood in blood vessels in known as ....
2.   Presence of blood in urine, sputum and faeces is known as........., ... and......, respectively.
3.   ....haemorrhages in large intestine is example of rinderpest in animals.
4.   ....is generalized oedema of body while ....is accumulation of fluid in tunica vaginalis.
5.   ....occurs in poultry due to accumulation of fluid in pericardial sac which is also known as..................
6.   Shock is circulatory disturbance characterized by decrease in..........., ...and by ....
7.   Agglutination of erythrocytes in blood vessels is known as ...., which may act as ....and leads to ...., ...and ....
8.   Discharge of blood from uterus in known as ....while the presence of blood in vomitus is called as ....

Q. 2.   *Write true or false against each statement. Correct the false statement.*
1.   ....Epistaxis is bleeding from mouth.
2.   ....Cardiac temponade is failure of heart due to excessive accumulation of blood in pericardial sac.
3.   ....In arteries the increased amount of blood as known passive hyperemia.
4.   ....Hydrocephalus is accumulation of blood in brain.
5.   ....Melena is the presence of blood in faeces.
6.   ....Laminated thrombi alternatively have red and grey colour deposits.
7.   ....Hematoma is the accumulation of blood in spherical shaped mass.
8.   ....Infarction is local area of necrosis as a result of oedema.
9.   ....Sludged blood is agglutination of RBC after haemorrhage.
10. ....Hydrothorax is accumulation of fluid in thoracic cavity.

Q. 3.   *Write short notes on.*
1.   Ischemia
2.   Infarction
3.   Primary shock
4.   Oedema
5.   Sludged blood

Q. 4.   *Define the followings.*
1.   Hemoptysis
2.   Suffusions
3.   Petechiae
4.   Hematoma
5.   Saddle thrombi
6.   Acute general active hyperemia
7.   Acute local passive hyperemia
8.   Hydrocephalus
9.   Valvular thrombi
10. Hydropericardium

Q. 5. *Select most appropriate word(s) from the four options given against each statement.*

1. Petechial haemorrhage are of .... size.
   (a) 1 mm   (b) 2 mm   (c) 5 mm   (d) 10 mm
2. Parasitic emboli are formed in dogs due to ....
   (a) *Strongylus* spp   (b) *Dirofilaria immitis*   (c) *Coccidia* spp.   (d)*Sarcoptes canis*
3. Metrorrhagia is haemorrhage from ....
   (a) Intestine   (b) Stomach   (c) Oviduct   (d) Uterus
4. Septic thrombus must have........................ in it.
   (a) Virus   (b) Parasite   (c) Fungi   (d) Bacteria
5. Presence of foreign material in blood vessels is known as ....
   (a) Thrombus   (b) Emboli   (c) Ischemia   (d) Infarction
6. Accumulation of fluid in peritoneal cavity is known as..........
   (a) Anasarca   (b) Hydropericardium   (c) Hydrothorax   (d) Ascites
7. Shock is circulatory disturbance characterized by ....
   (a) Reduced blood volume (b) Reduced blood flow (c) Hemoconcentration (d)All of the above
8. Active hyperemia is accumulation of blood in ....
   (a) Veins   (b) Lymphatics   (c) Arteries   (d) Intestines
9. Escape of all blood constituents through intact blood vessel is known as..........
   (a) Rhexis   (b) Ecchymosis   (c) Petechiae   (d) Diapedesis
10. Erythrophagocytosis is a feature of ....
    (a) Congestion   (b) Oedema   (c) Sludged blood   (d) Infarction

6

DISTURBANCES IN CELL METABOLISM

- **Cloudy Swelling**
- **Hydropic Degeneration**
- **Mucinous Degeneration**
- **Mucoid Degeneration**
- **Psuedomucin**
- **Amyloid Infiltration**
- **Hyaline Degeneration**
- **Fatty Changes**
- **Glycogen Infiltration**
- **Model Questions**

CLOUDY SWELLING

Swelling of cells occur with hazy appearance due to a mild injury. The cells take more water due to defect in sodium pump leading to swollen mitochondria which gives granular cytoplasmic appearance. It is the first reaction of cell to the mildest injury. Cloudy swelling is a reversible reaction (Figs. 6.1 & 6. 2).

Etiology
- Can be caused by even mildest injury.
- Any factor causing interference with metabolism of the cell like bacterial toxins, fever, diabetes, circulatory disturbances etc.

Macroscopic features
- Organ becomes enlarged and rounded.
- Weight of organ increases.
- Bulging on cut surfaces.
- Amount of fluid increases in organ.

Microscopic features
- Swelling of cells, edges become rounded.
- Increased size of cells.
- Cytoplasm of the cells becomes hazy/cloudy due to increased granularity.
- Can be seen in liver, kidney and muscles.

HYDROPIC DEGENERATION

Cells swell due to intake of clear fluid. Such cells may burst due to increased amount of fluid and form vesicle. Hydropic degeneration can be seen in epithelium of skin and /or mucous membranes of body (Figs. 6.3 & 6.4)

Etiology
- Mechanical injury.
- Burns.
- Chemical injury.
- Infections caused by virus like foot and mouth disease virus, pox virus etc.

Macroscopic features
- Vesicle formation.
- Accumulation of fluid under superficial layer of skin/mucus membrane.

- Heals rapidly within 2-4 days.
- No scar formation.
- Pyogenic organisms may convert it into *pustule*.

Microscopic features
- Cell size increases due to accumulation of clear fluid in cytoplasm.
- Droplets in cytoplasm as vacuoles.
- Cell bursts and epithelium protrudes leading to blister.
- Mostly affects prickle cell layer (Stratum spinosum) of skin.

MUCINOUS DEGENERATION

Excessive accumulation of mucin in degenerating epithelial cells. Mucin is a glassy, viscid, stringy and slimy is glycoprotein produced by columnar epithelial cells on mucus membranes. Such cells burst to release the mucin in lumen of organ and are called as *goblet cells*. When mucin is mixed with water, it is known as *mucus* (Figs. 6.5 & 6.6).

Etiology
- Any irritant to mucus membrane like chemicals and infection.
- Bacteria *e.g. E. coli.*
- Virus *e.g.* Rotavirus.
- Parasite *e.g.* Ascaris.

Macroscopic features
- Over production of mucus in intestines which covers intestinal contents/ stool.
- Over production of mucus in genital tract during oestrus characterized by mucus discharge from vulva.
- Nasal discharge during respiratory mucosa involvement.
- Mucus is mucin mixed with water and slimy and stringy in nature.

Microscopic features
- Increased number of goblet cells.
- Goblet cells are elliptical columnar cells containing mucus.

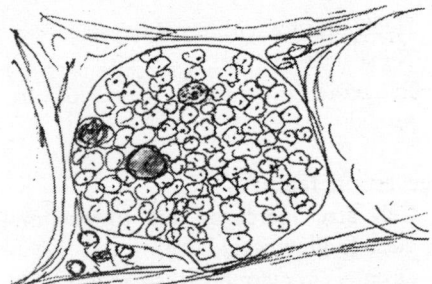

Fig. 6.1. Diagram showing cloudy swelling in liver

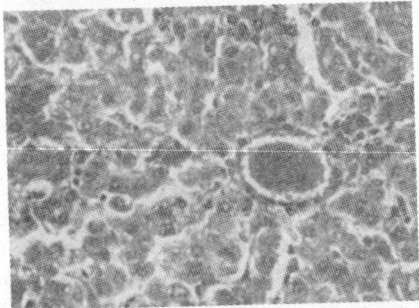

Fig. 6.2. Photomicrograph of liver showing cloudy swelling

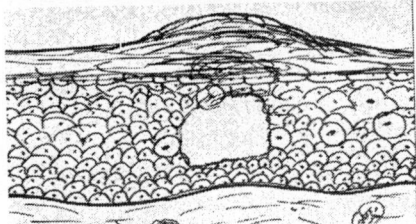

Fig. 6.3. Diagram showing hydropic degeneration and vesicle in skin

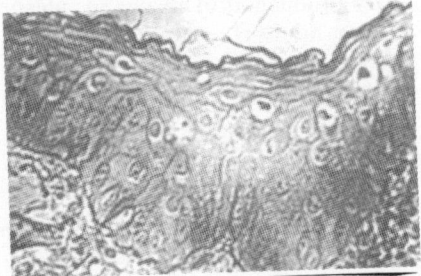

Fig. 6.4. Photomicrograph of hydropic degeneration in skin

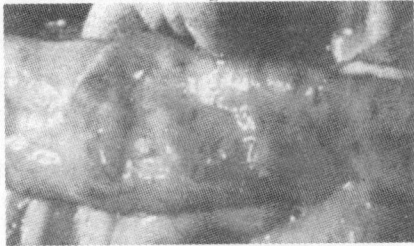

Fig. 6.5. Photograph of intestine showing mucous degeneration

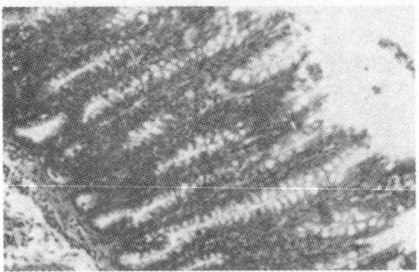

Fig. 6.6. Photomicrograph of intestine showing mucous degeneration

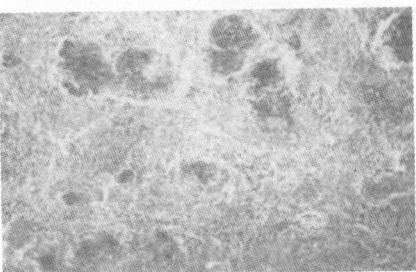

Fig. 6.7. Photomicrograph of spleen showing amyloid infiltration

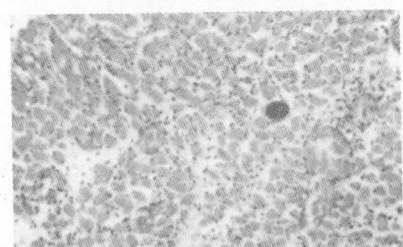

Fig. 6.8. Photomicrograph showing hyaline in muscles

- Mucin in lumen stains basophils through H & E staining.
- Seen on mucous surfaces only.

MUCOID DEGENERATION

Mucoid degeneration is mucin-like glycoprotein deposits in connective tissue.

Etiology

- In embryonic tissue *e.g.* umblical cord.
- In connective tissue tumors *e.g.* myxosarcoma.
- Myxedema due to thyroid deficiency.
- In cachexia due to starvation, parasitism or chronic wasting diseases.

Macroscopic features

- Shrunken tissue giving translucent jelly-like appearance.
- A watery, slimy and stringy material on cut surface.

Microscopic features

- Mucoid degeneration tissue stains blue
- Nuclei are hyperchromatic.
- Fibrous tissue is pale blue.
- Usually accompanied by fat necrosis.

PSEUDOMUCIN

Pseudomucin is secretion of ovaries and is observed in cystadenomas. However, it is not a disturbance of cell metabolism.

Etiology

- Cystadenoma, cystadenocarcinoma
- Paraovarian cysts.

Macroscopic features

- Transparent, slimy similar to mucin.
- It is not precipitated by acetic acid while mucin is precipitated.

Microscopic features

- Homogenous like plasma, stains pink with H&E stain.
- Extracellular.

AMYLOID INFILTRATION

Deposition of amyloid between capillary endothelium and adjacent cells. Amyloid is a starch like substance which stains brown/blue/black with iodine and chemically it is protein polysaccharide (Fig. 6.7).

Etiology

- Not exactly known.
- It is thought to be due to antigen-antibody reaction/deposition of immune complexes in between capillary endothelium and adjacent cells.

Macroscopic features

- Organ size increases with rounded edges, pits on pressure, cyanotic/yellow in colour and fragile.
- *Sago spleen* due to deposition of grey, waxy sago-like material.

Microscopic features

- Amyloid stains pink on H& E stain.
- It is a permanent effect in body and remains the whole life without causing much adverse effects.

HYALINE DEGENERATION

Glossy substance (glass-like) solid, dense, smoothly homogenous deposits in tissues. Tissue becomes inelastic. It is a permanent change. Hyaline is very difficult to distinguish macroscopically (Fig. 6.8).

Etiology

- Disturbance in protein metabolism.
- No specific cause.

Macroscopic and Microscopic features
Connective Tissue hyaline

- In old scars, due to lack of nutrients; homogenous, strong acidophilic and pink in colour. There are no nuclei and no fibrils.

Epithelial Hyaline

- Starch-like bodies in prostate, lungs, kidneys.

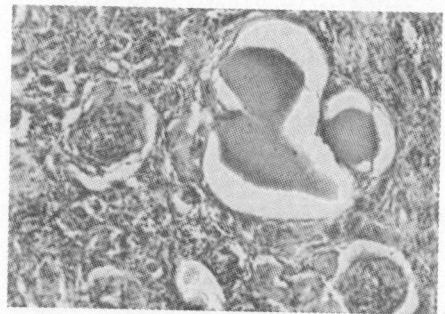

Fig. 6.9. *Photomicrograph of kidney showing hyaline*

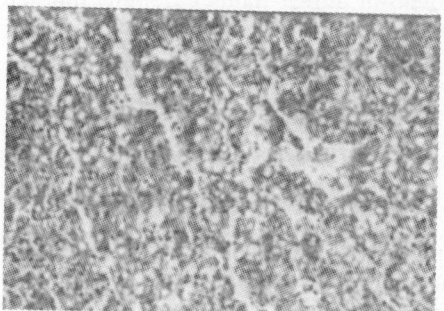

Fig. 6.11. *Photomicrograph of liver showing fatty changes*

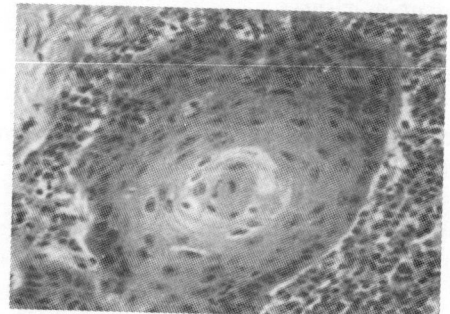

Fig. 6.10. *Photomicrograph of skin showing hyaline (epithelial pearl)*

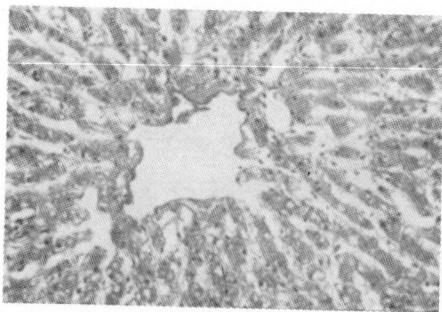

Fig. 6.12. *Photomicrograph of liver showing glycogen infiltration*

- Microscopically characterized by round, homogeneous, pink, within an alveolus of lung.
- Homogenous, pink in kidney tubules/glomeruli (Fig. 6.9).

Keratohyaline
- Occurs due to slow death of stratified squamous epithelial cells because of lack of nutrients. Keratinized epithelium is firm, hard and colourless. Microscopically, it is seen in epithelial pearls *e.g.* horn cancer, warts (Fig. 6.10).

FATTY CHANGES
Intracellular accumulation of fat in liver, kidneys and heart. It is a reversible change.

Etiology
- Increased release of fatty acids.
- Decreased oxidation of fatty acids.
- Lipotrope deficiency.
- In ketosis, diabetes, pregnancy toxaemia.

Macroscopic features
- Enlargement of organ.
- Cut surfaces are bulging and greasy.
- Organ colour becomes light.

Microscopic features
- Intracellular deposition of fat droplets. (Fig. 6.11)
- In cytoplasm clear round/oval spaces with eccentrically placed nucleus.
- Stains yellow orange with sudan III.

GLYCOGEN INFILTRATION (GLYCOGEN STORAGE DISEASE)

Glycogen accumulates when increased amount of glycogen enters in the cells of kidneys, muscles and liver (Fig. 6.12).

Etiology

- Diabetes mellitus.
- Impaired carbohydrate metabolism due to drugs *e.g.* corticosteroid therapy.

Macroscopic features

- Affected organ becomes enlarged.

Microscopic features

- Intracellular deposits of glycogen in cells of kidneys, liver and muscles.
- Small clear vacuoles seen in distal portion of proximal convoluted tubules, hepatocytes etc.
- It can be stained as bright red by Best's. Carmine and PAS and reddish brown by iodine.

MODEL QUESTIONS

Q. 1.   *Fill in the blanks with suitable word(s).*

1. Cells swell due to accumulation of clear fluid in ....which occurs in .... layers of epithelial cells or mucous membrane in case of .... disease.
2. Pyogenic bacteria invades the vesicle and may convert it into ....
3. Cloudy swelling is a .... reaction against .... injury/ irritant and it is the ....reaction of body.
4. Mucoid degeneration occurs due to .... deficiency and in .... due to .... , ... and ....
5. Pseudomucin appears in .... and .... and is characterized by appearance of .... and ....material like mucin.
6. Amyloid is ....like substance which stains ....with iodine and chemically it is ....
7. Connective tissue hyaline is seen in .... due to lack of ....and is characterized by..................., ... and pink in colour.
8. Keratohyaline is .... due to lack of nutrients and occurs in ....cancer.

Q. 2.   *Write True or False against each statement. Correct the false statements.*

1. ....Vesicle formation occurs as a result of breaking of cells due to cloudy swelling.
2. ....Amyloid is caused by antigen-antibody complexes.
3. ....Mucinous degeneration occurs in connective tissues with accumulation of slimy and stringy material.
4. ....Epithelial hyaline is characterized by the presence of epithelial pearls.
5. ....Diabetes mellitus may lead to glycogen storage disease.
6. ....Hydropic degeneration mostly occurs in prickle cell layer of skin or mucous membrane.
7. ....Cachexia due to starvation my lead to mucoid degeneration.
8. ....Cloudy swelling is characterized by hazy and cloudy cells due to swelling of mitochondria.
9. ....Mucin is mucus mixed with water and stringy in nature.
10. ....Glycogen is stained as redish brown by PAS.

Q. 3. **Write short notes on.**
1. Fatty changes
2. Keratohyaline
3. Glyocogen storage disease
4. Mucus
5. Cloudy swelling

Q. 4. **Define the following**

1. Pseudomucin
2. Mucin
3. Hyaline
4. Amyloid
5. Vesicle

6. Pustule
7. Goblet cells
8. Sago spleen
9. Epithelial pearl
10 Sodium pump

Q. 5. **Differentiate the followings**
1. Mucinous and mucoid degeneration.
2. Vesicle and Pustules.
3. Cloudy swelling and hydropic degeneration.
4. Hyaline and amyloid infiltration.
5. Fatty changes and glycogen infiltration.

Q. 6. **Select suitable word(s) from the four options to correct the following statements.**
1. Hydropic degeneration leads to ………….. formation in skin.
   (a) Vesicle   (b) Pustule   (c) Scab   (d) Papule
2. Cloudy swelling is characterized by hazy cytoplasm due to swollen ………
   (a) Endoplasmic reticulum (b) Golgi bodies   (c) Mitochondria   (d) Nucleus
3. The mucous containing cells in mucous membranes are known as …….
   (a) Epithelial cells   (b) Pearl cells   (c) Columnar cells   (d) Goblet cells
4. Mucin stains ………… by H&E stain.
   (a) Blue   (b) Pink   (c) Yellow   (d) Black
5. Sago spleen is observed in ………
   (a) Amyloid   (b) Mucin   (c) Hyaline   (d) Pseudomucin
6. Epithelial pearl is an example of ……….
   (a) Amyloid   (b) Mucin   (c) Hyaline   (d) Cell Swelling
7. Ketosis in cow may cause……………
   (a) Hyaline degeneration (b) Fatty change   (c) Amyloid   (d) Cell swelling
8. Mucous degeneration in intestine is caused by ………………
   (a) Rotavirus   (b) *E. Coli*   (c) Ascaris   (d)All of the above
9. Corticosteroid therapy may lead to ……………
   (a) Fatty changes   (b) Hyaline   (c) Glycogen   (d) Cell swelling
10. Amyloid occurs in body as a result of …………..
   (a) Immune complexes (b) Antigen   (c) Antibody   (d) Starch

7

NECROSIS, GANGRENE AND POST-MORTEM CHANGES

- **Necrosis**
  - **Coagulative Necrosis**
  - **Caseative Necrosis**
  - **Liquifactive Necrosis**
  - **Fat Necrosis**
- **Apoptosis**
- **Gangrene**
- **Post-mortem Changes**
  - **Autolysis**
  - **Putrefaction**
  - **Pseudomelanosis**
  - **Rigor Mortis**
  - **Algor Mortis**
  - **Livor Mortis**
  - **Hypostatic Congestion**
  - **Post-mortem Emphysema**
  - **Post-mortem Clot**
  - **Displacement of Organs**
  - **Imbibition of Bile**
- **Model Questions**

NECROSIS

Local death of tissue /cells in living body is known as necrosis, It is characterized by the followings.

- *Pyknosis* is condensation of chromatin material, nuclei becomes dark, reduced in size and deeply stained.
- *Karyorrhexis* is fragmentation of nucleus.
- *Karyolysis* is dissolution of nucleus into small fragments, basophilic granules/fragments.
- *Chromatolysis* is lysis of chromatin material.
- *Necrobiosis* is physiological cell death after completion of its function *e.g.* RBC after 140 days.

Necrosis is further classified into coagulative, caseative, liquifactive and fat necrosis which are different from apoptosis (Figs. 7.1 to 7.3).

COAGULATIVE NECROSIS

Local death of cells/tissue in living body characterized by loss of cellular details, while tissue architecture remains intact (Fig. 7.4).

Etiology
- Infections.
- Ischemia.
- Mild irritant *e.g.* toxins/chemical poisons.
- Heat, trauma.

Macroscopic features
- Organ becomes grey/white in colour, firm, dense, depressed with surrounding tissue.

Microscopic features
- Cellular outline present, which maintains the architecture of tissue/ organ.
- Nucleus absent or pyknotic.
- Cytoplasm becomes acidophilic.

CASEATIVE NECROSIS

Local death of cells/tissue in living body; the dead cells/tissues are characterized by presence of firm, dry and cheesy consistency. It occurs due to coagulation of proteins and lipids (Fig. 7.5).

Etiology
- Chronic infections *e.g.* *Mycobacterium tuberculosis*.
- Systemic fungal infections.

Macroscopic features
- Dead tissue looks like milk curd or cottage cheese.
- Tissue dry, firm, agranular, white/grey/ yellowish in colour

Microscopic features
- Disappearance of cells; no cell details/ architecture.
- Purplish granules on H&E staining, blue granules from nucleus fragments, red granules from cytoplasm fragments.

LIQUIFACTIVE NECROSIS

Local death of cells/tissues in living body characterized by rapid enzymatic dissolution of cells. The intracellular hydrolases and proteolytic enzymes of leucocytes play role in dissolution of cells (Fig. 7.6).

Etiology
- Pyogenic organisms.

Macroscopic features
- Liquifactive necrosed tissue present in a cavity "Abscess".
- It contains small/large amount of cloudy fluid, which is creamy yellow (Pus).

Microscopic features
- Areas of liquifactive necrosis stains pink.
- Infiltration of neutrophils.
- Sometimes empty spaces but infiltration of neutrophils at periphery.

FAT NECROSIS

Local death of adipose cells in living body.

Etiology
- Trauma.

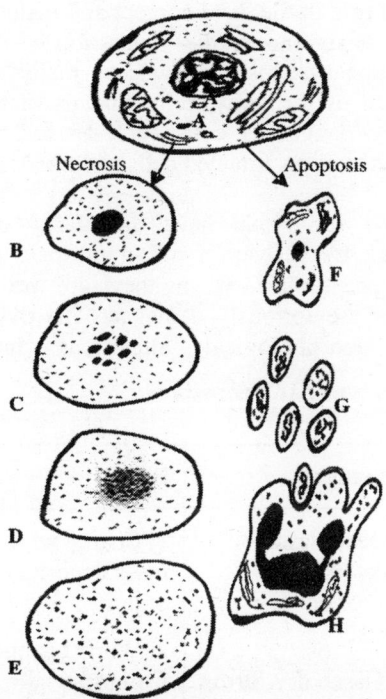

Fig. 7.1. Diagram showing pathogenesis of necrosis
(A) Normal (B) Pyknosis (C) Karyorrhexis
(D)Karyolysis (E) Chromatolysis,
(F) Apoptosis (G) Blebs and (H) Phagocytosis

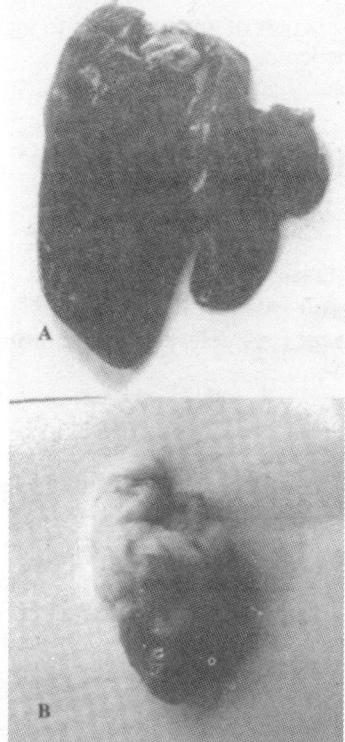

Fig. 7. 3. Photograph of (A) liver and (B) heart
showing necrosis

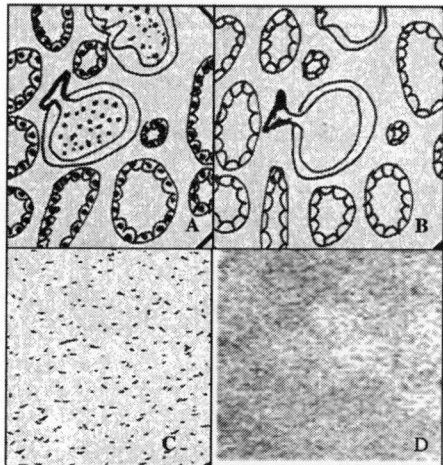

Fig. 7.2. Diagram showing necrosis (A) Normal
(B) Coagulative (C) Caseaative and (D)Liquifactive

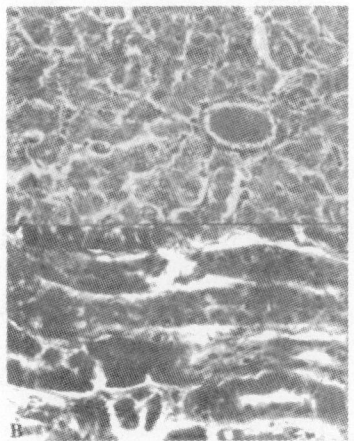

Fig. 7. 4. Photomicrograph of (A) liver and
(B) Kidney showing coagulative necrosis

67

- Increased action of enzymes due to leakage of pancreatic juice.
- Starvation

Macroscopic features
- Chalky white mass deposits in organ.
- White opaque firm mass.

Microscopic features
- Adipose cell without nucleus (Fig. 7.7).
- Macrophage giant cells contain fat droplets.

important role in the development and maintenance of homeostasis and in the maturation of nervous and immune systems. It is also a major defense mechanism of the body, removing unwanted and potentially dangerous cells such as self-reactive lymphocytes, virus infected cells and tumor cells.

Most cells in animal have the ability of self-destruction by activation of an intrinsic cellular suicidal programme when they are no longer needed or are seriously damaged. The dying cell exhibits morphological alterations including

Table 7.1 Differential features of various types of Necrosis

	Coagulative	Liquifactive	Caseative	Fat
Macroscopic features	1. Organ becomes gray/white in colour, firm, dense, depressed with surrounding tissue	1. Liquifactive necrosed tissue present in a cavity "Abscess" 2. It contains small/ large amount of cloudy fluid, which is creamy yellow (Pus)	1. Dead tissue looks like milk curd or cottage cheese 2. Tissue dry, firm, agranular, white/gray/ yellowish in colour	1. Chalky white mass deposits in organ 2. White opaque firm mass
Microscopic features	1. Cellular out line present, which maintains the architecture of tissue/ organ 2. Nucleus absent or pyknotic 3. Cytoplasm becomes acidophilic	1. Areas of liquifactive necrosis stains pink. 2. Infiltration of neutrophils 3. Sometimes empty spaces but infiltration of neutrophils at	1. Disappearance of cells; no cell details/ architecture 2. Purplish granules on H&E staining, blue granules from nucleus fragments, red granules from cytoplasm fragments.	1. Adipose cell without nucleus 2. Macrophages giant cells contain fat droplets. 3. Presence of lime salts in tissues.

- Presence of lime salts in tissues.

APOPTOSIS

Apoptosis is a finely tuned mechanism for the control of cell number in animals; the process is operative during foetal life, tumor regression and in the control of immune response. Apoptosis plays an

shrinkage of cell, membrane blebbing, chromatin condensation and fragmentation of nucleic acid. Cells undergoing apoptosis often fragment into membrane bound apoptotic bodies that are readily phagocytosed by macrophages or neighbouring cells without generating an inflammatory response.

These changes distinguish apoptosis from cell death by necrosis. Necrosis refers to the morphology most often seen when cells die from severe and sudden injury such as ischemia, sustained hyperthermia or physical and chemical trauma. In necrosis, there are early changes in mitochondrial shape and function; cell losses its ability to regulate osmotic pressure, swells and ruptures. The contents of the cell are spilled into surrounding tissue, resulting in generation of a local inflammatory response.

Necrosis is the consequence of a passive and degenerative process while the apoptosis is a consequence of an active process.

Execution of apoptosis requires the coordinated action of aspartate specific cysteine proteases (caspases) which are responsible for cleavage of key enzymes and structural proteins resulting in death of cell. Apoptosis is triggered by a variety of signals which activate the endogenous endonucleases to initiate the process of fragmentation of nuclear DNA into oligonucleosomal size fragments. Initially, the DNA fragments are large (50-300 Kb) but are later digested to oligonucleosomal size (multimers of 180-200 bp). The formation of this distinct DNA ladder is considered to be a biochemical hallmark of apoptosis.

There is rounding of nucleus with pyknosis and rhexis, chromatin coalesces to form a crescent along the nuclear membrane. Cell fragments to form blebs, which may have one or more organelles. Such changes occur in apoptotic cells within 20 min duration.

Apoptosis is generally synonymously used with "programmed cell death" but it differs from programmed cell death as apoptosis cannot be prevented by cycloheximide or actinomycin D, rather these chemicals accelerate the process of apoptosis while programmed cell death is prevented by these chemicals.

GANGRENE

Necrosis of tissue is followed by invasion of saprophytes. Gangrene is mainly divided into three types: Dry, moist and gas gangrene.

DRY GANGRENE

Dry gangrene occurs at extremities like tail, tip of ears, tip of scrotum, hoof etc. due to necrosis and invasion of saprophytes. The evaporation of moisture takes place resulting into dry lesions.

Etiology
- Mycotoxins from fungus *Fusarium equiseti* found on paddy straw in low lying areas with moisture (Degnala disease).

Macroscopic features
- Dry, fragmented crusts like lesions on tail, scrotum, ear (Figs. 7.8 & 7.9).
- Hoof becomes detached due to necrosis and gangrene, sloughing, exposing the red raw surface (Figs. 7.10 & 7.11).
- Blackening of the affected area.

Microscopic features
- Necrosis and invasion of saprophytes in skin of tail, ear or scrotum.

MOIST GANGRENE

Moist gangrene mostly occurs in internal organs of body like lungs, intestine, stomach etc. It occurs due to necrosis and invasion of saprophytes leading to dissolution of the tissues (Figs 7.12 & 7.13).

Etiology
- Drenching of milk, medicines etc. *e.g.* Aspiration pneumonia/ Drenching pneumonia.
- Volvolus/Intussusception or torsion in intestine.

Macroscopic features
- Greenish or bluish discolouration of the affected organ.
- Dissolution of affected part into fragments
- Presence of foreign material like milk, fibre, oil, etc.

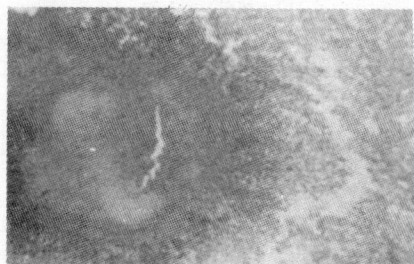

Fig. 7.5. Photomicrograph showing caseative
necrosis

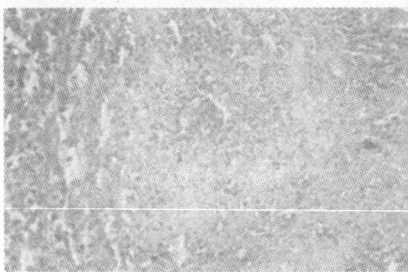

Fig. 7.6. Photomicrograph showing liquifacticve
necrosis

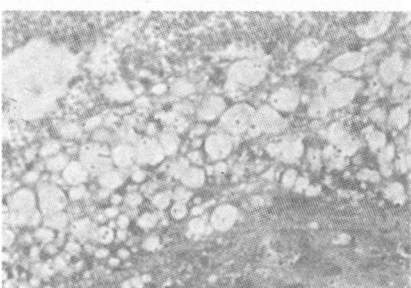

Fig. 7.7. Photomicrograph of fat showing necrosis

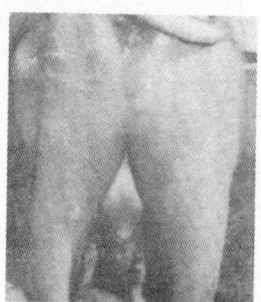

Fig. 7.8. Photograph of buffalo bull showing
dry gangrene in scrotum

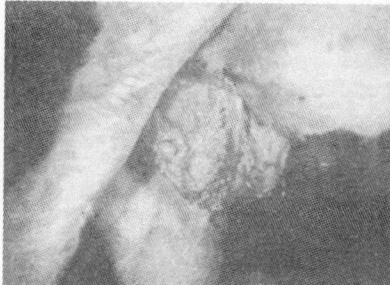

Fig. 7.9. Photograph of a cow showing gangrene
in udder

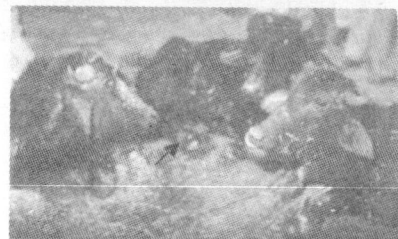

Fig. 7.10. Photograph of buffalo calves showing
sloughing of hoofs due to Degnala disease

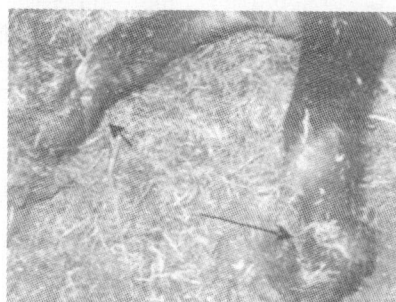

Fig. 7.11. Photograph of buffalo calf showing
sloughing of hoofs due to Degnala disease

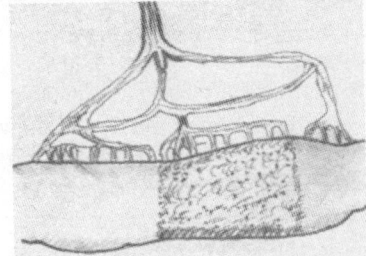

Fig. 7.12. Diagram showing moist gangrene
in intestine

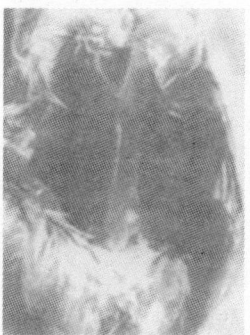

Fig. 7.13. Photograph showing moist gangrene in
poultry

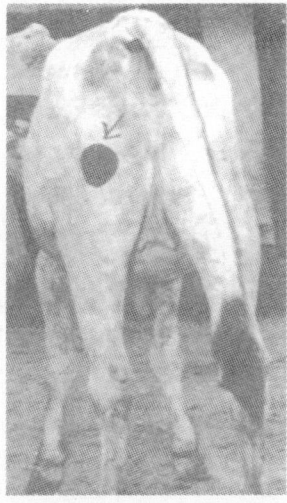

Fig. 7.14 Photograph showing gas
gangrene in heifer

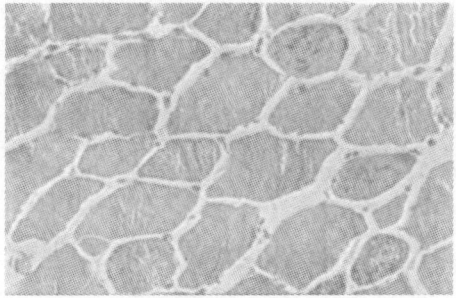

Fig. 7.15 Photomicrograph showing
myositis/gas gangrene

Microscopic features

- Necrosis and invasion of saprophytes
- Presence of foreign material like milk, fibres, oil etc.

GAS GANGRENE

Gas gangrene occurs in muscles particularly of thigh muscles of hind legs in heifers in case of black leg (Black Quarter; B.Q.) (Figs. 7.14 & 7.15).

Etiology

- *Clostridium chauvei*
- Gram positive, rod, anaerobe.
- Produces toxins under anaerobic conditions which cause disease.
- Stress, trauma, transportation predisposes animals.

Macroscopic features

- Oedema of Muscles in affected part particularly thigh region.
- Blackening of muscles due to production of H_2S by bacteria and its chemical reaction with iron of free hemoglobin producing iron sulphide.
- Presence of gas in the area giving *crepitating sound* on palpation.

Microscopic features

- Necrosis of muscles
- Presence of Gram positive rod shaped Clostridia
- Dissolution of muscle fibers due to saprophytes/ toxins of the organism.

71

Table 7.2 Differential features of various types of Gangrene

	Dry	Moist	Gas
Macroscopic features	1. Dry, fragmented crusts like lesions on tail, scrotum, ear 2. Hoof becomes detached due to necrosis and gangrene, sloughing, exposing the red raw surface. 3. Blackening of the affected area.	1. Greenish or bluish discoloration of the affected organ. 2. Dissolution of affected part into fragments 3. Presence of foreign material like milk, fiber, oil, etc.	1. Oedema of Muscles in affected part particularly thigh region. 2. Blackening of muscles due to production of H_2S by bacteria and its chemical reaction with iron of free hemoglobin producing iron sulphide. 3. Presence of gas in the area giving crepitating sound on palpation
Microscopic features	1. Necrosis and invasion of saprophytes in skin of tail, ear or scrotum	1. Necrosis and invasion of saprophytes 2. Presence of foreign material like milk, fibers, oil, etc.	1. Necrosis of muscles 2. Presence of Gram positive rod shaped Clostridia 3. Dissolution of muscle fibers due to saprophytes/ toxins of the organism

POST-MORTEM CHANGES

Alterations in cells/tissues occur after death of animal. The degree of such alterations and their speed depends upon the environmental temperature, size of animal, species of animal, external insulation and nutritional state of the animal. The postmortem changes occur rapidly in high environmental temperature, large, and fur/wool-bearing and fatty animals.

Autolysis

Autolysis is the digestion of tissue by its own enzymes and is characterized by uniform destruction of cells without any inflammatory reaction. After death, a state of hypoxia occurs leading to decreased ATP. The cell organelles degenerate and the membrane of lysosomes dissolve releasing the lysosomal enzymes in the cell responsible for digestion of cells/tissues. These enzymes cause disintegration of cell components into small granules in the cell. Microscopically, autolysis is characterized by uniform dead cells without any circulatory changes and inflammatory reaction.

Putrefaction

Putrefaction is decomposition of tissue after death by saprophytes leading to production of foul odour. After autolysis the saprophytes invade from external environment into the body, multiply and eventually digest the tissues with their enzymes. The tissue becomes fragile and produces foul odour.

Pseudomelanosis

Pseudomelanosis is greenish or bluish discolouration of tissues/organs after death. Saprophytes causing putrefaction also produce hydrogen sulfide which chemically reacts with iron portion of hemoglobin to produce iron sulfide. Iron sulfide is a black pigment and produces green, grey or black shades on combination with other tissue pigments.

Rigor mortis

Rigor mortis is the contraction and shortening of muscles after death of animal leading to stiffening and immobilization of body. It occurs 2-4 hours after death and remains till putrefaction sets in. Rigor mortis begins in cardiac muscles first and then in skeletal muscles of head and neck with a progression towards extremities. It is enhanced by high temperature and increased metabolic activity before death; while it is delayed by starvation, cold and cachexia. Rigor appears quickly in case animal has died due to strychnine poisoning as a result of depletion of energy source ATP. Muscle fibres shorten due to contraction and remain in contraction in the absence of oxygen, ATP and creatine phosphate. Rigor mortis remains till 20-30 hours of death, the duration depends on autolysis and putrefaction. It disappears in same order as it appeared from head, neck to extremities. It can be used to determine the length of time after the death of animal.

Algor mortis

Algor mortis is cooling of body. As after death there is no circulation of blood, which maintains the body temperature, body becomes cool. However, it takes 2-4 hours, depending on the species, environmental temperature and type of animal.

Livor mortis

Livor mortis is the staining of tissues with hemoglobin after death of animals. It gives pinkish discolouration to the tissues.

Hypostatic congestion

Due to gravitational force, the blood is accumulated in dependent ventral parts of body. It is helpful in establishing of the state of the body at the time of death.

Post-mortem emphysema

It occurs due to decomposition by gas producing organisms including saprophytes. The gas is mainly accumulated in gastrointestinal tract causing rupture of the organ.

Post-mortem clot

It is clotting of blood after death of animal mainly due to excessive release of thrombokinase from dying leucocytes and endothelial cells. It is smooth in consistency having glistening surface that is red or yellow in colour. Post-mortem clot is uniform in structure and it does not attach to the wall of blood vessel as thrombus does. In anthrax, post-mortem clot does not appear. Post-mortem clot is of two types: Red or current jelly clot forms when the components of blood are evenly distributed throughout the clot. It occurs due to rapid clotting of blood. The yellow or chicken fat clot occurs when the components of blood are not distributed evenly. The dorsal position is red and upper position in yellow due to WBC fibrin and serum. It occurs due to prolonged coagulation time of blood leading to sedimentation of red blood cells.

Displacement of organs

Displacement of internal organs due to rolling of dead animal. Mainly intestine/stomach and uterus are affected with displacement which can be differentiated from ante-mortem displacement by absence of passive hyperemia.

Imbibition of bile

Cholebilirubin present in the gall bladder diffuses to the surrounding tissues/organs and stains them with yellow/ greenish pigmentation.

MODEL QUESTIONS

Q. 1. *Fill in the blanks with suitable word(s) to answer the following.*
1. ………….. necrosis is caused by *Mycobacterium tuberculosis* and is characterized by ………….. material formed due to coagulation of ………….. and …………..
2. Chromatolysis is the lysis of ………….. material.
3. Necrosis is defined as death of cells/ tissue in ….. body and is characterized by ……, ….., and ……..
4. Abscess is an example of………….. necrosis caused by ………….. organisms.
5. Fat necrosis occurs by the action of enzymes of …….. and is characterized by …….. deposits on organs.
6. Aspiration pneumonia in calves is an example of ………….. gangrene.
7. Degnala disease is caused by ……… toxins found on paddy straw and is characterized by ……….. gangrene.
8. Gas gangrene is caused by ………….. in muscles of heifers and is characterized by ………………..………….. and ………….. sound on palpation.
9. Autolysis is ………….. of tissues by ………….. enzymes.
10. Greenish discolouration of tissues after death is known as ………….. as a result of ………….. action and production of ………….. which combines with ………….. of hemoglobin.

Q. 2. *Write true or false against each statement and correct the false statement.*
1. ………..Autolysis is the local death of tissue in living body.
2. ………..Algor mortis is cooling of body after death.
3. ………..necrosis invaded by saprophytes leads to putrefaction.
4. ………..Hypostatic congestion may reveal the time of death of the animal.
5. ………..Diffusion of cholebilirubin present in gall bladder to surrounding tissues is known as imbibition of bile.
6. ………..Apoptosis is programmed cell death.
7. ………..Karyorrhexis is rounding of cells, which takes a deep stain.
8. ………..In coagulative necrosis, cellular details are maintained.
9. ………..Ischemia may lead to necrosis.
10. ………Fat necrosis is characterized by the presence of creamy yellow liquefied material.

Q. 3. *Write short notes on.*
1. Caseative Necrosis
2. Abscess
3. Gas gangrene
4. Post-mortem changes
5. Lysosomal enzymes

Q. 4. *Define the following.*
1. Pyknosis
2. Karyolysis
3. Karyorrhexis
4. Chromatolysis
5. Gangrene
6. Apoptosis
7. Necrobiosis
8. Necrosis
9. Autolysis
10. Livor mortis

Q. 5. *Select appropriate word(s) from four options given against each statement.*

1. In liquifactive necrosis.............. cells are present.
   (a) Monocytes   (b) Lymphocytes   (c) Eosinophils   (d) Neutrophils
2. Programmed cell death is known as .... in living body.
   (a) Apoptosis   (b) Necrosis   (c) Autolysis   (d) None of the above
3. Chalky white deposits are observed in .... necrosis.
   (a) Coagulative   (b) Liquifactive   (c) Fat   (d) Caseative
4. Gangrene in lungs is an example of .... grangrene.
   (a) Dry   (b) Moist   (c) Gas   (d) All of the above
5. Degnala disease is an example of .... gangrene.
   (a) Dry   (b) Moist   (c) Gas   (d) None of the above
6. Digestion of cells/tissues by their own enzymes is known as ....
   (a) Necrosis   (b) Autolysis   (c) Gangrene   (d) Putrefaction
7. Greenish discolouration of tissues after death is also known as ....
   (a) Pseudomelanosis   (b) Melanosis   (c) Necrosis   (d) Imbibition of bile
8. Algor mortis is the .... of body.
   (a) Staining with hemoglobin   (b) Cooling   (c) Hardening   (d) Softening
9. Rigor mortis remains in body .... hrs
   (a) 12-15 hrs   (b) 20-30 hrs   (c) 35-48 hrs   (d) 5-10 hrs
10. Lysis of chromatin material is known as ....
    (a) Karyolysis   (b) Karyorrhexis   (c) Chromatolysis   (d) Caseation

8

DISTURBANCES IN CALCIFICATION AND PIGMENT METABOLISM

- **Calcification**
  - **Dystrophic**
  - **Metastatic**
- **Pigmentation**
  - **Endogenous pigments**
  - **Exogenous pigments**
- **Crystals**
  - **Gout (Urates and uric acids)**
- **Model Questions**

CALCIFICATION

Calcification is the deposition of calcium phosphates and calcium carbonates in soft tissues other than bones and teeth. It may be classified as dystrophic and metastatic calcification.

DYSTROPHIC CALCIFICATION

Dystrophic calcification is characterized by the deposits of calcium salts in necrosed tissue of any organ (Fig 8.1).

Etiology /Occurrence
- Necrosis.
- Parasitic infections.
- Tuberculous lesions.

Macroscopic features
- Organ becomes hard, nodular.
- Grey/white deposits in necrosed tissue looking like honey comb.
- Gritty sound on cutting.

Microscopic features
- Irregular deposits of calcium salts in necrosed tissue.
- Calcium takes black/purplish colour on H & E staining.

METASTATIC CALCIFICATION

Metastatic calcification is characterized by deposition of calcium salts in soft tissue as a result of hypercalcemia (Fig. 8.2).

Etiology/ Occurrence
- Hyperparathyroidism.
- Renal failure.
- Excess of vitamin-D.
- Increased calcium intake.

Macroscopic features
- Organ becomes hard.
- Wall of arteries becomes hard due to calcium deposits.

Microscopic features
- Deposition of calcium in soft organs like myocardium, arteries, muscles, etc.
- Purplish/black colour calcium surrounded by comparatively normal tissue.

MELANOSIS

Melanosis is the deposition of melanin, a brown/ black pigments in various tissues/ organs specially in lung, blood vessels and brain (Figs. 8.3 to 8.5).

Etiology/Occurrence
- Hyperadrenalism.
- Melanosarcoma.
- Melanoma.

Macroscopic features
- Organ/tissue involved becomes black in colour.
- Discolouration may be focal or diffused.

Microscopic features
- Brown/black colour pigment is seen in cells.
- The size, shape and amount of pigment vary.

HEMOSIDEROSIS

Hemosiderosis is characterized by deposition of hemosiderin pigment in spleen and other organs. Hemosiderin is a blood pigment with a shiny golden yellow colour and is usually found within the macrophages (Fig. 8.6).

Etiology/ Occurrence
- Extensive lysis of erythrocytes.
- Haemorrhage.
- Hemolytic anemia.

Macroscopic features
- Colour of organ becomes brownish.
- Brown induration of lungs.

Microscopic features
- Presence of golden yellow/golden brown pigment in red pulp of spleen, lungs, liver and kidneys.

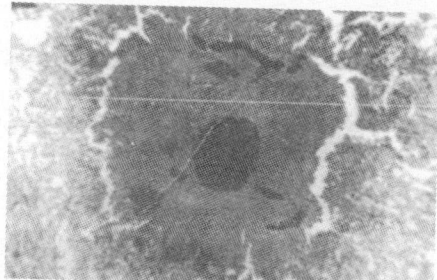

Fig. 8.1 Photomicrograph of lung showing dystrophic calcification in tuberculous granuloma

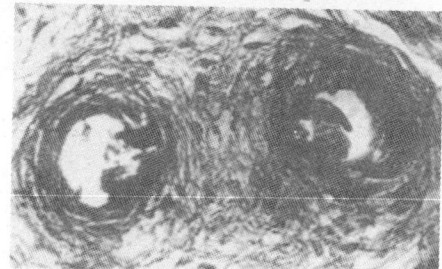

Fig. 8.2 Photomicrograph of arteries showing metastatic calcification

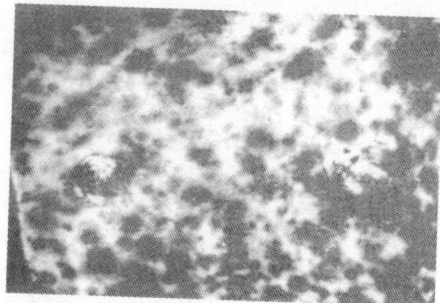

Fig. 8.3. Photograph showing melanosis

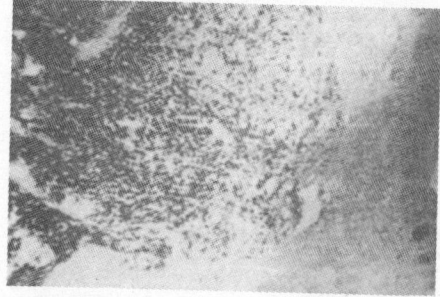

Fig. 8.4 Photomicrograph of skin showing melanosis

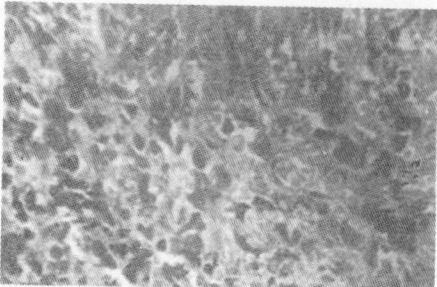

Fig. 8.5. Photomicrograph of skin showing melanosis.

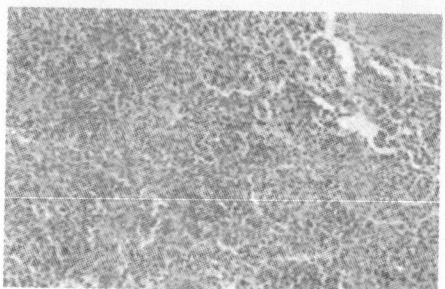

Fig. 8.6 Photomicrograph of spleen showing hemosiderosis

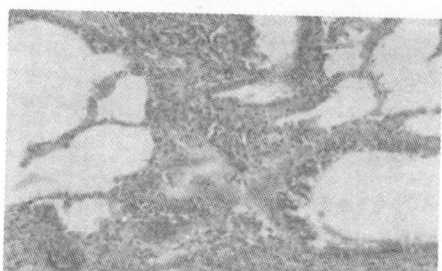

Fig. 8.7 Photomicrograph of lung showing pneumoconiasis

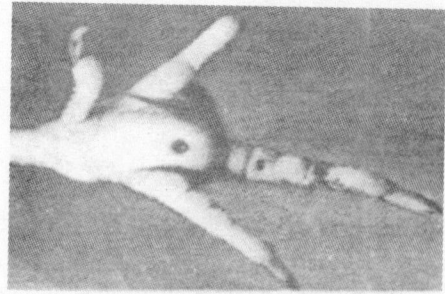

Fig. 8.8 Photograph of foot pad of a bird showing gout

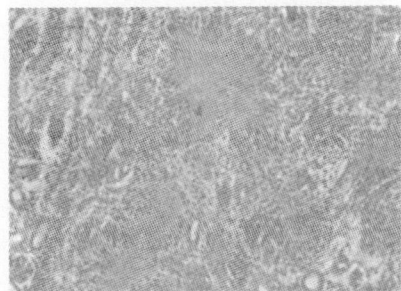

Fig. 8.9. *Photomicrograph of kidney showing urates (gout)*

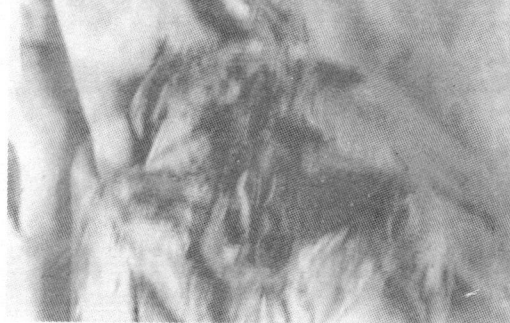

Fig. 8.10. *Photograph of a bird showing deposition of urates and uric acid in ureter (gout)*

- In most of the cases, the pigment is found intracellularly in macrophages.

BILE PIGMENTS

Bile pigments are derived from the breakdown of erythrocytes such as bilirubin and biliverdin. The icterus is hyperbilirubinemia as a result of either excessive lysis of erythrocytes or due to damage in liver or obstruction in the bile duct. The hemolysis results in iron, globin and porphyin; the latter being converted into biliverdin. Biliverdin is reduced to produce bilirubin, an orange-yellow pigment bound to albumin and transported by RE cells to liver. In hepatic cells, it is separated from albumin and conjugated with glucuronic acid and excreted in bile as bilirubin diglucuronide. In intestine, it is further reduced by bacteria to urobilinogen, which is reabsorbed into circulation and carried to liver for re-excretion in bile while a small amount enters in circulation and is excreted through urine. The unabsorbed urobilinogen is oxidized in lower intestine to form urobilin and stercobilin, which give normal pigment to faeces.

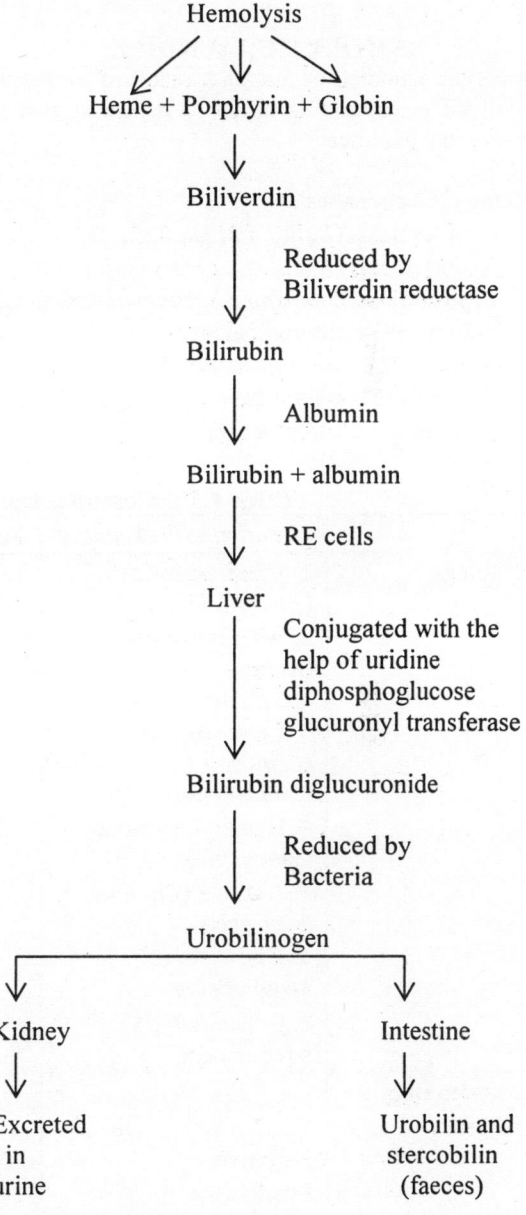

ICTERUS

Icterus is increased amount of bile pigments in blood and is often called as *hyper- bilirubinemia* or *jaundice*. It is of three types hemolytic, toxic and obstructive jaundice.

HEMOLYTIC JAUNDICE

Hemolytic jaundice occurs as a result of excessive hemolysis in circulating blood. It is also known as *pre-hepatic* jaundice.

Etiology/ Occurrence
- Piroplasmosis (*Babesia bigemina*).
- Anaplasmosis (*Anaplasma marginale*).
- Leptospirosis(*Leptospira ictehaemmorrhagae*).
- Equine infectious anemia virus.
- Anthrax (*Bacillus anthracis*).
- *Clostriduum hemolyticum.*
- β- haemolytic streptococci.

TOXIC JAUNDICE

Toxic jaundice occurs as a result of damage in liver leading to increased amount of unconjugated and conjugated bilirubin in blood. It is also known as *hepatic jaundice*.

Etiology
- Toxin/Poisons.
- Copper poisoning.
- Leptospirosis.

OBSTRUCTIVE JAUNDICE

Obstructive jaundice occurs as a result of obstruction in bile duct causing hindrance in normal flow of bile. It is also known as *post-hepatic jundice*.

Etiology
- Blocking of bile canaliculi by swollen hepatocytes.

Table 8.1 Differential features of various types of Jaundice

	Hemolytic (Prehepatic)	Toxic (Hepatic)	Obstructive (Post hepatic)
Etiology	1. Piroplasmosis (*Babesia bigemina*) 2. Anaplasmosis (*Anaplasma marginale*) 3. Leptospirosis (*Leptospira ictehaemmorrhagae*) 4. Equine infectious anemia virus 5. Anthrax (*Bacillus anthracis*) 6. *Clostriduum hemolyticum* 7. β- haemolytic streptococci	1. Toxin/Poisons 2. Copper poisoning 3. Leptospirosis	1. Blocking of bile canaliculi by swollen hepatocytes 2. Obstruction in bile duct (Liver flukes, tapeworms and ascaris) 3. Biliary cirrhosis, Cholangitis and Cholelithiasis 4. Pressure on bile duct due to abscess, neoplasm. 5. Inflammation and swelling at duct opening in duodenum.
Vanden Berg's reaction Direct Indirect	 Negative Positive	 Positive Positive	 Positive Negative

- Obstruction in bile duct (Liver flukes, tapeworms and ascaris).
- Biliary cirrhosis, Cholangitis and Cholelithiasis.
- Pressure on bile duct due to abscess, neoplasm.
- Inflammation and swelling at duct opening in duodenum.

Macroscopic features
- Mucous membrane yellow in colour.
- Omentum, mesentry, fat become yellow.
- Increased yellow colour in urine.
- Conjunctiva becomes yellow.

Microscopic features
- Brownish pigment in tubules of kidney.
- Bile pigments in spleen.
- Hemolysis, erythrophagocytosis.
- Hepatitis.

Diagnosis
- Van-den-Bergh reaction.
- Direct reaction detects bilirubin diglucuronide (Obstructive jaundice).
- Indirect reaction detects hemobilirubin (Hemolytic jaundice).
- Both reaction (Toxic jaundice).

Table 8.2 Vanden Berg's reaction

	Type of reaction	Type of jaundice	Type of pigment
1.	Direct reaction (+)	Obstructive	Cholibilirubin
2.	Indirect reaction (+)	Hemolytic	Hemobilirubin
3.	Biphasic reaction (+)	Toxic/ Hepato-cellular	Both present

PNEUMOCONIASIS
Pneumoconiasis is the deposition of dust/carbon particles in lungs through air inhalation. It is also known as anthracosis (carbon), silicosis (silica) or asbestoses (asbestos) (Fig 8.7).

Etiology/ Occurrence
- Dusty air containing carbon/silica/asbestous
- Near factory/coal mines.

Macroscopic features
- Hard nodules in lungs.
- Nodules my have black /brown /grey colour
- Nodules may produce cracking sounds on cut.

Microscopic features
- Presence of carbon/other exogenous pigment in intercellular spaces or in cytoplasm of alveolar cells and macrophages.
- Formation of granuloma around the foreign particles including the infiltration of macrophages, lymphocytes, giant cells and fibrous tissue proliferation.

CRYSTALS
Deposition of different kinds of crystals in tissues like uric acid, sulphonamides and oxalates etc. The uric acid and urates when deposited in tissues are known as *gout*.

GOUT (URATES & URIC ACIDS)
Gout is a disease condition in which urates and uric acid are deposited in tissues and is characterized by intense pain and acute inflammation (Figs. 8.8 to 8.10).

Etiology/Occurrence
- Common in poultry due to deficiency of uricase enzyme.
- Deficiency of vitamin A.
- Absence or inadequate amount of uricase.

Macroscopic features
- White chalky mass of urates and uric acid.
- Deposition of urates/uric acid on pericardium, kidneys etc.
- Dialation of ureter due to excessive accumulation of urates.

Microscopic features
- Presence of sharp crystals in tissue.

- Crystals are surrounded by inflammatory cells including macrophages, giant cells and lymphocytes.

MODEL QUESTIONS

Q. 1. *Fill in the blanks with suitable word(s).*
1. Metastatic calcification is characterized by deposition of calcium in soft tissues as a result of .... which is caused by ...., ..., ... and ...., ...
2. Hemosiderosis is the deposition of pigment in spleen which is seen as .... colour and usually found in the ....
3. Melanin is a ....colour pigment usually gives colour to ...., ...and ....
4. Bilirubin is a.................... pigment and occurs in body due to ...., ... and ...., which is characterized by .... colour of ....
5. In liver bilirubin is conjugated with............ to give rise to............. which is excreted in bile and reduced in intestine to.......... while unabsorbed portion is converted into............ and............

Q. 2. *Write true or false against each statement and correct the false statements.*
1. ......Bilirubin is produced as a result of reduction of biliverdin.
2. ......Hyperadrenalism may lead to melanosis.
3. ......Stercobilin gives colour to urine
4. ......Hemolytic anemia may give rise to hemosiderosis.
5. ......The swollen hepatocytes may cause the appearance of both conjugated and unconjugated biliruibin in blood.
6. ......Necrosed tissue is after some time calicified due to hypercalcemia.
7. ......Excessive hemolysis may cause jaundice.
8. ......Urobilin gives colour to urine and faeces.
9. ......Hemosiderin is green or red colour pigment.
10. ......Anaplasmosis may cause post-hepatic jaundice.

Q. 3. *Write short notes on.*
1. Dystrophic calcification
2. Hemosiderosis
3. Melanosis
4. Hemolytic jaundice
5. Gout
6. Toxic icterus
7. Van den Bergh reaction
8. Metastatic calcification
9. Pneumoconiasis
10. Obstructive jaundice

Q. 4. *Define the followings.*
1. Silicosis
2. Urobilinogen
3. Gout
4. Urobilin
5. Asbestoses
6. Anthracosis
7. Uricase
8. Stercobilin
9. Hemosiderin
10. Pneumoconiasis

Q. 5. *Select appropriate word(s) from four options given against each statement.*

1. Dystrophic calcification occurs in animals due to ....
   (a) Tuberculosis   (b) Parasitic infection   (c) Necrosis   (d)All of the above
2. Melanosis is the brown/black discolouration of tissue/organ as a result of excessive accumulation of melanin due to ....
   (a) Hyperadrenalism (b) Hyperthyroidism   (c)Hyperparathyroidism (d)Hypermelanemia
3. Hemosiderin is...............colour pigment.
   (a) Green   (b) Red   (c) Golden Yellow   (d) Blue
4. Urobilinogen is the ....form of bilirubin.
   (a) Unconjugated (b) Conjugated and reduced   (c) Conjugated (d) Conjugated and oxidised
5. Hemolysis may give rise to............
   (a) Pre-hepatic icterus (b) Post-hepatic icterus   (c) Toxic icterus   (d) None of the above
6. Obstructive jaundice occurs as a result of
   (a) Hemolysis   (b) Liver necrosis   (c) Cholangitis   (d) Prioplasmosis
7. Indirect Van den Bergh reaction is an indication of...............
   (a) Obstructive icterus (b) Hemolytic icterus   (c) Hepatic jaundice   (d) None of the above
8. Deposition of carbon particles in lungs is known as............
   (a) Silicosis   (b) Asbestoses   (c) Pneumoconiasis   (d) Anthracosis
9. Gout is the deposition of............... in tissues.
   (a) Uric acid crystals (b) Oxalate crystals   (c) Hemosiderin   (d) Urobilin
10. The absence of............... in poultry is the main cause of gout.
    (a) Trypsin   (b) Lymphnodes   (c) Amylase   (d) Uricase

9

INFLAMMATION AND HEALING

- **Inflammation**
- **Introduction and Terminology**
- **Pathogenesis of Inflammation**
  - **Vascular Changes**
  - **Cellular Changes**
  - **Chemical Changes**
- **Phagocytosis**
- **Types of Inflammation**
- **Healing**
- **Model Questions**

INFLAMMATION

Inflammation is a complex process of vascular and cellular alterations that occur in body in response to injury. The term inflammation has been derived from the Latin word *inflammare*, means to set on fire. Inflammation is considered as an important event in body that activates the existing defence mechanisms in circulating blood to dilute, naturalize or kill the irritant/ causative agent. Thus, it is said that immunity is the resistance of body, while inflammation is the activation of that immunity. It is beneficial to body except when chronic or immune origin. Inflammation starts with sublethal injury and ends with healing.

Etiology

- Any irritant/ injury.
- Bacteria, virus, parasite, fungus etc.
- Trauma.
- Physical or chemical injury.

Macroscopic features

- Inflammation is characterized by 5 cardinal signs;
- Redness;
- Swelling (Fig. 9.1);
- Heat;
- Pain;
- Loss of function

Microscopic features

- Acute inflammation is characterized by more intense vascular changes like congestion, oedema, haemorrhages, leakage of fibrinogen and leucocytes (Fig. 9.2).
- Chronic inflammation is characterized by more proliferative and/or regenerative changes such as proliferation of fibroblasts and regeneration of epithelium along with infiltration of leucocytes (Fig. 9.3).

INTRODUCTION AND TERMINOLOGY

Inflammation may occur in any organ/tissue depending upon the type of injury and irritant. The inflamed state of an organ is called most often with a suffix "itis" detailed nomenclature is as under for different organs/ tissues.

Abomasum	–	Abomasitis
Artery	–	Arteritis
Bileduct	–	Cholangitis
Bone & bone marrow	–	Osteomyelitis
Bone	–	Osteitis
Brain	–	Encephalitis
Bronchi	–	Bronchitis
Bursa	–	Bursitis
Caecum	–	Typhlitis
Cervix	–	Cervicitis
Colon	–	Colonitis
Conjunctiva	–	Conjunctivitis
Connective tissue	–	Cellulitis
Cornea	–	Keratitis
Crop	–	Ingluvitis
Durameter	–	Leptomeningitis
Ear	–	Otitis
Endocardium	–	Endocarditis
Eosophagus	–	Esophagitis
Epididymis	–	Epididymitis
Eustachian tube	–	Eustachitis
External ear	–	Otitis externa
Eyelid	–	Blepheritis
Eyes	–	Ophthalmitis
Fascia	–	Fascitis
Fat	–	Steatitis
Gall bladder	–	Cholecystitis
Glans penis	–	Balanitis
Gums	–	Gingivitis
Heart	–	Carditis
Inner part of uterus	–	Endometritis
Internal ear	–	Otitis interna
Intestine	–	Enteritis
Iris	–	Iritis
Joints	–	Arthritis
Kidney & pelvis	–	Pyelonephritis
Kidney	–	Nephritis
Lacrimal gland	–	Dacryadenitis
Larynx	–	Laryngitis
Ligament	–	Desmitis
Lip	–	Cheilitis
Liver	–	Hepatitis
Lungs	–	Pneumonitis/Pneumonia
Lymph nodes	–	Lymphadenitis

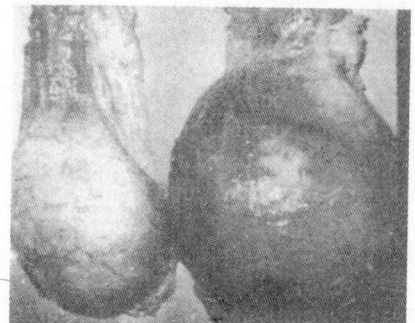

Fig.9.1. *Inflammation of testes showing redness and swelling*

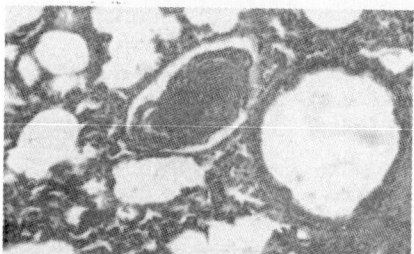

Fig. 9.2. *Photomicrograph of acute inflammation showing intense vascular changes*

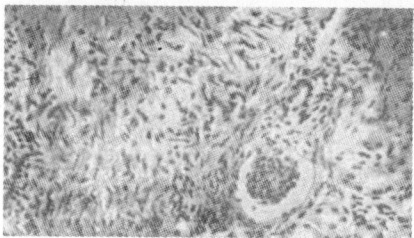

Fig.9.3. *Photomicrograph of chronic inflammation showing proliferative changes*

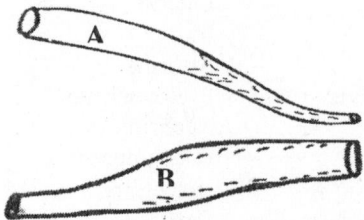

Fig.9.4. *Diagram of a blood vessel showing (a) Vasoconstriction and (b) Vasodilation.*

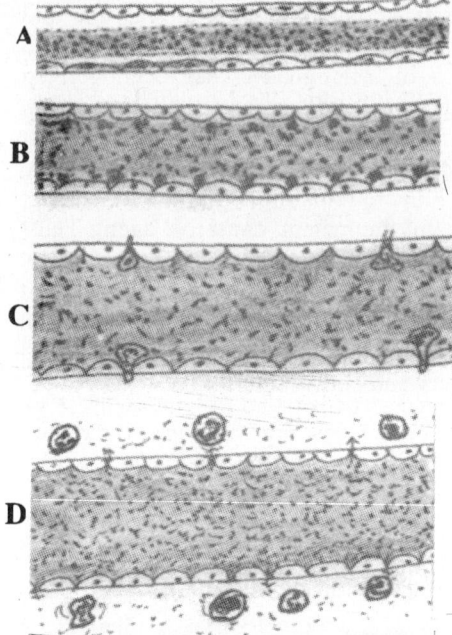

Fig. 9.5. *Diagram of blood vessel showing altered blood flow (a) Normal (b) Decreased blood flow (c) Pavementation and (d) increased permeability*

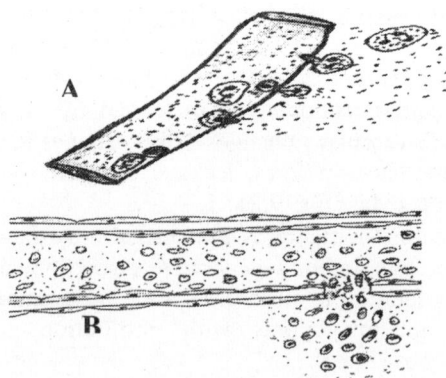

Fig. 9.6 . *Diagram of blood vessels showing (a) diapedesis and (b) rhexis*

86

Lymph vessels	–	Lymphangitis
Meninges	–	Meningitis
Middle ear	–	Otitis media
Mouth cavity	–	Stomatitis
Muscle	–	Myositis
Myocardium	–	Myocarditis
Nails	–	Onychia
Nasal passage	–	Rhinitis
Nerve	–	Neuritis
Omasum	–	Omasitis
Ovary	–	Oophoritis
Oviduct	–	Salpingitis
Palates	–	Lampas / palatitis
Pancreas	–	Pancreatitis
Pericardium	–	Pericarditis
Peritoneum	–	Peritonitis
Pharynx	–	Pharyngitis
Piameter	–	Pachymeningitis
Pleura	–	Pleuritis
Prepuce	–	Posthitis
Rectum	–	Proctitis
Reticulm	–	Reticulitis
Retina	–	Retinitis
Rumen	–	Rumenitis
Salivary glands	–	Sialadenitis
Sinuses	–	Sinusitis
Skin	–	Dermatitis
Spermatic cord	–	Funiculitis
Spinal cord	–	Myelitis
Spleen	–	Spleenitis
Stomach	–	Gastritis
Synovial membrane of joints	–	Sinovitis
Tendon	–	Tendinitis
Testes	–	Orchitis
Tongue	–	Glossitis
Trachea	–	Tracheitis
Ureter	–	Ureteritis
Urethra	–	Urethritis
Urinary bladder	–	Cystitis
Uterus	–	Metritis
Vagina	–	Vaginitis
Vein	–	Phlebitis
Vertebra	–	Spondylitis
Vessel	–	Vasculitis
Vulva	–	Vulvitis

PATHOGENESIS OF INFLAMMATION

Inflammation starts with sublethal injury and ends with healing; in between there are many events that take place which are described as under:

Transient vasoconstriction

The blood vessels of the affected part become constricted for movement of blood as a result of action of irritant (Fig. 9.4A).

Vasodialation and Increase in permeability

The blood vessels become dilated. Endothelium becomes more permeable and releases procoagulant factors and prostaglandins. Fluid and proteins come out due to leakage in endothelium. Fluid contains water, immunoglobulins, complement component, biochemical factors of coagulation and mediators of inflammation (Fig. 9.4B).

Blood flow decrease

Due to stasis of blood in blood vessel, there is increase in leakage of fluids /cells outside the blood vessels. It gives rise to congestion/ hyperemia. There is margination of leucocytes also known as *pavementation* (Figs. 9.5).

Cells in perivascular spaces

Due to pseudopodia movement, leucocytes come out from the dilated blood vessels through intact and swollen endothelium and this process is known as *"diapedesis"*. Cells also come out through break in blood vessel and this process is called as *"rhexis"* (Fig. 9.6).

Leucocytes degranulate in perivascular tissue spaces

When Leucocytes reach tissue spaces, they release chemical mediators of inflammation, antimicrobial factors in tissues such as cationic proteins, hydrogen peroxide, hydrolytic enzymes, lysozymes, proteases, kinins, histamine, serotonin, heparin, cytokines, and complement (Fig. 9.7).

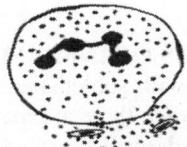

Fig. 9.7. Diagram of polymorphonuclear cell showing degranulation

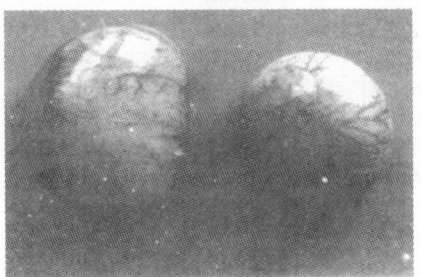

Fig 9.8. Photograph of testicles showing congestion

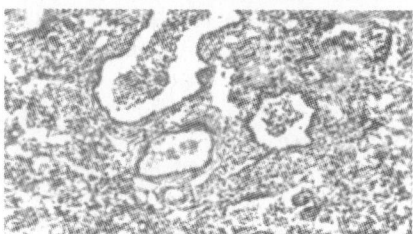

Fig. 9.9. Photomicrograph of lung showing acute inflammation

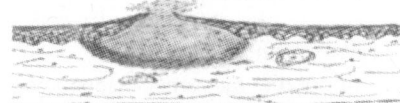

Fig. 9.10. Diagram of an abscess

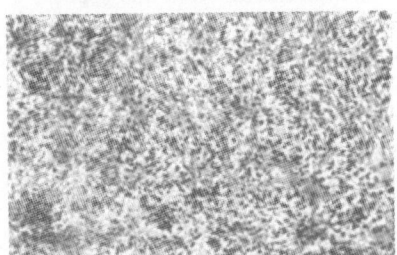

Fig. 9.11. Photomicrograph showing polymorphonuclear cells in fibrin network

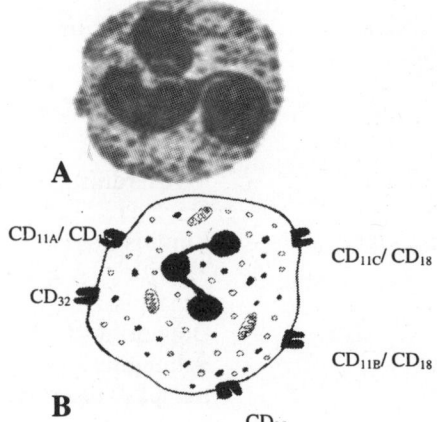

Fig. 9.12. A. Photomicrograph of polymorphonuclear cell B. diagram of polymorphonuclear cell showing different receptors

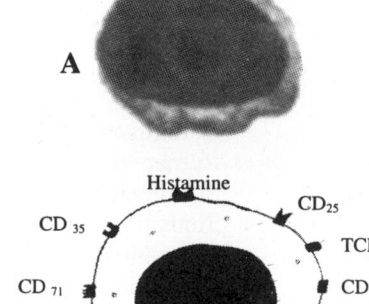

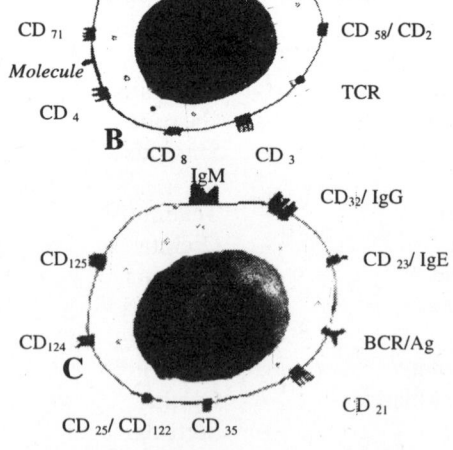

Fig.9.13. A. Photomicrograph of lymphocyte, B. Diagram of T-lymphocyte and C. B- lymphocyte showing different receptors.

Irritant is removed and damaged tissue healed

By the process of inflammation irritant is neutralized/removed or killed. Fluids are absorbed through lymphatics and debris is removed by phagocytosis. Blood vessel becomes normal.

If the irritant is strong and not normally removed by the inflammatory process, it remains at the site and gets covered by inflammatory cells and after some time by fibrous cells in order to localize the irritant. *e.g.* granuloma.

VASCULAR CHANGES

In inflammation, there is transient vasoconstriction followed by vasodilation increased capillary permeability and decrease in blood flow. Circulatory changes are more pronounced in acute inflammation (Figs. 9.8 to 9.11).

Etiology

• Any irritant/ injury causing inflammation.

Macroscopic features

• Congestion of the affected organ/tissue.
• Oedema.
• Haemorrhage.

Microscopic features

• Congestion of blood vessels.
• Oedema, presence of fibrin net work.
• Infiltration of leucocytes such as neutrophils, lymphocytes, macrophages, eosinophils etc.

CELLULAR CHANGES

In inflammation, there is infiltration of leucocytes in the inflamed area in order to provide defense to the body and to kill or neutralize the etiological factors.

Etiology/ Occurrence

• Any irritant/ injury causing inflammation.

Macroscopic features

• Formation of pus/ abscess if there is increased number of neutrophils in the inflamed area.
• Area becomes hard, painful, with swelling/ nodule.

Microscopic features

• Presence of leucocytes in the inflammation area.
• Presence of the type of cell may also determine the type of inflammation.

Cells of inflammation are polymorphonuclear cells, lymphocytes, macrophages, eosinophils, mast cells, plasma cells, giant cells, etc.

Polymorphonuclear cells

They are also known as neutrophils (mammals) and heterophils (birds). Size of these cells vary from 10μ to 20μ. They are attracted by certain chemotactic factors like bacterial proteins, C_3a, C_5a, fibrinolysin and kinins. These cells are produced in bone marrow and are short life of only 2-3 days. Mature cells have multilobed nucleus and two types of granules. Primary granules are the azurophilic granules present in lysosomes containing acid hydrolases, myeloperoxidases and neuraminidases. Secondary or specific granules have lactoferin and lysozymes. These cells degranulate through Fc receptor, binding with non-specific immune complexes or opsonins (Fig. 9.12).

Lymphocytes

Lymphocytes are produced in primary lymphoid organs like thymus, bursa of Fabricious and bone marrow and their maturation takes place in secondary lymphoid organs like spleen, lymphnodes, tonsils, and mucosa associated lymphoid tissue etc. These cells may survive for years and in some cases for whole life of an animal. There are two types of lymphocytes seen on light microscopy i.e. small and large. Small lymphocytes are mainly T-helper or T-cytotoxic cells having nuclear cytoplasm ratio (N:C). The larger lymphocytes have low N:C ratio and are mainly B cells and NK cells. There are large numbers of molecules present on cell surface of lymphocytes which are used to distinguish the type of cells. These are known as markers and are identified by a set of monoclonal antibodies and are termed as Cluster of Differentiation (CD system of

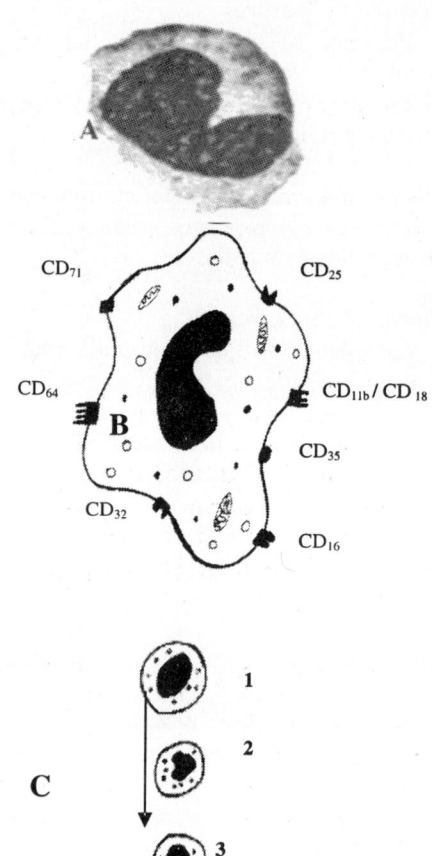

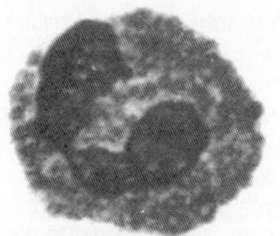

Fig. 9.15. Photomicrograph of eosinophil

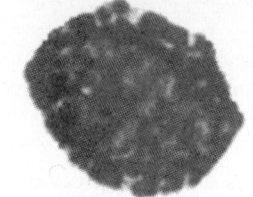

Fig. 9.16. Photomicrograph of basophil

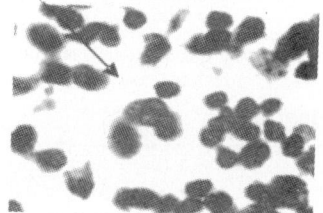

Fig. 9.17. Photomicrograph of plasma cell

Fig. 9.14. A. Photomicrograph of macrophage/ monocyte B. Diagram of macrophage showing different receptors and C. Diagram showing different stages and types of phagocytic cells: 1. Stem cell 2. Promonocyte 3. Monocyte 4. Microglia in brain 5. Histiocyte in connective tissue 6. Kupffer cell in liver 7. Alveolar macrophages and 8.Oosteoclasts in bone

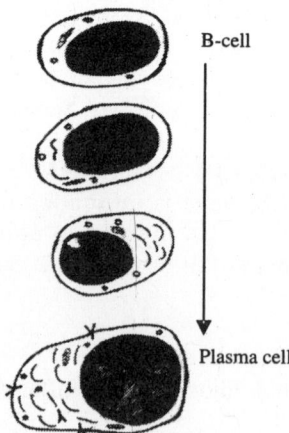

Fig. 9.18. Diagram of plasma cell

classification) *e.g.* CD_4 T-helper cells, CD_8 T-cytotoxic cell, CD_2 and CD_5 Pan-cell marker and CD_7 NK cells.

B-lymphocytes are characterized on the basis of presence of mature immunoglobulins (IgG, IgA, IgM, IgE, IgD) on their surface. They comprise only 5-15% of total peripheral blood lymphocytes. The B-cells having IgM, IgG, IgD are present in blood while IgA-bearing B-lymphocytes are present in large numbers on mucosal surfaces. The B-lymphocytes can be further divided into B_1 and B_2; B_1 are present predominantly in peritoneal cavity and are predisposed for autoantibody production while B_2-cells are conventional antibody-producing cells (Fig. 9.13).

Natural Killer (N.K.) cells are also present in 10-15% of total peripheral blood lymphocytes. These are defined as the lymphocytes which do not have any conventional surface antigen receptor i.e. TCR or immunoglobulin. In other words, they are neither T nor B cells. The NK cells do not have CD_3 molecule but CD_{16} and CD_{56} are present on their surface. These cells may kill tumor cells, virus containing cells and targets coated by IgG non specifically. They excrete gamma interferon interleukin 1 and GM- CSF.

Macrophages

The mononuclear macrophages are the main phagocytic and antigen presenting cells which develop from bone marrow stem cells and may survive in body till life. The professional phagocytic cells destroy the particulate material while antigen presenting cells (APC) present the processed antigen to the lymphocytes. They have horseshoe shaped nucleus and azurophilic granules. They have a well developed Golgi apparatus and many intracytoplasmic lysosomes which contain peroxidases and hydrolases for intracellular killing of microorganism. Macrophages have a tendency to adhere to glass or plastic surface and are able to phagocyte the bacteria and tumor cells through specialized receptors. These cells also have CD_{14} receptors for lipopolysaccharide (LPS) binding protein normally present in serum and may coat on Gram negative bacteria. There are CD_{64} receptor for binding of Fc portion of IgG responsible for opsonization, extracellular killing and phagocytosis. Antigen presenting cells (APC) are associated with immunostimulation, induction of T-helper cell activity and communication with other leucocytes. Some endothelial and epithelial cells may, under certain circumstances, also acquire the properties of APC when stimulated by cytokines. They are found in skin, lymphnodes, spleen and thymus (Fig. 9.14).

Eosinophils

Eosinophils comprise 2-5% of total leucocyte count in peripheral blood. They are responsible for killing of large objects which cannot be phagocytosed such as parasites. However, they may also act as phagocytic cells for killing bacteria but it is not their primary function. These cells have bilobed nucleus and eosinophilic granules. The granules are membrane-bound with crystalloid core. These granules are rich in major basic protein which also releases histaminase and aryl sulfatase and leucocyte migration inhibition factor (Fig. 9.15).

Mast cells/ Basophils

There are 0.2% basophils in peripheral blood which have deep violet blue coloured granules. The tissue basophils are known as mast cells. They are of two types, mucosal mast cells and connective tissue mast cells. Basophilic granules present in these cells are rich in heparin, SRS-A and ECF-A. When any antigen or allergen comes into contact with cells, it crosses links with IgE bound on the surface of mast cells and stimulates the cells to degranulate and release histamine which plays an active role in allergy (Fig. 9.16).

Platelets

Platelets are derived from bone marrow and contain granules. These cells help in clotting of blood and are involved in inflammation. When endothelial surface gets damaged, platelets adhere and aggregate on damaged endothelium and release

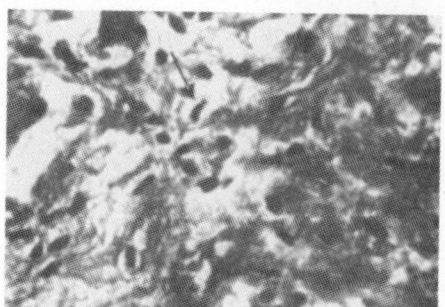

Fig. 9.19. Photomicrograph of epithelioid cells

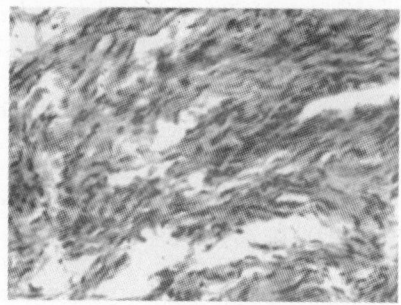

Fig. 9.22. Photomicrograph showing proliferation of fibroblasts

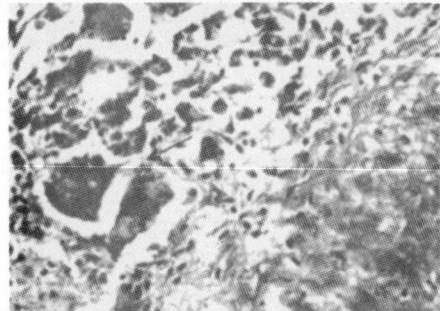

Fig. 9.20. Photomicrograph of giant cells

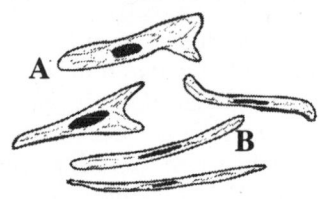

Fig. 9.23. Diagram of A. fibroblasts and B. fibrocytes

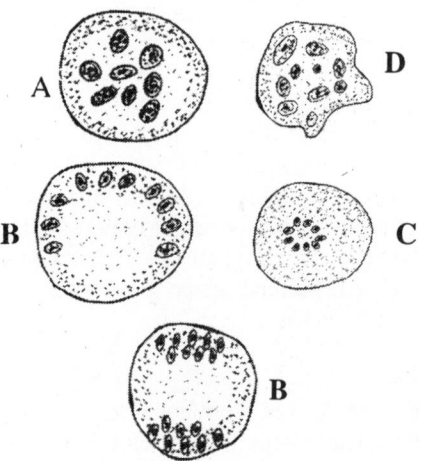

Fig. 9.21 Diagram of giant cells: A. foreign body B. Langhan's C .Touton, and D. Tumor giant cell

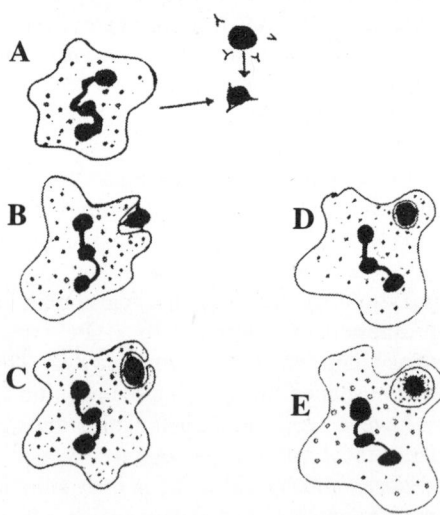

Fig. 9.24. Diagram showing phagocytosis. A. Opsonization and Chemotaxis B - C. Engulfment and D - E. Digestion.

substances to increase permeability, attract leucocytes and activate complement.

Plasma cells

The plasma cells are modified B-lymphocytes meant for production of immunoglobulins. Plasma cells have smooth spherical or elliptical shape with increased cytoplasm and eccentrically placed cart wheel-shaped nucleus. The cytoplasm stains slightly basophilic and gives a magenta shade of purplish red. In the cytoplasm, there is a distinct hyaline homogenous mass called **Russell body** which lies on the cisternae of the endoplasmic reticulum. This is the accumulation of immunoglobulin produced by these cells. Such cells are present in almost all types of inflammation (Figs. 9.17 & 9.18).

Epithelioid cells

They are the activated macrophages mostly present in granuloma when macrophages become large and foamy due to accumulation of phagocytosed material (bacteria) and degenerated tissue debris. These cells are considered as **hallmark of granulomatous inflammation**. They are elongated with marginal nucleus that looks like columnar epithelial cell and hence the name "Epithelioid" cells (Fig. 9.19).

Giant cells

The giant cells are multinucleated macrophages fused together to kill the microorganisms. They are formed by the fusion of many macrophages to phagocytose larger particles such as yeast, fungi and mycobacteria. They have usually more than one nucleus and abundant cytoplasm. Such cells are formed when macrophages fail to phagocytose the particulate material. They are of several types as listed blow (Figs. 9.20 & 9.21).

Foreign body giant cells: They have many nuclei, upto 100, which are uniform in size and shape and resemble the macrophage nucleus. The nuclei are scattered in the cytoplasm. Such cells are seen in chronic infectious granulomas of tuberculosis.

Langhan's giant cells: They are horseshoe shaped giant cells having many nuclei and are characteristically present in tubercle. The nuclei resemble that of macrophages and epithelioid cells. The nuclei are mostly arranged at periphery giving horseshoe shape.

Touton giant cells: They are multinucleated cells having vacuolation in the cytoplasm due to increased lipid content. They mostly occur in xanthoma.

Tumor giant cells: These are larger, pleomorphic and hyperchromatic cells having numerous nuclei with different size and shape. Nuclei of such cells do not resemble that of macrophages or epithelioid cells. They are not true giant cells and not formed from macrophages but are found in cancers as a result of fast division of nuclei in comparison to cytoplasm.

Fibroblasts

Fibroblast proliferates to replace its own tissue and others which are not able to regenerate. The new fibroblasts originate from fibrocyte as well as from the fibroblasts through mitotic division. Collagen fibres begin to appear on 6th day as an amorphous ground substance or matrix. They are characteristic of chronic inflammation and repair. Fibroblasts are elongated cells having long nuclei, sometimes looking like the smooth muscle fibres. The proliferation of fibroblasts is extremely active in neonates and slow and delayed in old animals. The fibroplasia can be enhanced by removal of necrosed tissue debris and by fever (Fig. 9.22 & 9.23).

CHEMICAL CHANGES

There is a long list of chemical mediators responsible for acute inflammation. These are endogenous biochemical compounds, which can increase the vascular permeability, vasodilation, chemotaxis, fever, pain and cause tissue damage. Such chemical mediators are released by cells, plasma or damaged tissue and are broadly classified as: cell and plasma derived chemical mediators of inflammation.

CELL DERIVED MEDIATORS

Vasoactive amines

Histamine

Histamine is found in basophilic granules of mast cells or basophils and in platelets. It is released through stimuli due to heat, cold, irradiation, trauma, irritant, chemical and immunological reactions and anaphylotoxins C3a, C5a and C4a. Histamine is also released due to action of histamine releasing factors from neutrophils, monocytes and platelets. It acts on blood vessels and causes vasodilation, increased vascular permeability, itching and pain.

Serotonin (5-Hydroxy-tryptamine)

It is present in tissues of gastrointestinal tract, spleen, nervous tissue, mast cells and platelets. It also acts on blood vessels to cause vasodilation and increased permeability but its action is mild in comparison to histamine.

Arachidonic acid metabolites

Arachidonic acid is a fatty acid, which either comes directly from the diet or through conversion of linoleic acid to arachidonic acid. Arachidonic acid is activated by C5a to form its metabolites through either cyclo-oxygenase or lipo-oxygenase pathways. Cyclo-oxygenase is a fatty acid enzyme which acts on arachidonic acid to form prostaglandin endoperoxidase (PGG) which is further transformed into prostaglandins like PGD_2, PGE_2, PGF_2, thromboxane A_2 (Tx A_2) and prostacyclin (PGI_2). Prostaglandins act on blood vessels to cause vasodilation, increased permeability bronchodilation except $PGF_2\alpha$, which is responsible for vasodilation and bronchoconstriction. Thromboxane A_2 is a vasoconstrictor, bronchoconstrictor, and causes aggregation of platelets leading of increased function of inflammatory cells. Prostacylin is found to be responsible for vasodilation, bronchodilation and inhibitory action on platelet aggregation.

Lipo-oxygnese acts on arachidonic acid to form hydroperoxy eico-satetraenoic acid (5HPETE) which is further converted into 5HETE, a chemotactic agent for neutrophils and leucotrienes (LT) or slow reacting substance of anaphylaxis (SRS-A). The leucotrienes include an unstable form leucotriene A (LTA), which is soon converted into leucotriene B (LTB), a chemotactic and adherence factor for phagocytic cells, and leucotriene C, D and E (LTC, LTD, LTE) causing contraction of smooth muscles leading to vasoconstriction, bronchoconstriction and increased vascular permeability.

Lysosomal components

Lysosomal granules are released by neutrophils and macrophages to cause degradation of bacterial and extracellular components, chemotaxis and increased vascular permeability. These lysosomal granules are rich in acid proteases, collagenases, elastases and plasminogen activator.

Platelet activating factor (PAF)

Platelet activating factor (PAF) is released from IgE sensitized mast cells, endothelial cells and platelets. It acts on platelets for their aggregation and release, chemotaxis, bronchoconstriction, adharence of leucocytes and increased vascular permeability. In low amount PAF causes vasodilation while in high concentration it leads to vasoconstriction.

Cytokines

Cytokines are hormone-like substances produced by activated lymphocytes (*Lymphokines*) and monocytes (*Monokines*). These are glycoprotein in nature with low molecular weight (8-75KD) and are composed of single chain. They differ from hormones which are specifically produced by endocrine glands to maintain homeostasis through endocrine action as cytokines are produced by many different cell types and act on different cells of body with very high functional activity. They cause autocrine, paracrine and endocrine action leading to tissue repair and resistance to infection. Cytokines are broadly classified as interleukins, interferon, cytotoxins and growth factors.

Interleukins (IL)

Interleukins are cytokines required for cell to cell interaction among immune cells. They are numbered serially in order of their discovery; however, their actions are different and not related with each other.

Table 9.1 Interleukins

Sl. No.	Type of interleukin	Size MW (KD)	Source	Target / Action
1.	Interleukin-1 (IL-1α, IL-1β and IL-1RA)	17	Macrophages, Langerhans cells, T-cells, B-cells, Vascular endothelium, Fibroblasts, Keratinocytes.	T-cells, B-cells, Neutrophils, Eosinophils, Dendritic cells, Fibroblasts, Endothelial cells, Hepatocytes, Macrophages.
2.	Interleukin-2 (IL –2)	15	T- helper-1 cells (Th-1).	T-cells, B-cells, NK cells.
3.	Interleukin-3 (IL-3)	25	Activated T-cells, Th-1 cells, Th-2 cells, Eosinophils, Mast cells.	Stimulates growth and maturation of bone marrow stem cells, Eosinophilia, Neutrophilia monocytosis, Increases phagocytosis, Promotes immuno-globulin secretion by B-cells.
4.	Interleukin-4 (IL-4)	20	Activated Th-2 cells.	B-cells, T-cells, Macrophages, Endothelial cells, Fibroblasts, Mast cells, IgE production in allergy, Down regulate IL1, IL6, and TNF-α.
5.	Interleukin-5 (IL-5)	18	Th-2 cells, Mast cells, Eosinophils.	Eosinophils, Increases T-cell cytotoxicity.
6.	Interleukin-6 (IL-6)	26	Macrophages, T-cells, B-cells, Bone marrow stromal cells, Vascular endothelial cells, Fibroblasts, Keratinocytes, Mesangial cells.	T-cells, B-cells, Hepatocytes, Bone marrow stromal cells, Stimulates acute phase protein synthesis, Acts as pyrogen.
7.	Interleukin-7 (IL-7)	25	Bone marrow, Spleen cells, Thymic stromal cells.	Thymocytes, T-cells, B-cells, Monocytes, Lymphoid stem cells, Generates cytotoxic T-cells.
8.	Interleukin-8 (IL-8)	8	Macrophages.	T-cells, Neutrophils.
9.	Interleukin-9 (IL-9)	39	Th-2 cells.	Growth of Th-cells, Stimulates B-cell, Thymocytes, Mast cells.
10.	Interleukin-10 (IL-10)	19	Th cells, B-cells, Macrophages, Keratinocytes, Th-2 cells.	Th-1 cells, NK cells, Stimulates B-cells, Thymocytes, Mast cells.
11.	Interleukin-11 (IL-11)	24	Bone marrow stromal cells, Fibroblasts.	Growth of B-cells, Megakaryocyte colony formation, Promotes the production of acute phase proteins.
12.	Interleukin-12 (IL-12)	75	Activated macrophages.	Th-1 cells activity, T-cell proliferation and cytotoxicity, NK cell proliferation and cytotoxicity Suppresses IgE production, Enhances B-cell immunoglobulin production.
13.	Interleukin- 13 (IL-13)	10	Th-2 cells	B-Cells, Macrophages, Neutrophils, Inhibits macrophage activity,

				Stimulates B-cell proliferation, Stimulates neutrophils.
14.	Interleukin 14 (IL-14)	53	T-cells, Malignant B-cells	Enhances B-cell proliferation, Inhibits immunoglobulin secretion.
15.	Interleukin- 15 (IL-15)	15	Activated macrophages, Epithelial cells, Fibroblasts.	T-cells, NK cells, Proliferation of both cytotoxic and helper T-cells, Generates LAK cells
16.	Interleukin- 16 (IL-16)	13	T-cells (CD$_8$ cells)	T cells, CD$_4$ cells, Chemotactic for lymphocytes
17.	Interleukin- 17 (IL-17)	17	CD$_4$ cells	Promotes the production of IL-6, IL-8.
18.	Interleukin–18 (IL-18)		Macrophage	Induces γ-interferon production
19.	Interleukin–19 (IL-19)		Macrophage	Inhibit inflammatory and immune responses, suppress activities of T$_h$1 and T$_h$2 cells
20.	Interleukin–20 (IL-20)		Activated keratinocytes	Proliferation of keratinocytes and their differentiation, modulate skin inflammation
21.	Interleukin–21 (IL-21)		Activated T-cells	Regulation of haematopoiesis and immune responses, promotes production of T-cells, fast growth and maturation of NK cells and B-cells population
22.	Interleukin–22 (IL-22)		Activated T-cells	Induction of acute phase responses and proinflammatory role
23.	Interleukin–23 (IL-23)		Monocytes, activated dendritic cells	Induces γ interferon production and T$_h$1 lymphocyte differentiation
24.	Interleukin–24 (IL-24)		T$_h$2 cells	Tumor suppression
25.	Interleukin–25 (IL-18)		T$_h$2 cells	Stimulates release of IL-4, IL-5 and IL-13 from non lymphoid accessory cells
26.	Interleukin–26 (IL-26)		T- cells	Proinflammatory role, cutaneous and mucosal immunity
27.	Interleukin–27 (IL-27)		CD$_4$ cells	Rapid clonal expansion of naïve T-cells and CD$_4$ cells, induces proliferative response and cytokines production by Ag specific effector/memory T$_h$1 cells
28.	Interleukin–28 (IL-28)		Virus induced peripheral blood mononuclear cells	Immunity to viral infection (antiviral activity)
29.	Interleukin–29 (IL-29)		Virus induced peripheral blood mononuclear cells	Immunity to viral infection (antiviral activity)

Interferons

Interferons are glycoproteins having antiviral action and inhibit the virus replication in cells. These are of five types like alpha (α), beta (β), gamma (γ), omega (ω), and tau (ι).

Table 9.2. Interferons

Sl. No.	Interferon	Source	Action
1.	Interferon alpha (IFN-α)	Lymphocytes, Monocytes, Macrophages	Inhibit viral growth, activates macrophages
2.	Interferon beta (IFN-β)	Fibroblasts	Inhibit viral growth, activates macrophages
3.	Interferon gamma (IFN-γ)	Th-1 cells, Cytotoxic T-cells, NK cells, Macrophages	Stimulates B-cells, production, enhances NK Cells activity activates macrophages and phagocytosis. Promotes antibody-dependent and cell-mediated cytotoxicity.
4.	Interferon Omega (IFN-ω)	Lymphocytes, Monocytes Trophoblasts	Virus infected cells to check viral growth Activate Macrophages
5.	Interferon tau (IFN-ι)	Trophoblasts	Virus growth, Immunity to faetus through placenta.

Tumor necrosis factor or cytotoxins

Tumor necrosis factor or cytotoxins are produced by macrophages and T-cells and are associated with apoptosis in tumors. Tumor necrosis factor beta (TNF-β) is produced by T-helper 1 cells and activates CD_8^+ T-cells, neutrophils, macrophages, endothelial cells and B-lymphocytes. Tumor necrosis factor alpha (TFN-α) is produced by macrophages, T- cells, B-cells and fibroblasts and it activates macrophages and enhances immunity and inflammatory reaction.

Chemokines

Chemokines are small proteins divided into two α and β subfamilies. Alpha-chemokines include IL-8, which is produced by fibroblasts, macrophages, endothelial cells, lymphocytes, granulocytes, hepatocytes and keratinocytes. It acts as chemotactic agent for basophils, neutrophils and T-cells. The neutrophils get activated and release their granules and leucotrienes. There is increased respiratory burst. Besides, it also acts on basophils and lymphocytes. Macrophage inflammatory protein MIP-1 of β-chemokines are produced by macrophages, T and B-lymphocytes, mast cells and neutrophils. It acts on monocytes, eosinophils, B and T-lymphocytes. Beta-chemokines include macrophage inflammatory protein (MIP-1), monocyte chemoattractant protein (MCP) and RANTES protein. The MCP is produced by macrophages, T-cells, fibroblasts, keratinocytes and endothelial cells and activates the monocytes, stimulating them for respiratory burst and lysosomal enzyme release. RANTES is released by T-lymphocytes and macrophages and it acts as chemotactic agent for monocytes, eosinophils, basophils and some T-cells.

Growth factors

Many cytokines are also known as growth factors which act on cells and stimulate them to proliferate. Thus they play a very important role in inflammation and healing. In nature these are glycoprotein which controls the proliferation and maturation of several blood cells. The growth factors also include interleukin 3, 7, 11, and 15. The granulocyte colony stimulating factor (G-CSF) is produced by fibroblasts, endothelial cells and macrophages. It acts on granulocyte progenitors and regulate their maturation and production of superoxide. Macrophage colony stimulating factors (M-CSF) are the glycoproteins released by lymphocytes, macrophages, fibroblasts, epithelial cells and endothelial cells. They act on monocyte progenitors for their proliferation and differentiation and promote their killing activity. Granulocyte macrophage colony stimulating factor (GM-CSF) is released from macrophages, T-lymphocytes, endothelial cells and fibroblasts and facilitates phagocytosis, antibody dependent cell cytotoxicity (ADCC) and superoxide production. It activates eosinophils to enhance superoxide production and macrophages for increased phagocytosis and tumoricidal activity. Transforming growth factor (TGF) are five related proteins (TGF-B$_1$, B$_2$, B$_3$ in mammals; B$_4$ and B$_5$ in poultry) released from neutrophils, macrophages, T-and B-lymphocytes and they inhibit the proliferation of macrophages, T - and B-lymphocytes and stimulates the proliferation of fibroblasts.

PLASMA DERIVED MEDIATORS

Plasma derived mediators of inflammation are kinins, clotting, fibrinolytic and complement systems; each of them has initiators and accelerators in plasma depending upon their need through feedback mechanism. During inflammation Hagman factor (Factor XII) is activated through leakage in endothelial gaps in increased permeability of blood vessels. The activated factor XII acts on kinin, clotting and fibrinolytic systems and end product of these systems activate complement to generate C3a and C5a, which are potent mediators of inflammation.

Kinin system

Through activation of factor XII, kinin system generates the bradykinin which causes contraction of smooth muscles. The activated factor XII (XIIa) acts on prekallikrein activator which in turn converts the plasma prekallikrein into kallikrein.

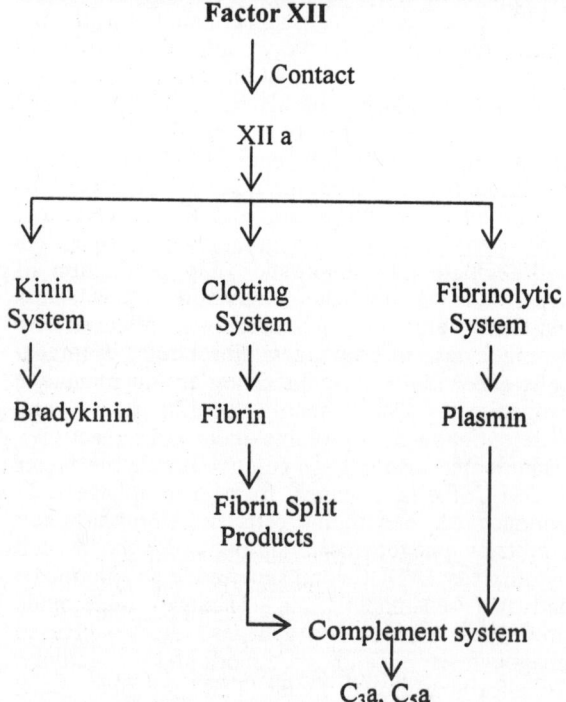

The bradykinin is formed from kininogen through the action of kallikrein. The bradykinin acts on smooth muscles leading to their contraction. Bradykinin is also found to be responsible for vasodilation, increased vascular permeability and pain.

Clotting mechanism

The activated Hagman factor (XIIa) initiates the cascade of clotting system and factor XI

Clotting system

(a) Extrisic mechanism

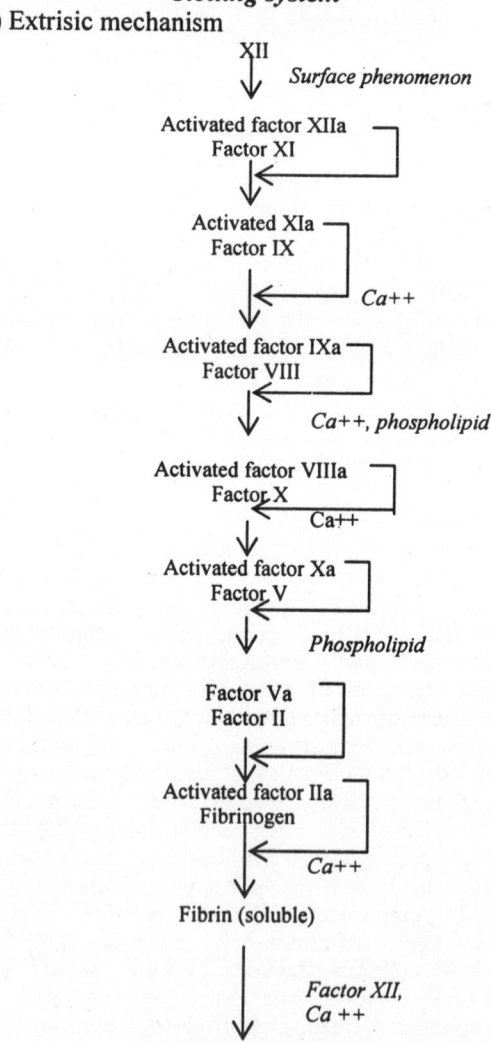

(b) Intrisic mechanism

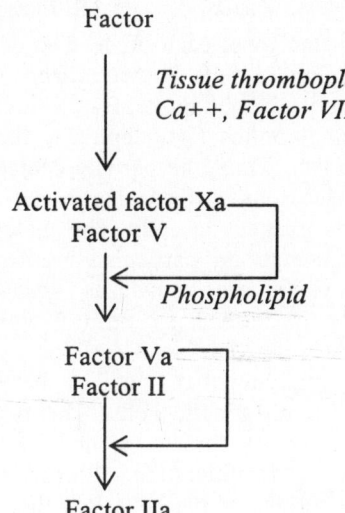

Factor

↓ *Tissue thromboplastin Ca++, Factor VII*

Activated factor Xa
Factor V

↓ *Phospholipid*

Factor Va
Factor II

↓

Factor IIa

into XIa which along with factor VIIa changes factor X into Xa. Factor Xa along with factor Va converts prothrombin into thrombin which acts on fibrinogen to form fibrin responsible for clotting of blood.

Fibrinolytic system

Plasminogen activator is released from endothelial cells and leucocytes and acts on plasminogen present as a component of plasma proteins to form plasmin. The plasmin is responsible for breakdown of fibrin into fibrinopeptides or fibrin split products, conversion of C_3 to C_{3a} and stimulates the kinin system to generate bradykinin.

Complement system

Complement is activated through classical and alternate pathways; the classical pathway includes activation of complement through antigen-antibody complexes while the alternate pathway gets activated via non-immunologic agents such as bacterial toxins. Complement system on activation generates 3 anaphylotoxin through either of pathway including C3a, C5a and C4a, which are responsible for release of histamine from the mast cells, increased vascular permeability and chemotaxis for leucocytes. The complement components are activated by antigen antibody complex and form AAC1423 which causes opsonization and enhances phagocytosis. C567 acts as chemotactic factor for phagocytic cells. AAC $_{1-7}$ renders the cell susceptible for lymphocytotoxicity by T-cell. The complement AAC $_{1-9}$ causes lysis of erythrocytes and Gram negative bacteria. However, Gram positive bacteria are resistant to complement lysis.

Antigen- antibody complex (AA)
On cell surface

↓ C_1

AAC_1

↓ C_4 ⟶ C_4a

$AAC_{14.}$

↓ C_2 ⟶ C_2x
Kinin-like product

AAC_{142}

↓ C_3 ⟶ C_3a
Anaphylotoxin

AAC_{1423}
C_5 ⟶ C_5a
C_6 *Anaphylotoxin*

AAC_{142356}

↓ C_7 ⟶ $C567$
Chemotactic factor

$AAC_{1423567}$

↓ C_8
AAC_{1-8}

↓ C_9

AAC_{1-9}

↓

Cell lysis

PHAGOCYTOSIS

Phagocytosis is the process of engulfment and digestion of particulate matter by certain cells of body (phagocytes; phagocytic cells). Mainly there are two types of the cells which perform the phagocytosis including polymorphonuclear neutrophils (PMN) or microphages and monocytes or tissue mononuclear cells also known as macrophages. The process of phagocytosis is almost similar by these micro and macrophages and involves 4 stages (Fig. 9.24):

I. Chemotaxis

The phagocytic cells, neutrophils and monocytes are present in circulating blood while there are several tissue macrophages found in inflammation. Vasodilation and decreased blood flow leads to disturbances in blood stream resulting in margination of leucocytes. At that time endothelial cells of blood vessels express certain proteins known as *selectins* and *integrins* that bind with neutrophils. Since they are attracted by certain chemical mediators, these cells are directed to migrate towards the chemical mediators. This directed migration of phagocytic cells is known as chemotaxis. Various chemotactic agents for different phagocytic cells are as under:

Chemotactic agents	Phagocytic cells
C_{3a}, C_{5a}, C_{567}, Leucotriene B_4, Bacterial proteins, LPS.	Neutrophils
C_{3a}, C_{5a}, C_{567}, Bacterial products	Macrophages/ monocytes
Neutrophilic cationic protein Cytokines, Kinins	
ECF-A, Parasitic proteins, Complement C_{3a}, C_{5a}.	Eosinophils

The chemotactic agents diffuse at the site of tissue damage to attract the phagocytic cells. However, large dose of chemotactic molecules may make the phagocytic cells insensitive to chemoattraction and such non-responsive cells may migrate from the damaged area after completion of phagocytosis.

II. Adherence and opsonization

The phagocytic cells and foreign particle like bacteria are suspended in body fluid with negative charge that repel each other. The negative charge on foreign particle is neutralized by coating of positively charged protein and such proteins are immunoglobulins (IgG) and C_{3b}, the complement component. Thus, the particle coated with IgG or C_{3b} reduces its surface charge and it is attracted towards phagocytic cells. The molecules (IgG or C_{3b}) coatings on particulate matter to facilitate phagocytosis are known as *opsonins* and this process is termed as *opsonization*. The word opsonin is derived from Greek language and means *sauce*, implying that it makes the particles more tastier to phagocytic cells. The phagocytic cells have receptors for Fc portion of IgG and C_3b protein that facilitates the adherence of the particles on the surface of the cells. Another mechanism is trapping of particulate material through pseudopodia movement of the phagocytic cells.

III. Ingestion

The phagocytic cell forms pseudopodia around the particles to cover it from outside. The particle is bound to the surface of cells through opsonization and is drawn inside the cytoplasm through engulfment. The phagocytic cell forms vacuole by enveloping the particle which is known as *phagocytic vacuole*. The plasma membrane covering phagocytic vacuole breaks and the ingested particle lies free in cytoplasm of phagocytic cell. The lysosome present in cell cytoplasm binds with phagocytic vacuoles to form *phagolysosome* or *phagosome*.

There is degranulation on the particle and liberation of hydrolytic enzymes and antibacterial substances to kill the ingested particle.

IV. Digestion

The ingested particles are destroyed by the phagocytic cells through two separate mechanisms, the respiratory burst and by action of lysosomal enzymes

Respiratory Burst

Soon after the ingestion of particulate material phagocytic cell increases its oxygen consumption nearly 100 fold and also activates the cell surface enzyme NADPH-oxidase. This activated enzyme converts NADPH to $NADP^+$ with release of electrons.

$$NADPH + O_2 \xrightarrow{\text{NADPH-Oxidase}} NADP^+ + 2\ O^- + H^+$$

One molecule of oxygen accepts a single donated electron, leading to the generation of one molecule of superoxide anion. $NADP^+$ increases the hexose monophosphate shunt and converts sucrose to a pentose, carbon dioxide and energy for utilization of the cellular functions. Two molecules of superoxide anions interact to generate one molecule of hydrogen peroxide under the influence of enzyme superoxide dismutase.

$$2(2O^-) + 2\ H^+ \xrightarrow{\text{Superoxide dismutase}} H_2O_2 + O_2$$

Superoxide anions do not accumulate in the cell because under the influence of dismutase enzyme they rapidly convert into hydrogen peroxide. However, there is accumulation of hydrogen peroxide in the cells which is also converted into bactericidal compounds the hypohalids through the action of myeloperoxidase.

$$H_2O_2 + Cl^- \xrightarrow{\text{Myeloperoxidase}} H_2O_2 + OCl^-$$
$$\text{(Hypochloride)}$$

Hypochloride kills bacteria by oxidizing their proteins and enhancing the bactericidal activities of the lysosomal enzymes.

Lysosomal enzymes

Once the phagolysosomes are formed, the lysosomal enzymes are released in the particulate matter that can kill the bacteria. Many Gram positive and Gram negative bacteria are destroyed by the lysosomal enzymes. However, there are certain bacteria like Brucella, Listeria which are so resistant that they even grow inside the cell and may become fatal to the cell. Dying neutrophils release elastases and collagenase which act as chemotactic factors for macrophages. The macrophages destroy the particulate material/ bacteria by both oxidative and non-oxidative mechanisms. In cattle, macrophages, after activation, synthesize the nitric oxide synthatase. This enzyme acts on L-arginine by using oxygen and NADPH to produce nitric oxide and citrulline. Nitric oxide is not highly toxic but it reacts with superoxide anions released during respiratory burst to produce very toxic derivatives such as NO_2, N_2O_3 ONOO and NO_3 which can kill the ingested bacteria and cause severe tissue damage. Macrophages are also used by the body as scavenger cells to remove the dead or dying cells.

When the foreign particulate material persists for longer period, macrophages accumulate in large number around it to kill and remove from the system. The phagocytosed particles are so potent that they kill the macrophages also. Then after destruction of macrophages it is rephagocytosed. This continuing destruction of macrophages leads to excessive release of lysosomal enzymes and reactive oxygen and nitric oxide metabolites resulting in chronic tissue damage and chronic inflammation. In such situation, macrophages become elongated looking like epithelial cells and such cells are termed as *epithelioid cells*. If these cells are also unable to destroy the ingested material then they combine/ fuse together to form multinucleated giant cells.

TYPES OF INFLAMMATION

Inflammation is classified according to the duration as of acute, subacute and chronic form. The acute inflammation is characterized by the presence of more vascular alterations while chronic inflammation is identified on the basis of presence of more proliferative changes, fibrosis and less vascular alterations (Fig. 9.25-I & II).

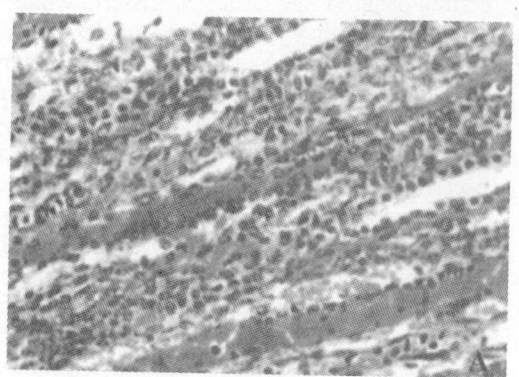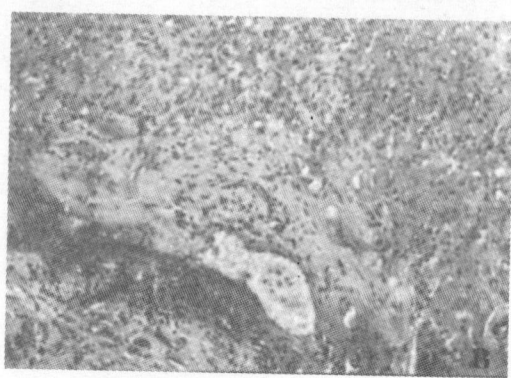

Fig. 9.25-I. Photomicrograph showing A. acute and B. Chronic inflammation

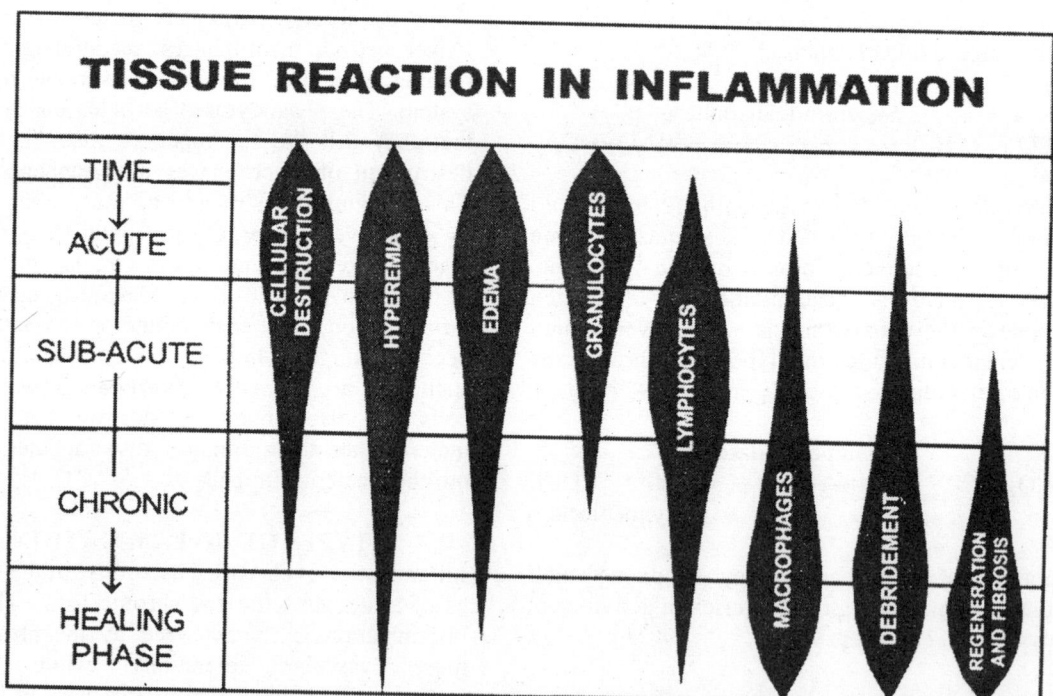

Fig. 9.25-II. Diagram showing tissue reaction in inflammation

Sl. No.	Changes	Acute	Subacute	Chronic
1.	Vascular changes	+++	++	+
2.	Proliferative changes	+	++	+++

On the basis of the presence of exudate, the inflammation is divided into catarrhal, serus, fibrinous, suppurative, eosinophilic, lymphocytic, haemorrhagic, granulomatous etc., described as under:

CATARRHAL INFLAMMATION

Catarrhal inflammation occurs on mucus surfaces and is characterized by the presence of increased amount of mucin as principal constituent of exudates *e.g. catarrhal enteritis, catarrhal rhinitis* (Figs. 9.26 & 9.27).

Etiology

- Mild irritant on mucous membrane *e.g.* Rotavirus infection in calves.
- Cold exposure causes excessive mucous discharges from nasal mucosa.

Macroscopic features

- Congestion.
- Presence of increased amount of slimy, stringy mucin along with stool.
- Mucus nasal discharge, if respiratory mucosa is involved.
- Mucous vaginal discharges in uterine disorders or as physiological phenomenon.

Microscopic features

- Increased number of goblet cells on mucous surface.
- Increased amount of mucin, which takes basic stain.
- Hyperplasia of epithelial cells on mucous surface.
- Infiltration of neutrophils, lymphocytes and macrophages.

SERUS INFLAMMATION

Serus inflammation occurs due to any mild irritant and is characterized by the presence of serum/plasma as main constituent of the exudates (Figs. 9.28 & 9.29).

Etiology

- Mild irritants *e.g.* chemicals.
- Physical trauma.
- Infection:
  - Virus *e.g.* Pox, FMD
  - Bacteria *e.g. Pasteurlla multocida*

Macroscopic features

- Congestion.
- Watery exudate in cavity/vesicle/in intercellular spaces.
- On rupture of vesicle clear fluid comes out.

Microscopic features

- Congestion.
- Presence of serus exudate-acidophilic in tissue.
- Infiltration of neutrophils/lymphocytes/mononuclear cells.

FIBRINOUS INFLAMMATION

Fibrinous inflammation is characterized by the presence of fibrin as main constituent of the exudates (Figs. 9.30 & 9.31).

Etiology

- Chemicals.
- Thermal injury.
- Bacteria *e.g. Corynebacterium diphtheriae.*
- Viruses *e.g.* Herpes virus, influenza virus.

Macroscopic features

- Organ becomes firm and tense.
- Surface of organ loses its shine.
- Produces adhesions in between two layers or two organs.

False membrane/crupous membrane present, which can be removed easily *e.g.* fibrinous membrane over heart and liver due to colisepticemia in birds.

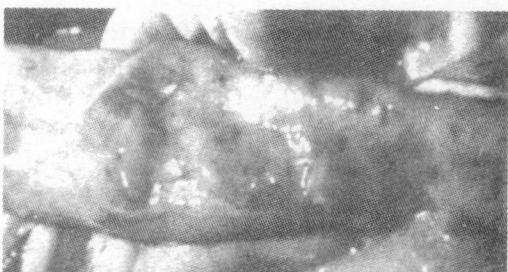

Fig 9.26. Photograph of intestine showing catarrhal inflammation

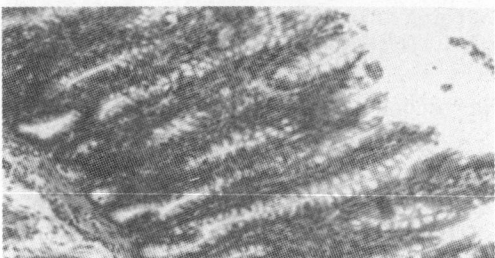

Fig 9.27. Photomicrograph of intestine showing catarrhal inflammation

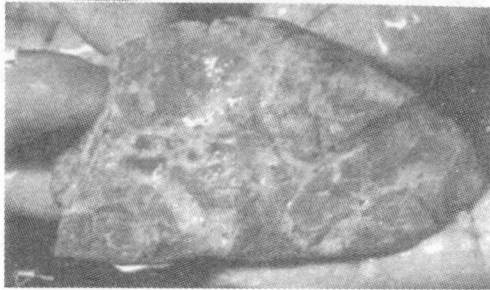

Fig 9.28. Photograph of lung showing serus inflammation

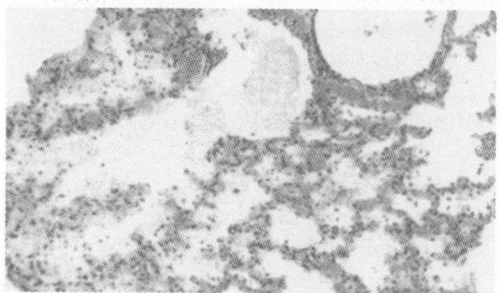

Fig 9.29. Photomicrograph of lung showing serus inflammation

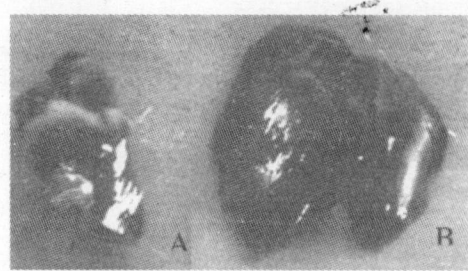

Fig 9.30. Photograph of A. heart and B. Liver showing fibrinous inflammation

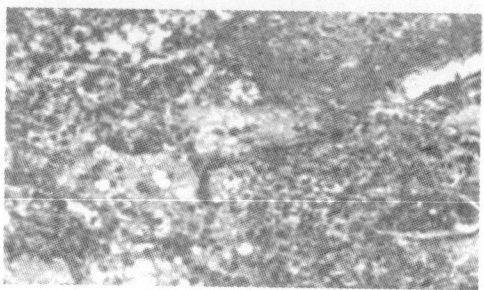

Fig 9.31. Photomicrograph showing fibrinous inflammation

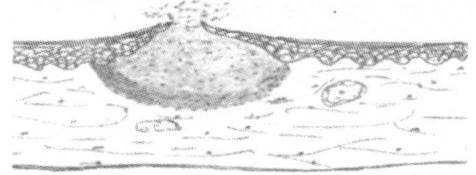

Fig 9.32. Diagram of an abscess (suppurative inflammation)

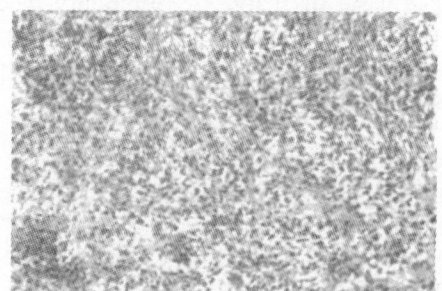

Fig 9.33. Photomicrograph showing suppurative inflammation

Microscopic features

- Congestion.
- Presence of fibrin network (thread-like) on the surface or in the organ.
- Infiltration of inflammatory cells like neutrophils, lymphocytes and macrophages.

SUPPURATIVE INFLAMMATION

Suppurative inflammation is characterized by the presence of neutrophils (polymorphonuclear cells) as principal constituent of the exudates (Figs. 9.32 & 9.33).

Etiology

- Bacterial infection *e.g.* Staphylococci.
- Chemicals *e.g.* turpentine.

Macroscopic features

- Presence of pus in lesion
- Pus is white yellow/greenish, thin, watery or viscid/material.
- When pus present in a cavity it is known as *abscess* while the presence of pus diffusely scattered throughout the subcutaneous tissue is known as *Phlegmon* or *cellulitis.*

Microscopic features

- Congestion.
- Presence of neutrophils as main constituent of the exudate.
- Liquifactive necrosis of the cells / tissue.

HAEMORRHAGIC INFLAMMATION

Haemorrhagic inflammation is characterized by the presence of erythrocyte as principal constituent of the exudate (Figs. 9.34 & 9.35).

Etiology

- Extremely injurious chemicals *e.g.* phenol.
- Bacterial infection *e.g.* Anthrax, H.S.
- Viral infection *e.g.* R.P., Blue tongue.

Macroscopic features

- Colour of organ/tissue becomes red/cyanotic.
- Exudate contains clots of blood.

- Petechial, echymotic haemorrhages on the surfaces of organs.
- Mucous membranes become pale / anemic.

Microscopic features

- Presence of erythrocytes outside the blood vessels in extracellular spaces along with neutrophils/ lymphocytes/ macrophages.
- Serus/serofibrinous exudates.

LYMPHOCYTIC INFLAMMATION

Lymphocytic inflammation is characterized by the presence of lymphocytes as principal constituent of the exudate (Fig. 9.36).

Etiology

- Viral / Bacterial infections.
- Toxic conditions.

Macroscopic features

- No characteristic gross lesion; sometimes there is formation of small modules on serosa of the affected organ.
- Enlargement of lymphnodes.
- Congestion.
- Presence of white/grey lymphoid nodules in organ.

Microscopic features

- Presence of lymphocytes in abundant number as principal constituent of the exudate.
- Congestion.
- Accumulation of lymphocytes around the blood vessels, "Peri vascular cuffing"
- Aggregation of lymphocytes leading to lymphofollicular reaction.

GRANULOMATOUS INFLAMMATION

Granulomatous inflammation is a chronic condition, characterized by the presence of granuloma in the organs. The granuloma consists of central caseative necrosis surrounded by lymphocytes, macrophages, epithelioid cells, giant cells and fibrous connective tissue (Figs. 9.37 & 9.38).

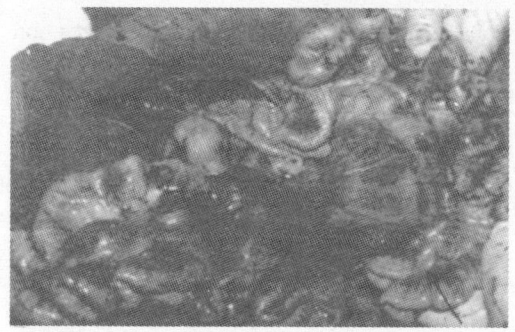

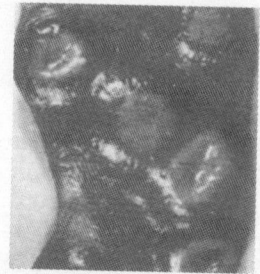

Fig. 9.37. Photograph of spleen showing granulomatous inflammation(ARS/USDA)

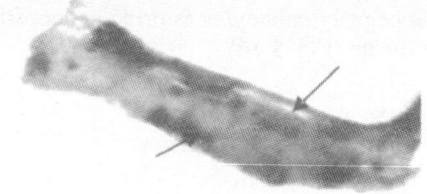

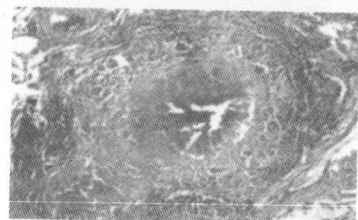

Fig. 9.38. Photomicrograph of lung showing granulomatous inflammation

Fig. 9.34. Photographs of intestines showing haemorrhagic inflammation

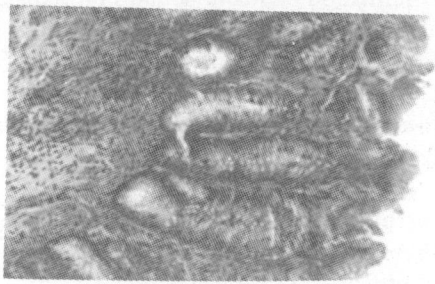

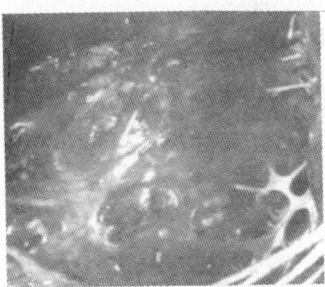

Fig. 9.39 Photograph of heart showing eosinophilic inflammation (ARS/USDA).

Fig. 9.35. Photomicrograph of intestine showing haemorrhagic inflammation

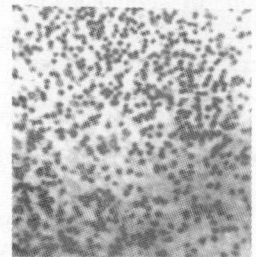

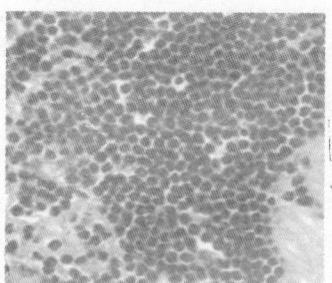

Fig. 9.36. Photomicrograph of brain showing lymphocytic inflammation

Fig. 9.40. Photomicrograph of heart showing eosinophilic inflammation (ARS/USDA).

Etiology

- Chronic bacterial infection *e.g.* tuberculosis.
- Fungal infections *e.g.* blastomycosis.

Macroscopic features

- Presence of hard, tiny, nodules in the organ.
- Lungs become hard, patchy.
- Lymphnodes become hard and fibrus.
- Later the affected organ is calcified and gives cracking sound on cut.

Microscopic features

- Presence of granuloma in the tissue/ organ.
- Central caseative necrosis, surrounded by epithelioid cells, macrophages, lymphocytes, giant cells and covered by fibrous connective tissue capsule.
- Caseative area contains causative organisms also, which can be demonstrated by special staining *e.g.* Tuberculous organisms by Acid-fast staining.
- Calcification of necrosed area at later stage looking black/ violet colour on H & E stain.

Table 9.2 Differential features of various types of inflammation

	Catarrhal	Serus	Fibrinous	Suppurative	Haemorr-hagic	Lymphocytic	Granulo-matous	Eosinophilic
Macroscopic features	1. Congestion 2. Presence of increased amount of slimy, stringy mucin along with stool. 3. Mucus nasal discharge, if respiratory mucosa is involved 4. Mucous vaginal discharges, in uterine disorders or as physiological phenomenon.	1. Congestion 2. Watery exudate in cavity/vesicle /in intercellular spaces 3. On rupture of vesicle clear fluid comes out	1. Organ becomes firm and tense. 2. Surface of organ lost its shine. 3. Produces adhesions in between two layers or two organs. 4. False membrane/ crupous membrane present, which can be removed easily e.g. fibrinous membrane over heart and liver due to colisepticemia in birds.	1. Presence of pus in lesion 2. Pus is white yellow/ greenish, thin, watery or viscid/ material. 3. When pus present in a cavity it is known as abscess. While the presence of pus diffusely scattered throughout the subcutaneous tissue is known as Phlegmon or cellulitis.	1. Colour of organ/tissue becomes red/cyanotic. 2. Exudate contains clot of blood. 3. Petechial, echymotic haemorrhages on the surfaces of organs. 4. Mucous membranes become pale / anemic.	1. No characteristic gross lesion; sometimes there is formation of small modules on serosa of the affected organ. 2. Enlargement of lymphnodes 3. Presence of white/gray lymphoid nodules in organ.	1. Presence of hard, tiny, nodules in the organ. 2. Lungs become hard, patchy. 3. Lymphnodes become hard and fibrous. 4. Later the affected organ calcified and gives cracking sound on cut.	1. Congestion 2. No characteristic gross lesion

Microscopic features	1. Increased number of goblet cells on mucous surface.\n\n2. Increased amount of mucin, which takes basic stain.\n\n3. Hyperplasia of epithelial cells on mucous surface.\n\n4. Infiltration of neutrophils, lymphocytes and macrophages.	1. Congestion\n\n2. Presence of serus exudate-acidophilic in tissue.\n\n3. Infiltration of neutrophils/ lymphocytes/ mononuclear cells	1. Congestion\n\n2. Presence of fibrin network (thread like) on the surface or in the organ.\n\n3. Infiltration of inflammatory cells like neutrophils, lymphocytes and macrophages.	1. Congestion\n\n2. Presence of neutrophils as main constituent of the exudate.\n\n3. Liquifactive necrosis of the cells / tissue.	1. Presence of erythrocytes out side the blood vessels in extracellular spaces along with neutrophils/ lymphocytes/ macrophage.\n\n2. Serus/ serofibrinous exudates.	1. Presence of lymphocytes in abundant number as principal constituent of the exudate.\n\n2. Accumulation of lymphocytes around the blood vessels, "Peri vascular cuffing"\n\n3. Aggregation of lymphocytes leading to lymphofollicular reaction.	1. Presence of granuloma in the tissue/ organ.\n\n2. Central caseative necrosis, surrounded by epithelioid cells, macrophages, lymphocytes, giant cells and covered by fibrous connective tissue capsule.\n\n3. Caseative area contains causative organisms also, which can be demonstrated by special staining e.g. Tuberculous organisms by Acid-fast staining.\n\n4. Calcification of necrosed area at later stage looking black/ violet colour on H&E stain.	1. Presence of eosinophils in abundant numbers\n\n2. Congestion\n\n3. Accumulation of eosinophils around the parasites and/ or blood vessels.

EOSINOPHILIC INFLAMMATION

It is characterized by the presence of eosinophils as the main constituents of the exudate (Figs. 9.39 & 9.40).

Etiology

- Allergy/ Hypersensitivity.
- Parasitic diseases.

Macroscopic features

- Congestion.
- No characteristic gross lesion.

Microscopic features

- Presence of eosinophils in abundant numbers
- Congestion.
- Accumulation of eosinophils around the parasites and/ or blood vessels.

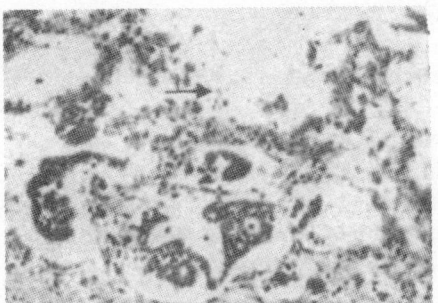

Fig. 9.41. Photomicrograph of lung showing
regenerative changes

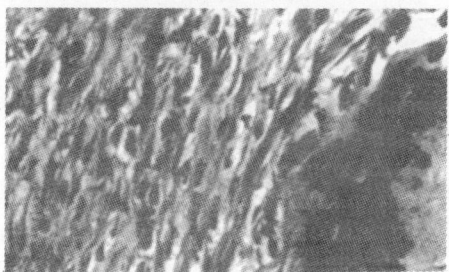

Fig. 9.42. Photomicrograph showing healing of
fracture

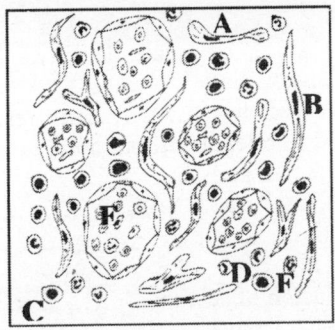

Fig. 9.43. Diagram showing granulation
tissue in repair

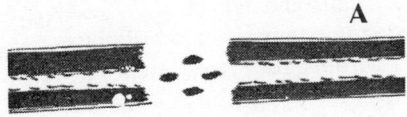

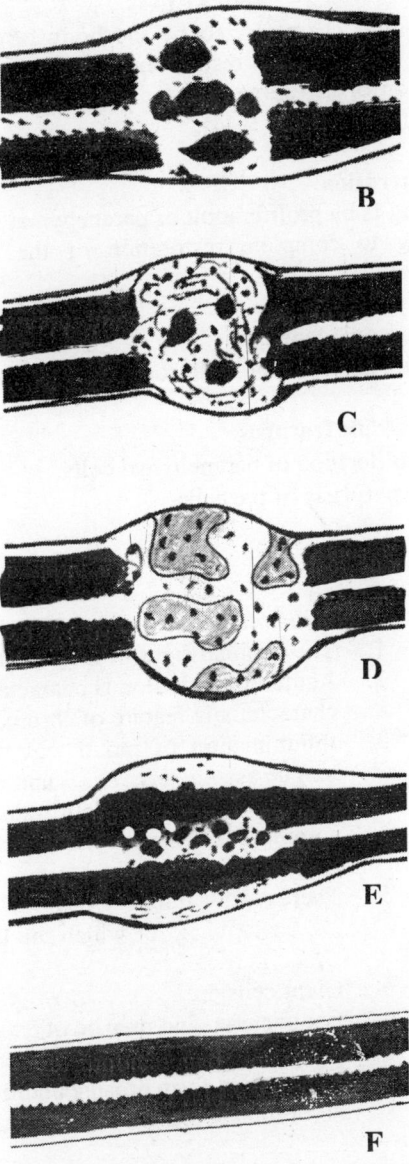

Fig. 9.44. Diagram showing fracture repair
A. Hematoma B. Inflammatory reaction C. Growth
of granulation tissue and formation of soft callus
D. Formation of procallus E. Formation of osseous
callus and F. Remodeled bone with complete
healing

HEALING

Healing is characterized by the body response to injury in order to restore normal structure and function of the damaged organ/tissue. It is of two types (Figs. 9.41 to 9.44).

Regeneration

Healing is by proliferation of parenchymatous cells leading to complete restoration of the original tissue.

Macroscopic features

• No significant gross lesion.

Microscopic features

• Proliferation of parenchymal cells.
• Hyperplasia of the cells.

Repair

Repair is the replacement of injured tissue by proliferation of fibrous tissue.

Macroscopic features

• Pink/red granules (granulation tissue) appear on healing part. These are the indication of formation of new blood vessels.
• It can be seen just beneath the scab.

Microscopic features

• Formation of granulation tissue *i.e.* fibroblasts, angioblasts, histiocytes, macrophages and parenchymal cells of organ.
• Fibroblasts are elongated fibrillar cells with ovoid hyperchromatic nuclei.
• Mitosis is frequently observed.

MODEL QUESTIONS

Q. 1. *Fill in the blanks with suitable word(s) to answer the followings.*

1. The cardinal signs of inflammation are ...., ..., ..., ... and ....
2. Acute inflammation is characterized by ...., while .... changes are the characteristic feature of chronic inflammation.
3. Inflammation of mouth cavity is known as ...., of palate as ...., tongue as .... and of salivary gland as ....
4. Inflammation starts with transient ...., followed by ...., resulting in coming out of leucocytes which reaches in tissues spaces to release antimicrobial factors such as ...., ..., ..., ..., ... and ....
5. There are three types of lymphocytes viz. ...., ..., and ...., of which the later is further classified as ....,.................. and ....
6. Giant cells are .... and formed with fusion of several .... to kill acid fast bacteria, and may be of ....and .... types.
7. Arachidonic acid is an acid formed in body by conversion of .... which is activated by .... to form prostaglandin through ....and............... pathway.
8. Serotonin is also known as .... and it is present in tissues of ...., ..., ... and .... cells and acts on .... to cause .... and .... but is mild in action in comparison to histamine.
9. Lysosomal granules of neutrophils and macrophages are rich in ...., ...,..................... and..................
10. Cytokines are .... like substances produced by .... and ....mostly and are of .... in nature.
11. Chemokines are .... proteins produced by ....,.................., ...,.................., ..., ... and....... and act as chemotactic factor for ...., ... and ....
12. Repair is the substitution of tissue by .... and is characterized by the presence of...........

Q. 2. *Write true or false against each statement and correct the false statement.*

1. ...... Keratitis is the inflammation of eyelid.
2. ...... Inflammation of gums is known as gingivitis.
3. ...... Salpingitis is the inflammation of salivary glands.
4. ...... Inflammation of pituitary gland is known as posthitis.
5. ...... Densinitis is the inflammation of lamina densa of glomerular basement membrane.
6. ...... Polymorphonuclear cells are first line of defence in body.
7. ...... Giant cells are multinucleated neutrophils formed to kill the bacteria.
8. ...... Mast cells have basophilic granules rich in histamine
9. ...... Arachidonic acid is activated by C_{5a} to form prostaglandin.
10. ...... Interleukins are those cytokines which are required for cell to cell interaction among the immunocytes.
11. ...... Bacteria are phagocytosed by macrophages and are destroyed by lysosomal enzymes.
12. ...... Nitric oxide produced in phagocytic cells is not toxic to phagocytosed material.
13. ...... Catarrhal inflammation is characterized by increased mucous as principal constituent of the exudate on the nucous surface.
14. ...... In colisepticemia, there is false membrane formation over liver and heart composed of fibrous cells.
15. ...... Suppurative inflammation is characterized by the presence of liquifaction and neutrophils.
16. ...... Granuloma consists of central caseative necrosis surrounded by lymphocytes, macrophages, epithelioid cells and giant cells.
17. ...... Eosinophilic inflammation is met with bacterial infections.
18. ...... Granulation tissue is composed of fibroblasts and small blood vessels.
19. ...... Fibrinous inflammation is seen in herpes virus infection.
20. ...... Perivascular cuffing is accumulation of neutrophils around the blood vessels.

Q. 3. *Define the followings.*

1. Lampas
2. Glossitis
3. Blepheritis
4. Rhinitis
5. Encephalomyelitis
6. Nephritis
7. Salpingitis
8. Proctitis
9. Typhlitis
10. Cheilitis
11. Abscess
12. Phlebitis
13. Cystitis
14. Carditis
15. Densinitis
16. Steatitis
17. Posthitis
18. Funiculitis
19. Orchitis
20. Leptomeningitis
21. Fascitis
22. Spondylitis
23. Balanitis
24. Neuritis
25. Pavementation
26. Diapedesis
27. Giant cells
28. Plasma cells
29. Monokines
30. Lymphokines
31. Chemokines
32. Chemotaxis
33. Phlegmon
34. Granuloma
35. Granulation tissue

Q. 4. *Write short notes on.*

1. Cells in inflammation
2. Chemical mediators of inflammation
3. Cytokines
4. Phagocytosis
5. Healing

Q. 5. *Select appropriate word(s) from four options given with each question.*

1. Inflammation is activation of ....
   (a) Cardinal signs   (b) Blood vascular changes (c) Immunity   (d) Fibroplasia

2. Which one of the following is not a cardinal sign of inflammation ....
   (a) Redness   (b) Pain   (c) Oedema   (d) Heat

3. Inflammation of gums in known as.........
   (a) Cheilitis   (b) Gingivitis   (c) Glossitis   (d) Orchitis

4. Inflammation of ovary is known as ....
   (a) Uveitis   (b) Urethritis   (c) Oopheritis   (d) Metritis

5. Primary granules of neutrophils contain.........
   (a) Lactoferin   (b) Lysozyme   (c) Myeloperoxidase   (d) Lipase

6. Lecucocytes marginate during vasodilation and come out from blood vessels through pseudopodia movement; the process is known as.........
   (a) Diapedesis   (b) Rhexis   (c) Pavementation   (d) Leucopenin

7. Macrophages become elongated with marginal nuclei to kill the acid fast bacteria and are known as ....
   (a) Giant cells   (b) Epithelial cells   (c) Epithelioid cells   (d) Plasma cells

8. Langhans type of giant cells are observed in lesions in.............
   (a) Tuberculosis   (b) Neoplasms   (c) Leukemia   (d) Rinderpest

9. Lymphocytes modified to produce antibodies are known as ....
   (a) T- helper cells   (b) T-cytotoxic cells   (c) Plasma cells   (d) Epithelioid cells

10. Fibroblasts proliferate in ....inflammation.
    (a) Acute   (b) Subacute   (c) Per acute   (d) Chronic

11. C_3a, C_5a and C_4a are the complement components which are also known as .....
    (a) Anaphylotoxin   (b) Prostaglandins   (c) Vasoactive amines   (d) None of the above

12. Cytokines are ....in action.
    (a) Autocrine   (b) Paracrine   (c) Endocrine   (d) All of the above

13. Tumor necrosis factor or cytotoxins are produced by macrophages and T-cells and are associated with ....in tumor.
    (a) Necrosis   (b) Necrobacillosis   (c) Degeneration   (d) Apoptosis

14. Coating of foreign particles / bacteria by immunoglobulins to make it more readily palatable by phagocytic cells is known as ....
    (a) Opsonization   (b) Adherence   (c) Chemotaxis   (d) Digestion

15. Catarrhal inflammation is characterized by increased number of.........
    (a) Goblet cells   (b) Neutrophils   (c) Giant cells   (d) Epithelial cells

16. Fibrinous inflammation is characterized by the presence of ....as principal constituent of exudates.
    (a) Serum   (b) Neutrophils   (c) Fibrin   (d) Fibroblasts

17. The principal constituent of purulent exudates is ....
    (a) Serum   (b) Plasma   (c) Neutrophils   (d) Eosinophils

18. Granulomatous inflammation is chronic in nature and is found in ....
    (a) Tuberculosis   (b) Rinderpest   (c) Canine distemper   (d) H.S.

19. In parasitic and allergic diseases, ...inflammation is mostly seen.
    (a) Fibrinous   (b) Haemorrhagic   (c) Eosinophilic   (d) Granulomatous

20. Granulation tissue is found in ....
    (a) Tuberculosis   (b) John's disease   (c) Repair   (d) Rinderpest

10
CONCRETIONS

- **Concretions**
  - **Calculi**
    - **Urinary Calculi**
    - **Biliary Calculi**
    - **Salivary Calculi**
    - **Pancreatic Calculi**
    - **Enteric Calculi**
  - **Piliconcretions**
  - **Phytoconcretions**
  - **Polyconcretions**
- **Model Questions**

CONCRETIONS

Concretions are solid, compact mass of material, endogenous or exogenous in origin, found in tissues, body cavities, ducts or in hollow organs. Concretions are stone-like bodies commonly occur in urinary system, gall bladder and gastrointestinal tract. Concretions of endogenous origin are known as *calculi* while those formed from exogenous material are known as *piliconcretion* (Hair), *phytoconcretion* (plant fibres) and *polyconcretion* (polythenes).

Calculi

Calculi are formed due to deposition of salts around the nucleus/nidus consisting of either fibrin, mucus, desquamated epithelial cells or clumps of bacteria. Due to the gradual and repeated precipitation of salts, calculi becomes laminated. In the process of calculi formation, the inner structural arrangement gets shrinked, producing a rough superficial surface. Calculi formation is more common in urinary system and in gall bladder of man and animals; however, they may also occur in salivary gland, pancreas and intestines.

URINARY CALCULI

Urinary calculi are formed in renal tubules, pelvis or in urinary bladder which may be carried away by urine and may cause obstruction in ureter or urethra. Urinary calculi is also known as urolith and the process of formation of calculi is termed as **urolithiasis** (Figs. 10.1 & 10.2).

Etiology
- Vit A deficiency.
- Bacterial infection *e.g. E. coli*, Micrococci, Streptococci.
- Sulfonamide therapy.
- Hormonal therapy.
- Hyperparathyroidism.

Macroscopic features
- May vary in size from 1 mm to several mm.
- Mostly rounded, pearl-like, laminated.
- Brown, grey and yellowish in colour.
- Enlargement and fibrosis of kidneys.

Microscopic features
- In kidney sections tiny, laminated bodies of concretion.
- Hydronephrosis.
- Chemical composition of urinary calculi may vary in various species of animals.
- *Horse:-* Calcium carbonate, calcium phosphate, magnesium carbonate.
- *Ruminants:-* Calcium phosphate, magnesium phosphate, aluminium phosphate, calcium oxalate.
- *Pigs:-* Ammonium phosphate, magnesium phosphate, calcium carbonate, magnesium carbonate, magnesium phosphate, magnesium oxalate.
- *Dogs:-* Calcium carbonate, calcium phosphate, sodium urate, ammonium urate.

BILIARY CALCULI

Biliary calculi are formed in gall bladder and bile ducts and are also known as cholelith. These are common in man; however, in cattle and pigs gall stones are also seen. They are semisolids but become hard and brittle on drying.

Etiology
- Bacteria.
- Sand particles.
- Particles of ingesta / intestinal contents.
- Desquamated epithelium.

Macroscopic features
- In gall bladder and bile duct.
- 1 mm to 3-4 cm in diameter.
- Numbers vary from 1 to many.
- Obstructive jaundice.
- Cholecystitis and cholangitis.

Microscopic features
- In sections, concentric layers of cholesterin, bilirubin, calcium carbonate and coagulated material.
- Cholecystitis, cholangitis.

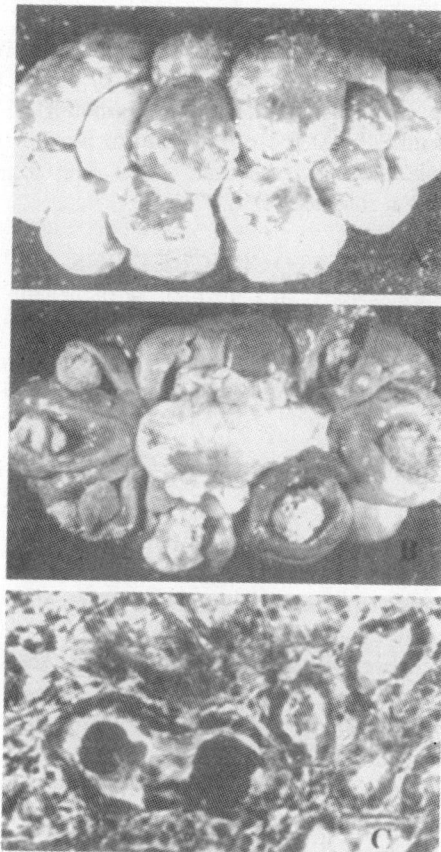

Fig. 10.1. Photograph of kidney of bullock showing presence of calculi A. Gross intact kidney B. Cross section of kidney and C. Microscopic structure of kidney having concretion.

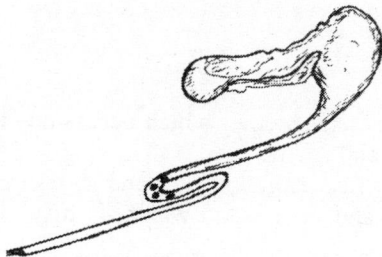

Fig. 10.2. Diagram showing predilection site of calculi in sigmoid flexure of urethra in bullocks

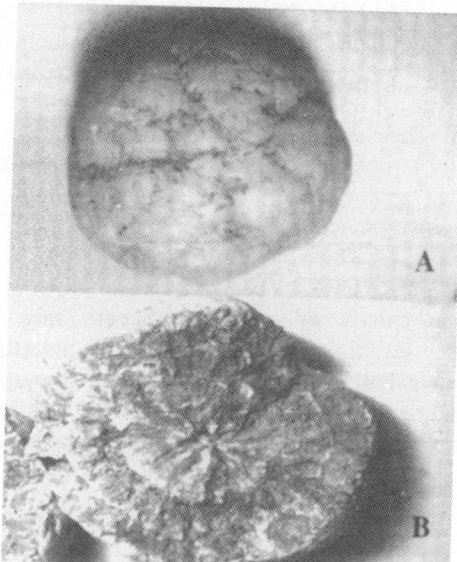

Fig. 10.3. Photograph of enterolith A. Intact B. Cross section of enterolith

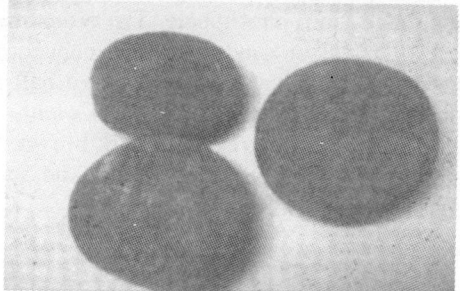

Fig. 10.4. Photograph of Piliconcretion

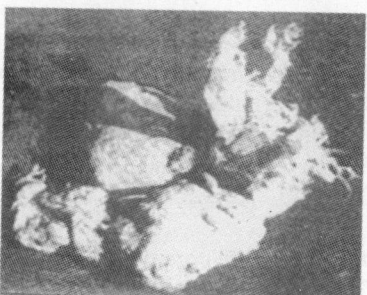

Fig. 10.5. Photograph of Polyconcretion

115

SALIVARY CALCULI

Salivary calculi are formed in excretory ducts of the parotid, sublingual and submaxillary salivary glands. Size of such calculi vary upto 25-30 mm diameter. They are made up of salts like calcium carbonate, calcium phosphate, magnesium carbonate, sodium carbonate, around the plant fibres. Salivary calculi also known as sialolith.

PANCREATIC CALCULI

Pancreatic calculi or pancrealolith are rare in occurrence in animals but may be found in cattle. Pancreatic calculi is grey in colour with size upto few centimeter. They are made up of calcium carbonate, calcium oxalate and calcium phosphate around a nidus of cholesterol or fatty acids.

ENTERIC CALCULI

Enteric calculi or enterolith are common in horses, and occur mostly in large intestine 'colon'. In horse, a nidus is surrounded by wheat and rye bran containing magnesium phoshphate. The nidus may be a piece of metal or sand on which concentric layers are deposited. They may look like a ball of round or oval in shape (Fig. 10.3). Colour of enterolith may vary from greyish to dark brown. In dogs, bone in diet may provide a nidus and such concretions are known as *coproliths*.

PILICONCRETIONS

Piliconcretions are hair balls, that occur in calves or in adults due to excessive licking of skin. Due to licking, animals swallow large amount of hairs which take the shape of ball due to movements of stomach. Mostly, the hair balls are found in stomach or in colon (Fig. 10.4).

PHYTOCONCRETIONS

Phytoconcretions are formed around the food materials and may occur in stomach and intestine of animals and in crop of poultry. They may cause obstruction of bowel. They are also known as *phytobezoars*.

POLYCONCRETIONS

They are made up of polythenes and excessive deposition of salts around them. They may vary in size from a few centimeters to several centimeters and weigh upto kilograms. They cause obstruction leading to death of animals (Fig. 10.5).

Such concretions are observed in cattle wandering on street in cities and in zoo animals. The polythene containing vegetable waste or green leaves and food materials are thrown away on roads, and are easily available to the animals. Polythene is not degraded in stomach and remains there to form a nidus, around which the salts are deposited and take the shape of calculi leading to obstruction of digestive tract passage.

MODEL QUESTIONS

Q. 1.   *Fill in the blanks with suitable word(s).*
1.   Concretions of endogenous origin are known as .... which occurs due to nidus provided by ...., ... ,.............. and ....
2.   In ruminants, the urinary calculi is made up of ...., ..., ... and ....
3.   Gall stones may cause.................,............... and .... which may lead to ....
4.   Enterolith commonly occurs in .... in horses.
5.   Coprolith occurs in .... due to eating of ....

Q. 2. *Write true or false against each statement and correct the false statement.*
1.   ....Vitamin B deficiency may lead to formation of urinary calculi.
2.   ....Polyconcretions are made up of polythenes.

3. .... Hair balls are also known as phytobezoars.
4. .... Choleliths may lead to toxic jaundice.
5. .... Uroliths may cause hydronephrosis.

Q. 3. **Write short notes on.**
1. Urolithiasis
2. Piliconcretions
3. Enteroliths
4. Polyconcretions

Q. 4. **Define the followings.**
1. Phytobezoars
2. Coproliths
3. Piliconcretions
4. Sialolith
5. Pancrealolith
6. Nidus
7. Cholecystitis
8. Cholangitis
9. Hydronephrosis
10. Obstructive jaundice

Q. 5. **Select appropriate word(s) from the four options given with each statement.**
1. Calculi are stone-like bodies which have ....origin.
   (a) Endogenous　　(b) Hematogenous　　(c) Exogenous　　(d)None of the above
2. Piliconcretions are made up of ....
   (a) Plant fibres　　(b) Polythenes　　(c) Hairs　　(d) Desquamated cells
3. Urinary calculi are formed in renal tubules and in horse they are made up of ....
   (a) Calcium carbonate　(b) Calcium phosphate　(c) Magnesium carbonate　(d)All of the above
4. Choleliths may cause ....
   (a) Toxic jaundice (b) Post-hepatic Jaundice　(c) Pre-hapatic jaundice (d)Hemolytic jaundice
5. Sialoliths occur in ....
   (a) Pancreas　　(b) Salivary gland　　(c) Sinus　　(d)Seminal vesicle
6. Coprolith may occur in dogs due to presence of ....in food.
   (a) Sand　　(b) Muscles　　(c) Plant fibers　　(d) Bones
7. Cholelithiasis may lead to inflammation of ....
   (a) Gall bladder　　(b) Intestine　　(c) Stomach　　(d) Pancreas
8. Enteric calculi are more common in horse due to feeding of ....
   (a) Grams　　(b) Wheat bran　　(c) Grass　　(d) Beans
9. Polyconcretions are formed due to accumulation of .... in G.I. Tract.
   (a) Hairs　　(b) Polysaccharides　　(c) Polyuria　　(d) Polythenes
10. Vitamin .... deficiency may lead to formation of urinary calculi.
    (a) A　　(b) B　　(c) D　　(d) K

11
IMMUNITY AND IMMUNOPATHOLOGY

- **Immunity**
- **Immunopathology**
  - **Hypersensitivity**
    - **Type I**
    - **Type II**
    - **Type III**
    - **Type IV**
  - **Autoimmunity**
  - **Immunodeficiency**
    - **Congenital**
    - **Acquired**
- **Model Questions**

IMMUNITY

Immunity is the resistance of body against extraneous etiological factors of disease, which is afforded by the interaction of chemical, humoral and cellular reactions in body. This is an integral part of the body without, which one cannot think of life. During the process of evolution, nature has provided this defence mechanism in the bodies of all living creatures particularly of higher animals and man, that protects them from physical, chemical and biological threats. It can be classified as natural or paraspecific and acquired or specific immunity.

Natural/paraspecific immunity

There are some species which are resistant to particular diseases due to presence of natural resistance against them *e.g.* horse, pig, cat are resistant to canine distemper virus; dogs are resistant to feline panleucopenia virus, chickens are resistant to anthrax. Even within species, there is natural resistance that protects some individuals while others are susceptible *e.g.* Indian deshi cattle Zebu (*Bos indicus*) is quite resistant to piroplasmosis in comparison to *Bos taurus*. Besides, there are the mechanisms or barriers in body provided by nature. These are:

- *Skin and mucous membrane* prevent organisms from gaining entrance in body.
- **Mucous** prevents from infections by trapping and keeping them away.
- *Saliva, gastric juice and intestinal enzymes* kill bacteria.
- *Tears, nasal and GI tract secretions* are bactericidal due to presence of lysozymes.
- *Phagocytic cells* such as neutrophils kill bacteria through phagocytosis.
- *Macrophages* kill organisms through phagocytosis.
- *Natural antibodies* act as opsonins and help in phagocytosis.
- *Interferons* have antimicrobial properties. They are host/species specific and arrest viral replication.

- *Interleukins, cytotoxins and growth factors* stimulate the immune reactions and inflammation.
- *Natural killer cells* kill targets coated with IgG.

Acquired/specific immunity

Acquired immunity develops in body as a result of prior stimulation through antigen. It is specific to a particular antigen against which it was developed. It can be restimulated on second or subsequent exposure with antigen and thus, it has memory for a particular antigen. It differs from natural immunity in respect of prior stimulation, specificity and memory. It can be classified as humoral and cell mediated immunity.

Humoral immunity

This is the immunity present in fluids of body mainly in blood. There are antibodies in serum of blood, which protect body from diseases. It is specific to particular antigen. Antibodies are formed in blood as a result of exposure of the foreign substances including bacteria, virus, parasite and other substances.

Antigen is foreign substance, which is able to stimulate the production of antibodies in body. They may be of high molecular weight protein, polysaccharides, and nucleic acids. Simple chemicals of low molecular weight are not able to induce immunity. However, they may be conjugated with large molecular weight molecules such as protein to become antigenic and induce antibody production, such substances are termed as *haptens.*

Antibodies are protein in nature present in serum and produced as a result of antigen. Antibodies are specific to antigen. Most of the microorganisms have several antigenic determinants and antibodies are produced against each antigenic determinant specifically. The antibody response to antigen can be enhanced if the antigen is released slowly in body. There are several substances like oils, waxes, alum, aluminium hydroxide, which may be added with antigen so that it is released slowly in body to

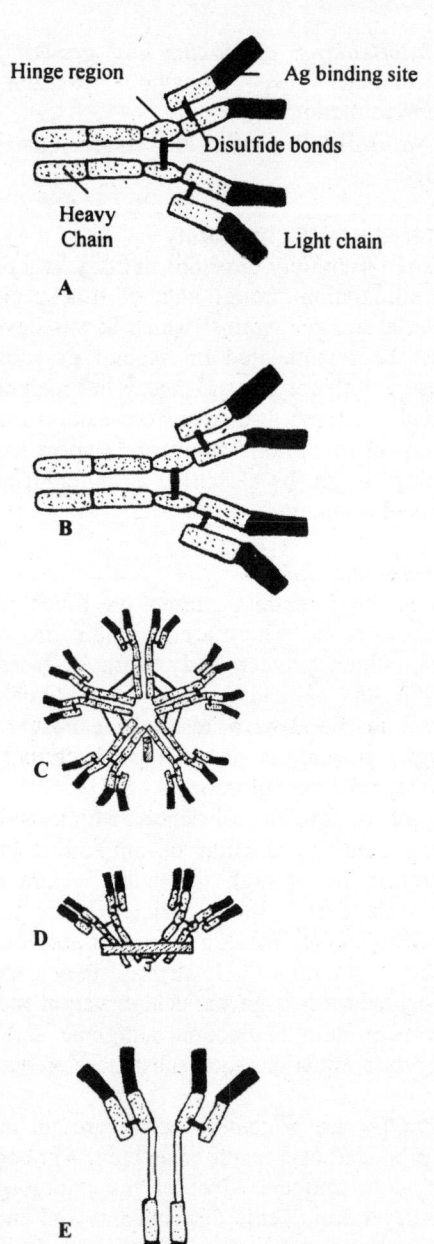

Fig.11.1. Diagram showing A, Structure of antibody with its different parts B. Immunoglublin–G (IgG), C. Immunoglobulin-M (IgM), D. Immunoglobulin-A (IgA) and E. Immunoglobulin-E (IgE).

increase the antibody production. Such substances are known as *adjuvants*. Antibodies are also known as *immunoglobulins* as they are the part of globulins. They are glycoprotein in nature and are of 5 types IgG, IgA, IgM, IgD and IgE.

Immunoglobulin G (IgG)

It is the main antibody found in high concentration (75%) in serum with a mw 150 KD. It is produced by plasma cells in spleen, lymphnodes and bone marrow. It has two identical light chains and two gamma heavy chains. The light chains may be of kappa or lamda type. IgG is the smallest immunoglobulin which may pass through blood vessels with increased permeability. It has the capacity to quickly bind with foreign substances leading to opsonization. Its binding with antigen may also activate the complement.

Immunoglobulin M (IgM)

This is about 7% of total serum immunoglobulins. It is also produced by plasma cells in spleen, lymphnodes and bone marrow. It is pentamer, five molecules of conventional immunoglobulin with mw 900 KD. These five molecules are linked through disulfide bonds in a circular form. A cysteine rich polypetide of 15KD mw binds two of the units to complete circle and is known as 'J' chain. It is produced in body during primary immune response. It is considered to be more active than IgG for complement activation, neutralization of antigen, opsonization and agglutination. IgM molecules are confined to the blood and have no or little effect in tissue fluids, body secretions and in acute inflammation.

Immunoglobulin A (IgA)

It is secreted as dimmer (mw 300 KD) by plasma cells present under body surfaces like intestinal, respiratory and urinary system, mammary gland and skin. Its concentration is very little in blood. IgA produced in body surfaces is either secreted on surface through epithelial cells or diffuse in blood stream. IgA is transported through intestinal epithelial cells having a receptor of 71 KD which binds with the secretory component covalently to form a secretory IgA. This secretory component protects IgA in the intestinal tract from digestion. It cannot activate the complement and cannot perform the opsonization. IgA can neutralize the antigen and agglutinate the particulate antigen. IgA prevents adherence of foreign particles/antigen on the body surfaces and it can also act inside the cells. It is about 16% of total immunoglobulins present in serum.

Immunoglobulin E (IgE)

It is also present on body surfaces and produced by plasma cells located beneath the body surfaces. It is in very low concentration in serum. It can bind on receptors of mast cells and basophils. When any antigen binds to these molecules, it causes degranulation from mast cells leading to release of chemical mediators to cause acute inflammation. It mediates hypersensitivity type I reaction and is responsible to provide resistance against invading parasitic worms. It is of shortest half life (2-3 days) and thus is unstable and can be readily destroyed by mild heat treatment. It is 0.01% of total immunoglobulin in serum with 190 KD molecular weight.

Immunoglobulin D (IgD)

IgD is absent in most domestic animals. However, it is present in very minute amount in plasma of dog, non-human primates and rats. IgD can be detected in plasma. However, it cannot be found in serum due to lysis by proteases during clotting. It is only 0.2 % of total immunoglobulin in serum with mw 160 KD.

On the basis of their function, antibodies are classified as:

Antitoxins have the property to bind with toxins and neutralise them.

Agglutinins are those antibodies, which can agglutinate the RBCs and/or particulate material such as bacterial cells.

Precipitins can precipitate the proteins by acting with antigen and inhibit their dissemination and chemical activity.

Lysins can lyse the cells or bacteria through complement.

Opsonins have the property to bind with foreign particles, non specifically leading to opsonization, making the foreign material palatable to phagocytic cells.

Complement fixing antibodies bind with antigen and fix the complement for its lysis.

Neutralizing antibodies are those, which specifically neutralize/destroy the target /antigen; merely binding with antigen cannot be considered as neutralizing antibodies.

Immune response

When the antigen enters thebody of an animal is trapped, processed and eliminated by several cells, including macrophages, dendritic cells and B-cells. There are two types of antigen in body i.e. exogenous and endogenous. The exogenous or extracellular antigens are present freely in circulation and are readily available for antigen processing cells.

The endogenous or intracellular antigens are not free and are always inside the cells such as viruses. But when these viruses synthesize new viral proteins using biosynthetic process of the host cells, these proteins also act as antigen and are termed as endogenous or intracellular antigens.

The processing of antigen by macrophages is comparatively less efficient as most of the antigen is destroyed by the lysosomal proteases. An alternate pathway of antigen processing involves antigen uptake by a specialized population of mononuclear cells known as *dendritic cells* located throughout the body specially in lymphoid organs. Such dendritic cells have many long filamentous cytoplasmic processes called dendrits and lobulated nuclei with clear cytoplasm containing characteristic granules (Fig. 11.2).

Antigen presenting cells process the exogenous antigen and convert into fragments to bind with MHC class II molecules. Such processed antigen along with MHC class II molecule and certain cytokines such as IL-1 is presented to antigen recognizing cells (T-helper cells). Macrophages also regulate the dose of antigen to prevent inappropriate development of tolerance and provide a small dose of antigen to T- helper cells. However,

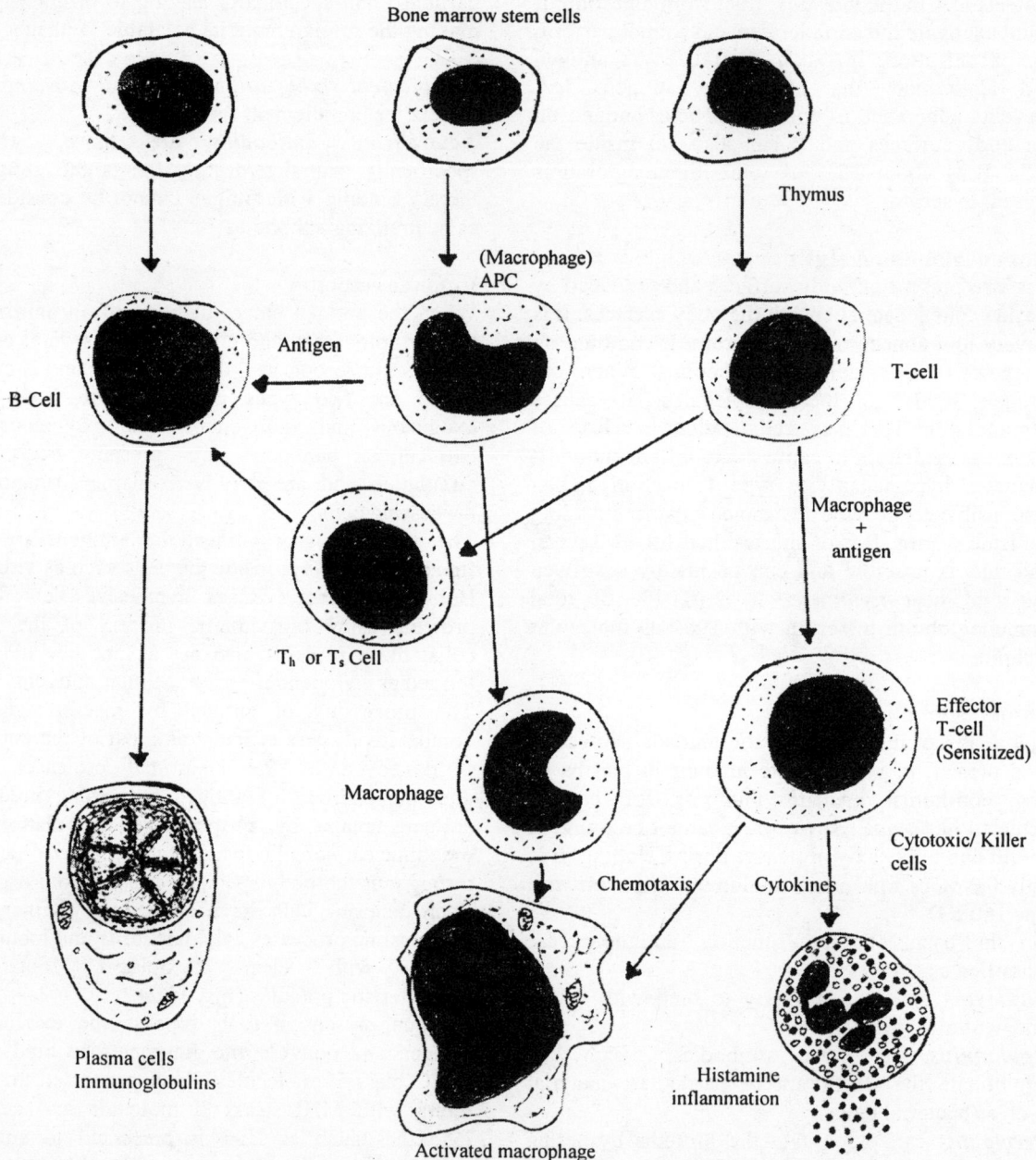

Bone marrow stem cells

(Macrophage)
APC

Antigen

B-Cell

Thymus

T-cell

T$_h$ or T$_s$ Cell

Macrophage
+
antigen

Macrophage

Effector
T-cell
(Sensitized)

Cytotoxic/ Killer
cells

Chemotaxis

Cytokines

Plasma cells
Immunoglobulins

Activated macrophage

Histamine
inflammation

Fig. 11.2. Diagram showing mechanism of induction of immunity in body

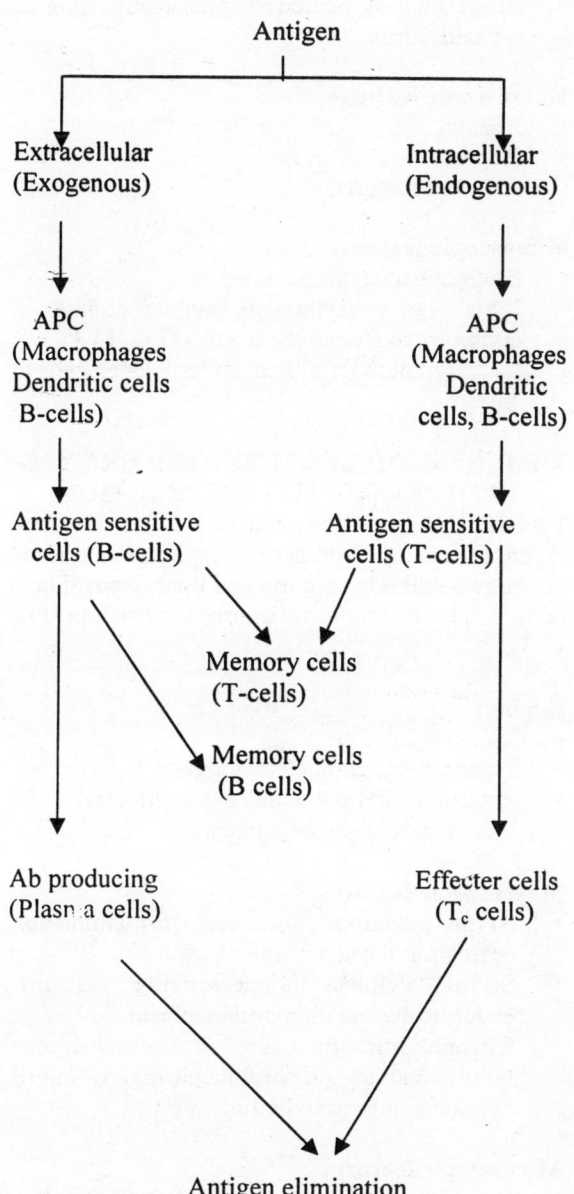

Antigen

Extracellular (Exogenous) — Intracellular (Endogenous)

APC (Macrophages Dendritic cells B-cells)

APC (Macrophages Dendritic cells, B-cells)

Antigen sensitive cells (B-cells)

Antigen sensitive cells (T-cells)

Memory cells (T-cells)

Memory cells (B cells)

Ab producing (Plasma cells)

Effecter cells (T_c cells)

Antigen elimination

if the antigen is presented to T-cells without MHC class II molecule, the T-cells are turned off resulting into tolerance. On an average, an antigen presenting cell possesses about 2×10^5 MHC class II molecules. A T-cell requires activation by 200-300 peptide-MHC class II molecules to trigger an immune response. Thus, it is estimated that an antigen-presenting cell may present several epitopes simultaneously to T-helper cells. A counterpart of T-helper cell also exists and is known as suppressor T-cell (T_s cell) which suppresses the immune response. The viral encoded proteins, endogenous antigens are handled in a different manner from exogenous antigens. Such antigens are bound to MHC class Ia molecules and transported to the cell surface. Such antigen and MHC class Ia molecule complex triggers a lymphocytic response *i.e.* T-cytotoxic cells (Tc-cells). These cytotoxic T-cells recognize and destroy virus infected cells. However, there is some cross priming leading to cell mediated immune response by exogenous antigens and humoral immune response by endogenous antigens. Some lymphocytes also function as memory cells to initiate secondary immune response.

On antigen exposure, there is a latent period of about four to six days and only after that serum antibodies are detectable. The peak of antibody titre is estimated around 2 weeks after exposure to antigen and then declines after about 3 weeks. During this primary immune response, majority antibodies are of IgM type whereas in secondary immune response, it is always predominated by IgG.

IMMUNOPATHOLOGY

Immunopathology includes the disorders of immune system characterized by increased response or hypersensitivity, response to self antigens (autoimmunity) and decreased responses (immunodeficiencies).

HYPERSENSITIVITY

It represents an accelerated immune response to an antigen (allergen), which is harmful to body rather than to provide protection or benefit to the body. Such violent reactions may lead to death. This condition is also known as *allergy* or *atopy*. The hypersensitive reactions can be classified into four classical forms including anaphylaxis (Type I), cytotoxic hypersensitivity (Type-II), Immune complex mediated hypersensitivity (Type III) and delayed type hypersensitivity (Type-IV) reaction.

ANAPHYLAXIS OR TYPE-I HYPERSENSITIVITY

Anaphylaxis or type I hypersensitivity reaction is rapidly developing immune response to an antigen characterized by humoral antibodies of IgE type (*reagin*). These reagins sensitize basophils/mast cells to release chemical mediators (Histamine, Serotonin, Prostaglandins, CFA for neutrophils and eosinophils) of inflammation leading to acute inflammatory reaction (Fig. 11.3).

Etiology
- Administration of drugs.
- Administration of serum.
- Bite of insects, bee etc.
- Dust, pollens etc.

Macroscopic features
- Bronchial asthma.
- Wheel and flare reaction on skin.
- Oedema, congestion, erythema, itching on skin.
- Rhinitis.

Microscopic features
- Congestion, pulmonary oedema, emphysema, constriction of bronchioles.
- Oedema, congestion, haemorrhage on skin.

CYTOTOXIC OR TYPE II HYPERSENSITIVITY REACTION

Cytotoxic reactions are characterized by lysis of cells due to antigen-antibody reaction on the surface of cells in the presence of complement.

Etiology/Occurrence
- Blood transfusion.
- Hemolytic anemia.
- Infections such as Equine infectious anemia, rickettsia, parasites (trypanosomiosis, babesiosis).
- Thrombocytopenia.

- Drugs such as penicillin, phenacetin, quinine cephalosporins.

Macroscopic features
- Anemia.
- Jaundice.
- Haemoglobinuria.

Microscopic features
- Erythrophagocytosis.
- Lysis of erythrocytes/agglutination of erythrocytes Hemolytic anemia (Fig. 11.4).
- Increased number of hemosiderin laden cells in spleen.

IMMUNE COMPLEX MEDIATED OR TYPE-III HYPERSENSITIVITY REACTION

Type-III hypersensitivity reaction is characterized by the formation of immune complexes as a result of antigen-antibody reaction and their deposition in body tissues leading to inflammatory reaction (Fig. 11.5).

Etiology
- Immunoglobulins.
- Tumor antigens, nuclear antigens.
- Environmental pollutants *e.g.* pesticides.
- Infections such as Leishmaniasis.

Macroscopic features
- **Arthus reaction** is focal area of inflammation, necrosis at the site of infection.
- **Serum sickness** is necrotizing vasculitis, endocarditis and glomerulonephritis.
- **Chronic immune complex disease** is renal failure due to glomerulonephritis, vasculitis, chroiomeningitis and arthritis.

Microscopic features
- Deposition of immune complexes in wall of blood vessels.
- Deposition of immune complexes in glomeruli (Fig. 11.6).

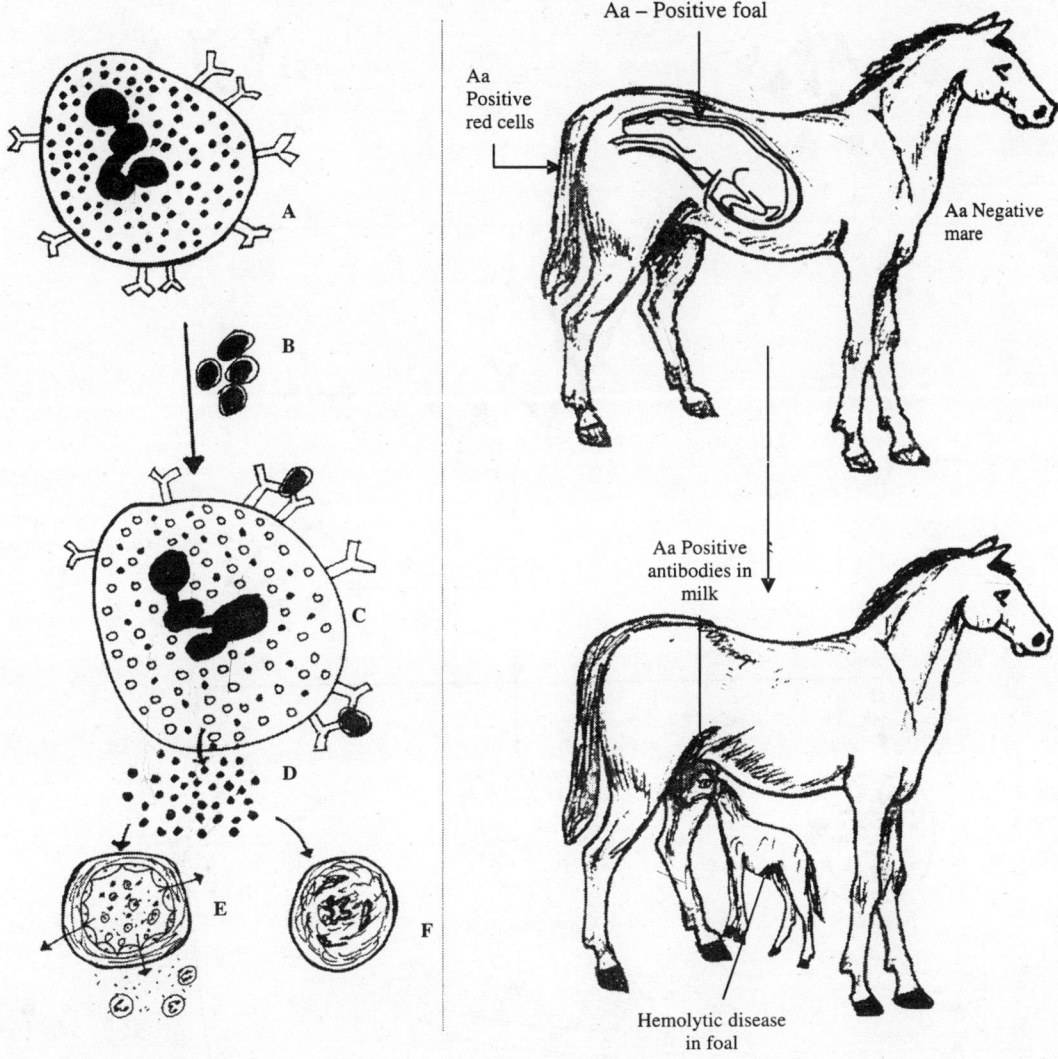

Fig.11.3. Diagram showing IgE mediated Type-I hypersensitivity reaction A. Mast cell B. Allergen, C. Allergen binds with two IgE molecules D. Degranulation and release of histamine, serotonin, mediators of inflammation IL-2,3,4,5,6,7,13.,TN-α, LTB4, LTC4, PAF and PGD₂, E. Increased vascular permeability and F. Bronchoconstriction.

Fig.11.4. Diagram showing type II hypersensitivity (hemolytic disease in foal)

125

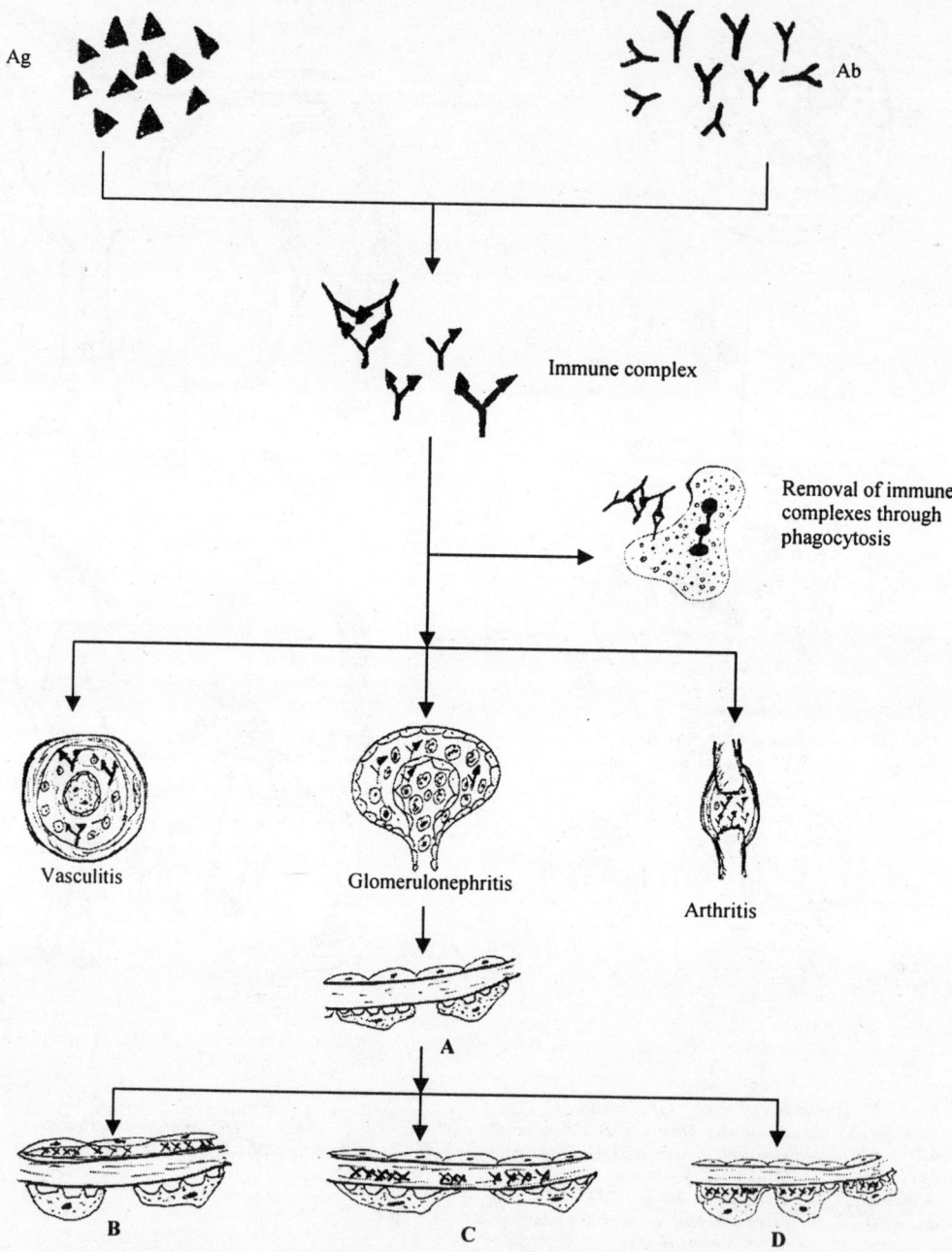

Ag

Ab

Immune complex

Removal of immune
complexes through
phagocytosis

Vasculitis

Glomerulonephritis

Arthritis

A

B

C

D

*Fig. 11.5. Diagram showing Type-III hypersensitivity reaction. A. Normal architecture of glomeruli B. Type I,
C. Type II and D. Type III Membrano proliferative glomerulonephritis (MPGN).*

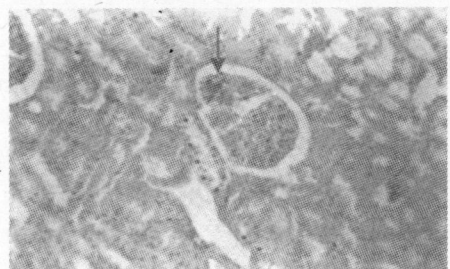

Fig. 11.6. Photomicrograph of immune complex mediated glomerulonephirtis

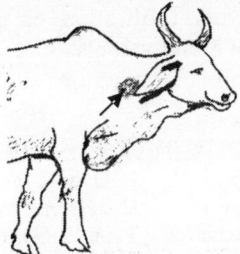

Fig. 11.7. Diagram showing of tuberculin reaction

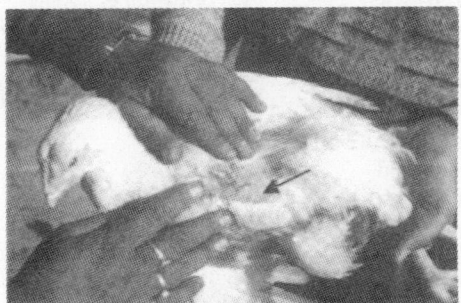

Fig. 11.8. Diagram showing DTH reaction of DNCB

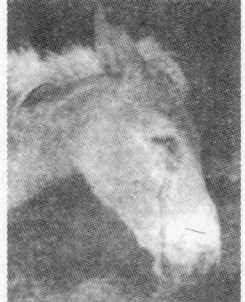

Fig. 11.9. Photograph showing mallein reaction

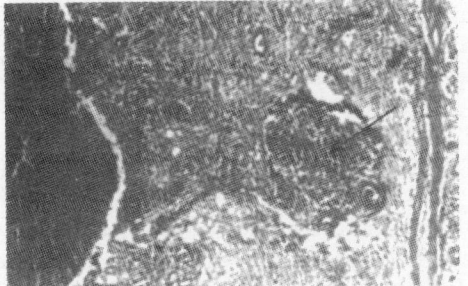

Fig. 11.10. Photomicrograph showing DTH reaction-lymphofollicular lesions

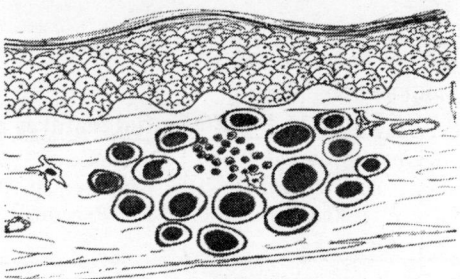

Fig. 11.11. Diagram showing microscopic picture of DTH reaction

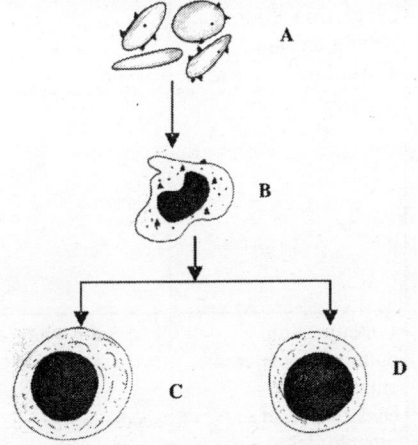

Fig. 11.12. Diagram Showing autoimmunity A. RBC showing presence of auto antigens B. Recognition of auto antigen by APC and their processing C. B-cells for antibody production and D. T-cells for cytotoxicity

- Infiltration of inflammatory cells such as neutrophils, macrophages and lymphocytes.
- Lesions of glomerulonephritis, polyarthritis.

DELAYED TYPE HYPERSENSITIVITY (DTH) OR TYPE IV HYPERSENSITIVITY REACTION

DTH reaction is mediated by sensitized T-lymphocytes and is the manifestation of cell-mediated immune response (Figs. 11.7 to 11.11).

Etiology
- Tuberculin reaction.
- Graft versus host reactions.
- Granulomatous reaction.

Macroscopic features
- Formation of nodules, which are hard, painful to touch.
- Rejection of transplants/grafts.

Microscopic features
- Heavy infiltrations of mononuclear cells particularly of T-lymphocytes and macrophages.
- Congestion and oedema.
- Lymphocytic infiltration is more common around the blood vessels.
- Lymphofollicular reaction.

Table 11.1 Differential features of various types of Hypersensitivity Reaction

	Anaphylaxis or Type-I Hypersensitivity Reaction	Cytotoxic or Type II Hypersensitivity Reaction	Immune Complex Mediated or Type-III Hypersensitivity Reaction	Delayed Type Hypersensitivity (DTH) or Type IV Hypersensitivity Reaction
Macroscopic features	1. Bronchial asthma. 2. Wheel and flare reaction on skin. 3. Oedema, congestion, erythema, itching on skin. 4. Rhinitis	1. Anemia 2. Jaundice 3. Haemoglobinuria	1. Arthus reaction is focal area of inflammation, necrosis at the site of infection. 2. Serum sickness is necrotizing vasculitis, endocarditis and glomerulonephritis. 3. Chronic Immune complex disease is renal failure due to glomerulonephritis, vasculitis, chroiomeningitis and arthritis.	1. Formation of nodules, which are hard, painful to touch. 2. Rejection of transplants/ grafts.
Microscopic features	1. Congestion, pulmonary oedema, emphysema, constriction of bronchioles. 2. Oedema, congestion, haemorrhage on skin	1. Erythrophago-cytosis 2. Lysis of erythrocytes/ agglutination of erythrocytes. 3. Increased number of hemosiderin laden cells in spleen.	1. Deposition of immune complexes in wall of blood vessels. 2. Deposition of immune complexes in glomeruli 3. Infiltration of inflammatory cells such as neutrophils, macrophages and lymphocytes. 4. Lesions of glomerulonephritis, polyarthritis.	1. Heavy infiltrations of mononuclear cells particularly of T-lymphocytes and macrophages. 2. Congestion and oedema 3. Lymphocytic infiltration is more common around the blood vessels 4. Lymphofollicular reaction.

AUTOIMMUNITY

In autoimmunity (auto=self) the immune response is generated against self antigens. It is an aberrant reaction that serves no useful purpose in body. Rather, the immunity developed against self antigens destroys the tissues of body and causes inflammation leading to death.

Etiology/Occurrence
*   Hidden antigens *e.g.* spermatozoa.
*   Alteration of antigens *e.g.* infections, mutations, chemicals bind with normal body proteins recognized as foreign (FIg. 11.12).
*   Cross reaction between antigens of self and foreign nature.
*   Forbidden clones of immunocytes.

Macroscopic features
*   Autoimmune hemolytic anemia (Fig. 11.4).
*   Anti-glomerular basement membrane (GBM) nephritis.
*   Lymphocytic thyroditis.
*   Lupus erythematosus- antinuclear antibodies.

Microscopic features
*   Hemolytic anemia.
*   Leukopenia.
*   Presence of antinuclear antibodies.
*   Infiltration of lymphocytes/ macrophages (Lymphocytic thryroditis).
*   In anti-GBM nephritis, there is immune complex mediated glomerulonephritis.

IMMUNODEFICIENCY

The alterations in immune system, which decrease the effectiveness or destroy the capabilities of the system to respond to various antigens are designated as immunodeficiency. This precarious situation may be attributed to poorly developed immunocompetence or depressed immunity as a result of genetic and environmental factors.

Immunodeficiences are thus classified as congenital or primary and acquired or secondary.

Congenital immunodeficiency
In this type of immunodeficiency, the defect in immunity is genetically determined and is present in animals since their birth.

Etiology/Occurrence
*   Defect in basic cellular components *e.g.* stem cells.
*   Defective genes.
*   Defect in enzymes.
*   Defective expression of cell components.

Types
Combined immunodeficiency syndrome (CIS)
*   Absence of stem cells of immunocytes.
*   Agammaglobulinemia.
*   Absence of T and B cells in blood, leucopenia.
*   Occurs due to autosomal recessive gene.
*   Aplasia or hypoplasia of thymus, lymphnodes, spleen.

Defects in T-lymphocytes
*   Thymic hypoplasia.
*   B-cells are normal and adequate amount of immunoglobulins present in blood.
*   Absence of T-dependent regions in lymphnodes.
*   In Danish cattle, exanthema, alopecia, parakeratosis occurs due to T-cell defect with A- 46 lethal trait gene.

Defects in B-lymphocytes
*   In equines – equine agammaglobulinemia
*   Normal T-cell count, absence of B-cells, absence of all classes of immunoglobulins.
*   'X' linked defects in gene occurs in males.
*   Absence of primary lymphoid follicles in germinal centres in spleen and lymphnodes.
*   Selective IgA, IgM and IgG deficiency may also occur.
*   Transient hypogammaglobulinemia in new born calves.

Partial T and B cell defects
*   Partial presence of T and B lymphocytes.
*   Recurrent infections, eczema, purpura.

- Due to 'X' chromosome-linked genetic defect.
- Poor platelet aggregation.

Deficiency of complement
- Rare, associated with abnormal regulation of immune responses leading to autoimmunity.
- Complement component C_1 C_2 and C_3 are deficient and deficiency is associated with systemic lupus erythematosus, polyarteritis nodosa, glomerulonephritis, rheumatoid arthritis.
- C_5, C_6, C_7 and C_8 deficiency leads to recurrent infections.
- Absence or deficiency of C_3 makes animal susceptible to bacterial infections due to lack of opsonization, chemotaxis and phagocytosis.

Defects in phagocytosis
- Neutropenia, leucopenia.
- Defects in neutrophils, macrophages, platelets, melanocytes and eosinophils.
- Defective chemotaxis, phagocytosis and bactericidal activity.
- Persistent bacterial infections, pyogenic infections.
- Associated with autosomal recessive gene defect and is also known as "Chediak Higashi syndrome".

ACQUIRED OR SECONDARY IMMUNODEFICIENCY

An animal can acquire the suppression of immune system due to drugs, diseases, deficiency of nutrition, neoplasm or environmental pollution. This is clinically manifested by increased susceptibility to infections, vaccination failures, recurrent infections and occurrence of new diseases and neoplasms.

Etiology/ Occurrence
Drugs
- Corticosteroids, azathioprines, alkalating agents, cyclophosphamide, cyclosporin A, antibiotics.
- Azathioprines used to suppress graft rejection
- Cyclophosphamides and chlorambucil affect the DNA reduplication of T- and B-lymphocytes leading to immunosuppression with no affect on macrophages.
- Cyclosporin A depresses CMI responses.
- Aspirin decreases phagocytosis and lymphocyte functions.
- Antibiotics like gentamicin, chloramphenicol, cephalosporin etc. cause decrease in immunity.

Infections
- Bovine herpes virus-1 (BHV-1) decreases CD_4^+ and CD_8^+ cells in blood.
- Equine herpes virus (EHV-1) causes reduction in T-cell functions.
- Marek's disease virus acts as lymphocytolytic agent in lymphoid follicles of spleen, bursa and thymus.
- Bovine viral diarrhoea virus reduces CD_4^+ and CD_8^+ T-lymphocytes, B-lymphocytes, neutrophils and IL- 2 in cattle.
- Respiratory syncytial virus inhibits lymphoproliferative responses in sheep and cattle leading to increased susceptibility to *Pasteurella multocida* infection.
- Blue tongue virus infects CD_4^+ and CD_8^+ lymphocytes and causes their destruction.
- Canine parvovirus causes depletion of lymphoid cells. Canine distemper virus activates the T-suppresser cells (T_s cells) leading to suppression of immunity.
- Infectious bursal disease virus selectively affects B- lymphocytes leading to increased susceptibility of birds.
- Infectious laryngotracheitis virus infects macrophages and causes their destruction.

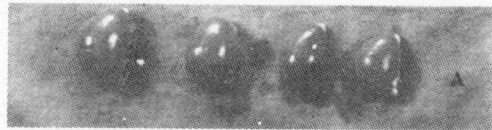

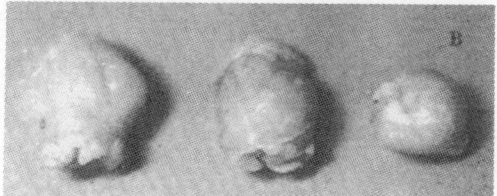

Fig. 11.13. Photograph showing atrophy of lymphoid organs due to A. Pesticide and B. heavy metals in birds

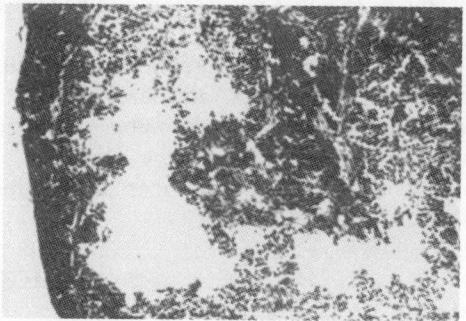

Fig. 11.15. Photomicrograph of thymus showing depletion of lymphoid tissue

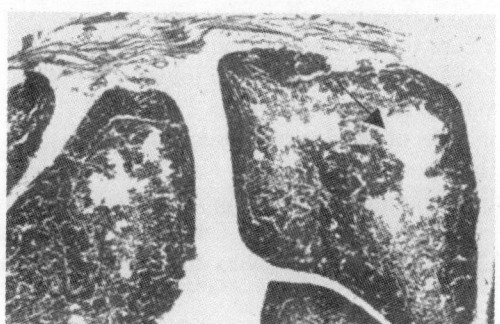

Fig. 11.14. Photomicrograph of bursa showing depletion of lymphoid tissue

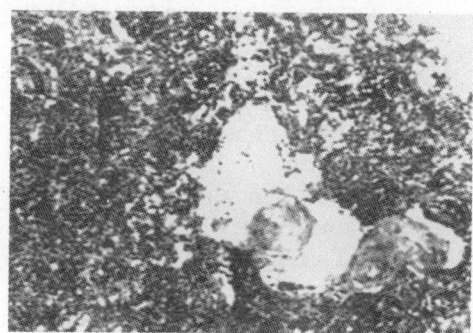

Fig. 11.16. Photomicrograph of spleen showing depletion of lymphoid tissue

- Feline leukemia virus causes lymphoid depletion, glomerulonephritis, defects in macrophages and complement.
- Feline immunodeficiency virus causes neutropenia, lymphopenia and inhibits the T- and B- cells' co-operation.
- Bovine immunodeficiency virus replicates in macrophages and CD_4^+ lymphocytes leading to their destruction and immunosuppression. It also causes lymphadenopathy, lymphocytolysis, reduction in lymphokine production.

Trauma/surgery
- Trauma or surgical interventions reduce specific immune responses and functional capacity of phagocytic cells.
- Such defects are transient and may reverse after healing of trauma/ surgery.
- Surgical operation/trauma increases the number of T- suppressor cells (T_s cells), which in turn depresses the immunity.

Environmental pollution (Fig. 11.13 to 11.16)
- Pesticides used in agriculture, animal husbandry and public health operations remain in ecosystem and food items for longer period and enter in body of animals and man through food, air, water and affect the immune system

leading to its depression and increased susceptibility to infections.

• Heavy metals are common contaminants of pesticides, fertilizers and are inadvertently accumulated in soil, plant, water, which enters directly or indirectly in the animal's body. These heavy metals (lead, mercury, cadmium) may exert their immunotoxic effects leading to immunosuppression.

• Mycotoxins such as aflatoxin, ochratoxin, zearalenone etc. also affect the immune system of animals leading to its suppression resulting increased susceptibility to infectious diseases.

MODEL QUESTIONS

Q. 1. *Fill in the blanks with suitable word(s).*

1. Due to presence of natural resistance in body ...., ... and .... are resistant to canine distemper virus infection.

2. Adjuvants such as ....,........................, ..., and .... are absorbed slowly in body and thereby .... the production of antibodies.

3. IgM antibodies constitute.................... per cent of total serum immunoglobulins with mw of about .... KD and are made up of .... molecules joined with ....; this antibody is produced during .... immune response of body.

4. Immunoglobulin D (IgD) is .... in most of the domestic animals.

5. Dendritic cells have .... filamentous cytoplasmic processes known as .... and ....nuclei with clear cytoplasm containing....................

6. A counterpart of T-helper cells is .... cells, which .... the immune response.

7. A T-cells require .... peptide- MHC class II molecules to trigger an immune response.

8. In secondary immune response, the main immunoglobulin is .... while in primary response it is ....

9. Immunopathology is defined as .... in immunity and characterized by ......, ...or ....

10. Acquired immunodeficiency is characterized by............. of immune system due to ...., ..., ..., ... and/or .... which is clinically manifested by ...., ..., ..., ... and ....

11. Deficiency of complement component C_1, C_2 and C_3 may lead to........, ..., ... and .... while absence of C_3 results in lack of ...., ..., and ....

12. Bovine immunodeficiency virus replicates in .... and ...., cells leading to their .... and .... which also causes ...., ... and ....

13. Surgical operation may increase the number of .... cells.

14. Infectious laryngotracheitis virus causes destruction of ....

15. Pesticides include ...., ..., ... and ....; residues of which cause .... in animals leading to ...., ... and ....

Q. 2. *Write true or false against each statement and correct the false statement.*

1. ......Chickens are resistant to anthrax.

2. ......Feline panleucopenia virus causes decrease in all cell types of leucocytes in dogs.

3. ......Indian cow (*Bos indicus*) is quite susceptible to piroplasmosis.

4. ......Haptens are low molecular weight substances, which are not able to induce immune response.
5. ......IgM is the main antibody found in serum.
6. ......IgA antibodies are mostly present on mucosal surfaces secreted in the form of dimmer.
7. ......IgE is also known as reagin.
8. ......Precipitins are those antibodies which precipitate the antigen and thereby enhances the activity of antigen.
9. ......Dendritic cells are more efficient in antigen processing in comparison to macrophages.
10. ......The latent period in antibody production on antigen exposure is 8 days.
11. ......Cyclosporin - A depresses humoral immunity.
12. ......Cyclophosphamide has no effect on phagocytosis by macrophages.
13. ......RSV infection makes animals more resistant to pasteurellosis.
14. ......Acquired immunodeficiency occurs in animals due to pesticides.
15. ......Feline immunodeficiency virus selectively affects only T-cells.
16. ......Trauma reduces activity of T-suppressor cells.
17. ......Blue tongue virus causes destruction of CD_4^+ and CD_8^+ cells.
18. ......Infectious bursal disease virus activates T-suppressor cells to cause immunosuppression.
19. ......Pesticides are also responsible to cause immune complex mediated glomerulonephritis.
20. ......Cadmium is immunotoxic and nephrotoxic.

Q. 3. *Define the following*

1. Natural killer cells
2. Antibodies
3. Antigen
4. Adjuvant
5. Haptens
6. Secretory antibody
7. J-chain
8. Agglutinin
9. Precipitin
10. Opsonins
11. Antigen presenting cells
12. Dendritic cells
13. T-helper cells
14. T-suppressor cells
15. T-cytotoxic cells
16. Hypersensitivity
17. Autoimmunity
18. Immunosuppression
19. Chediak Higashi syndrome
20. Immunotoxicity

Q. 4. *Write short notes on the followings.*

1. Paraspecific immunity.
2. Immune complex mediated glomerulonephritis.
3. Infections causing immunodeficiency in animals.
4. Immunoglobulins.
5. Immune response.
6. Autoimmunity.
7. Anaphylaxis.
8. Humoral immunity.
9. Cell mediated immunity.
10. Drugs induced immunosuppression.

Q. 5. *Select appropriate word(s) from the four options given with each statement to answer.*

1. This animal is not resistant to feline panleucopoenia virus infections.
   (a) Dog   (b) Cattle   (c) Cat   (d) Pig
2. Natural or paraspecific immunity does not include ....
   (a) Tears   (b) NK cells   (c) Cytokines   (d) Sensitized Tc cells
3. A foreign material capable of inducing the production of antibodies in animal is known as ......
   (a) Agglutinin   (b) Antigen   (c) Antipyretic   (d) Antidote

4. Antibodies are chemically .... in nature.
    (a) Lipopolysaccharide (b) Lipid   (c) Glycoprotein   (d) Protein
5. Which of the following is not an adjuvant.
    (a) Oil   (b) Wax   (c) Alum   (d) Glucose
6. Serum contains mainly this antibody..............
    (a) IgG   (b) IgM   (c) IgA   (d) IgD
7. IgD is found abundantly in ....
    (a) Cow   (b) Rat   (c) Sheep   (d) Horse
8. IgE is found in very low concentration in serum which has the property to bind with receptors present on ....cells.
    (a) Neutrophils   (b) Eosinophils   (c) T- lymphocytes   (d) Mast cells
9. IgD in not found in serum due to lysis by ....during clotting
    (a) Bacteria   (b) Proteaes   (c) Endonucleases   (d) Peroxidases
10. Processing of antigen by macrophages is comparatively less efficient due to lysis of antigen by ....
    (a) Proteases   (b) Peroxidases   (c) Endonucleases   (d) Lipases
11. There is a latent period in antibody production on exposure to any antigen which is ....
    (a) 6 days   (b) 20 days   (c) 25 days   (d) 4 weeks
12. The peak antibody titres are found at ....
    (a) 2 days   (b) 20 days   (c) 2 weeks   (d) 4 weeks
13. The exogenous antigen is processed in dendritic cells/macrophages and along with ....molecule it is presented to Th cells.
    (a) MHC class Ia   (b) MHC class II   (c) MHC class III   (d) MHC class Ib
14. T-cytotoxic cells recognize ....specifically to destroys them.
    (a) Bacteria   (b) Virus   (c) Antigen containing cells (d) Fungi
15. Anaphylaxis is also known as ....hypersensitivity
    (a) Type I   (b) Type II   (c) Type III   (d) Type IV
16. Equine infectious anemia virus may cause ....hypersensitivity
    (a) Type I   (b) Type II   (c) Type III   (d) Type IV
17. Reagin type of antibody is ......
    (a) IgA   (b) IgD   (c) IgM   (d) IgE
18. DTH reaction is mediated by ....
    (a) IgA   (b) IgG   (c) IgM   (d) Sensitised T–cells
19. Combined immunodeficiency syndrome occurs as a result of absence of ....
    (a) Stem cells   (b) B-cells   (c) T-cells   (d) Macrophages
20. Autoimmunity developes in body when immune mechanisms are directed towards .... antigens.
    (a) Self   (b) Foreign   (c) Protein   (d) Bacterial
21. In respiratory mucosa secretions, this antibody is mainly found................
    (a) IgG   (b) IgM   (c) IgA   (d) IgE
22. Corticosteroids bind with receptors present on ....cells leading to decrease in antibody production.
    (a) T- helper   (b) Macrophages   (c) B-cells   (d) T-suppressor
23. Canine distemper virus activates the ....cells.
    (a) T-helper cells   (b) T-suppressor cells   (c) B-cells   (d) Macrophages

24. Surgery may enhance the activity of ....cells and therefore modulate the immune response.
    (a) T- helper cells   (b) T-suppressor cells   (c) T- cytotoxic cells   (d) Macrophages

25. Pesticides are common contaminants of environment and may induce .... in animals.
    (a) Immunosuppression (b) Autoimmunity   (c) Hypersensitivity   (d)All of the above

26. Lead, mercury and cadmium are .... leading to immunosuppression.
    (a) Immunotoxic   (b) Nephrotoxic   (c) Hepatotoxic   (d) Neurotoxic

27. Aflatoxin may cause ....in animals.
    (a) Immunopotentiation   (b) Immunosuppression
    (c) Activation of macrophages   (d) Reduction of complement

28. Aspirin decreases ....
    (a) Antibody production (b) Phagocytosis   (c) All of the above   (d) None of the above

29. Bovine viral diarrhoea virus reduces..........................
    (a) T-suppressor cells (b) IL-1   (c) IL-2   (d) Interferon

30. Equine herpes virus (EHV-1) causes reduction in ......
    (a) B-cell   (b) T-cells   (c) Macrophages   (d) NK cells

Part B
Systemic Pathology

12
PATHOLOGY OF CUTANEOUS SYSTEM

- **Developmental anomalies**
- **Acanthosis nigricans**
- **Dermatitis**
  - **Vesicular dermatitis**
  - **Parasitic dermatitis**
  - **Allergic dermatitis**
  - **Gangrenous dermatitis**
- **Equine cutaneous granuloma**
- **Miscellaneous lesions of skin**
- **Model Questions**

DEVELOPMENTAL ANOMALIES

Congenital icthyosis

Congenital icthyosis is scaly epidermis which resembles the skin of fish and occurs due to a simple autosomal recessive homozygous gene in calves. This condition is characterized by scaly, horny, thick epidermis divided into plates by deep fissures. Microscopically, there is thick keratin layer over the epidermis.

Epitheliogenesis imperfecta

Epitheliogenesis imperfecta is a congenital defect characterized by discontinuity of epithelium on skin leaving patches without squamous epithelium mostly at feet, claws and oral mucosa. Such defect may occur in calves which succumb to infection after birth or such foetus may abort. This disease condition is inherited as an autosomal recessive trait.

Congenital alopecia

Alopecia or hairlessness on the skin with complete lack of hair follicles has been observed in dog and other animals. Such hairless sites may follow a regular pattern or occurs in patches. This is a hereditary defect recognized in certain breeds.

Congenital albinism

Albinism is absence of melanin pigmentation due to deficiency of tyrosinase. This congenital abnormality is encountered sporadically due to a recessive trait in most species. The melanocytes are present but there is lack of melanin synthesis due to tyrosinase deficiency.

Congenital cutaneous asthenia

The collagen fibres are irregular in size and orientation and become fragmented due to disorganization of fibrils within the fibres. This condition occurs due to a deficiency in procollagen peptidase responsible for formation of collagen. This condition leads to hyperelasticity and fragility of skin and hypermotility of joints in cattle, sheep and dogs.

ACANTHOSIS NIGRICANS

This is increased amount of melanin in skin along with hyperkeratosis. This condition commonly occurs in dogs, at ventral abdomen and medial surface of legs.

Etiology

• Hormonal imbalance.
• Tumors of testicles and pituitary gland.

Macroscopic features

• Colour of skin becomes black.
• Dry and scaly skin due to hyperkeratosis.

Microscopic features

• Proliferation of melanocytes and melanoblasts.
• Black/brown colour pigment intracellular/ extracellular.
• Cells appear as black or brown globular mass.
• Melanin granules are minute, dirty brown in colour and spherical in shape.
• Hyperkeratinization.

DERMATITIS

Dermatitis is the inflammation of skin characterized by hyperemia, erythema, serus exudation and infiltration of neutrophils and mononuclear cells (Figs. 12.1 to 12.4).

Etiology

• Bacteria, viruses, chemicals, allergy, trauma, fungi and their toxins.

Macroscopic features

• Erythematous patches on skin.
• Swelling of skin, itching sensation leads to damage/scratch due to rubbing.
• Loss of hairs, patches on skin, alopecia.

Microscopic features

• Hyperemia.
• Serus exudate.
• Infilteration of neutrophils and mononuclear cells.
• Presence of fungus in skin scrapings.

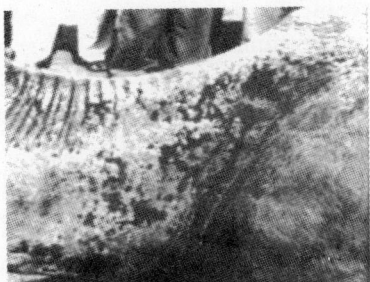

Fig 12.1. Photograph of a camel showing skin patches of fungal dermatitis

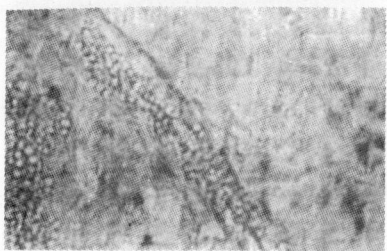

Fig 12.2.Photomicrograph of skin scraping showing presence of fungus (Ttrichophyton metagraphite)

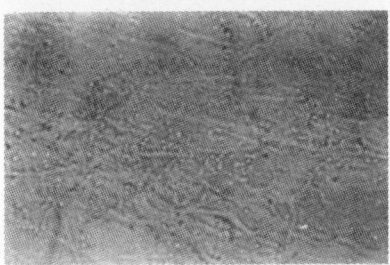

Fig 12.3. Photomicrograph of skin scraping showing presence of fungus (Trichophyton vericosum)

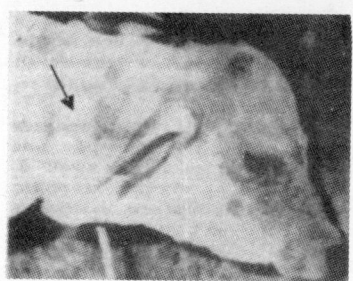

Fig 12.4. Photograph of a calf showing ringworm on face

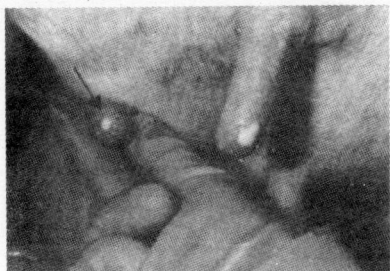

Fig 12.5. Photograph showing vesicle on teat.

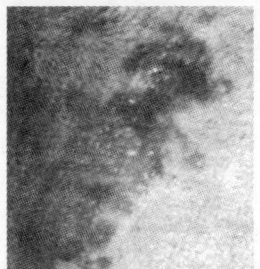

Fig 12.6. Photograph showing vesicles on skin (ARS/USDA)

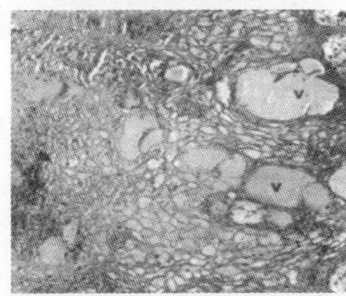

Fig 12.7. Photomicrograph showing hydropic degeneration and vesicle formation (v) (ARS/USDA)

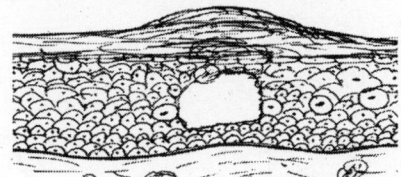

Fig 12.8. Diagram of vesicle in skin

VESICULAR DERMATITIS

Vesicular dermatitis is excessive accumulation of clear fluid in dermis and epidermis leading to vesicle/blister formation. It is also known as hydropic dermatitis (Figs. 12.5 to 12.8).

Etiology

- Sunburn.
- Heat.
- Foot and Mouth Disease virus.
- Pox virus.

Macroscopic features

- Oedematous fluid in dermis and epidermis resulting in thickening of skin.
- Hyperemia, vesicles.
- Break of vesicles leads to clear fluid discharge.

Microscopic features

- Hyperemia.
- Accumulation of clear fluid in epidermis and dermis, which is characterized by clear spaces or takes light pink stain of eosin.
- Some cells show hydropic degeneration.
- Infiltration of leucocytes.

PARASITIC DERMATITIS (ACARIASIS)

Acariasis or mange is caused by mites and is characterized by hyperkeratosis and inflammation of skin leading to itching, rubbing and scratching (Figs. 12.9 to 12.18).

Etiology

- Mites
  - *Sarcoptes scabei*
  - *Psoroptic* sp.
  - *Demodectic* sp.
  - *Chorioptic* sp.

Macroscopic features

- Hyperkeratosis of skin, dry and scaly appearance of skin.
- Haemorrhage/trauma due to rubbing/scratching as a result of intense itching.
- Absence of hairs on lesions.

Microscopic features

- Hyperkeratinization of skin.
- Hyperemia
- Infilteration of neutrophils, lymphocytes, macrophages, eosionophils
- Presence of mites at the site of lesions

ALLERGIC DERMATITIS

This is the inflammation of skin sensitized to certain substances, known as allergens. Such inflammation can be seen as a result of delayed type hypersensitivity (DTH) reaction.

Etiology

- Chemicals (DNCB/DNFB) (Figs. 12.19 & 12.20).
- Tuberculin reaction (Figs. 12.21 & 12.22).
- Allergic reaction.
- Soaps, detergents, organic chemicals.
- Parasites- fleas.

Macroscopic features

- Hyperemia, erythema
- Oedematous/nodular swelling, hard to touch.
- Hot, painful.
- Atopy with vesicular rash, pruritus, serus exudate.

Microscopic features

- Infilteration of eosinophils and mononuclear cells, macrophages, lymphocytes.
- Hyperemia, oedema, necrosis.

GANGRENOUS DERMATITIS

Gangrenous dermatitis is the inflammation of skin along with formation of gangrene caused by fungal toxins and characterized by sloughing of skin, dry gangrene with break in epidermis.

Etiology

- *Fusarium* sp. toxins
- Rice straw feeding – Degnala disease.

Macroscopic features

- Presence of gangrenous inflammation on extremities such as legs, udder, ears, tail, scrotum (Figs. 12.23 to 12.25).

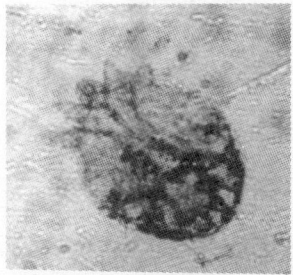

Fig 12.9. Photomicrograph of Sarcoptes scabei

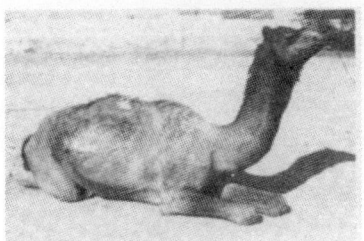

Fig 12.10. Photograph showing mange due to
S. scabei in a camel

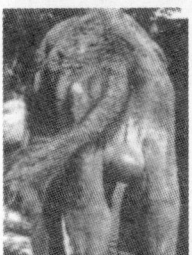

Fig 12.11. Photograph of camel showing
orchitis due to mange

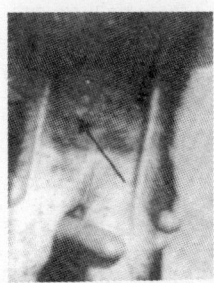

Fig 12.12. Photograph of a dog showing
pustular dermatitis due to demodectic mange

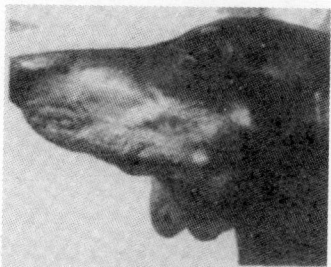

Fig 12.13. Photograph of dog showing
demodectic mange

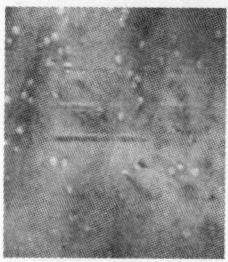

Fig 12.14. Photograph showing pustular dermatitis
due to demodectic mange (ARS/USDA).

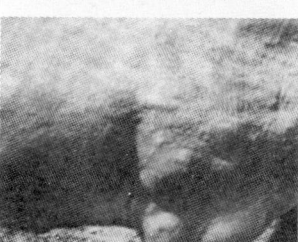

Fig 12.15. Photograph of cow showing
demodectic mange (ARS/USDA).

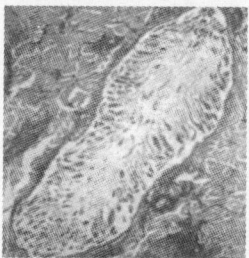

Fig 12.16. Photomicrograph showing
demodectic mites in cyst (ARS/USDA).

141

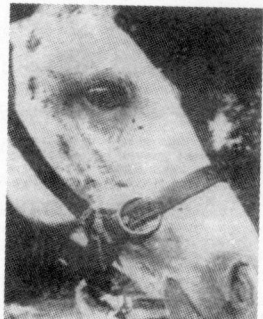

Fig 12.17. Photograph of horse showing chorioptic mange

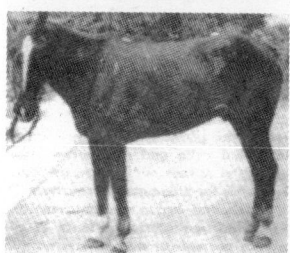

Fig 12.18. Photograph of horse showing chorioptic mange

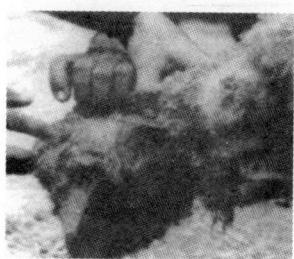

Fig 12.19. Photograph of sheep showing DTH reaction

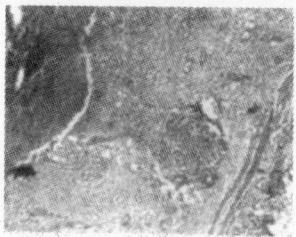

Fig 12.20. Photomicrograph showing DTH reaction in skin

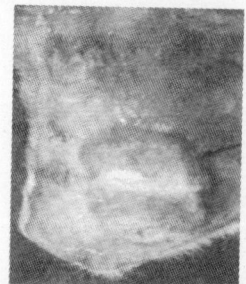

Fig.12.21. Photograph of tuberculoid dermatitis (ARS/USDA)

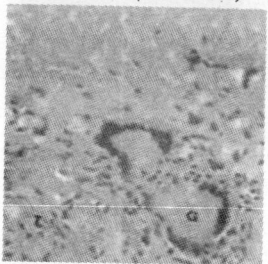

Fig.12.22. Photomicrograph of tuberculoid dermatitis (ARS/USDA)

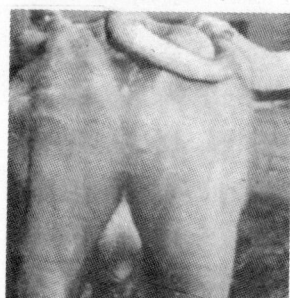

Fig.12.23. Photograph showing dry gangrene on scrotum of a buffalo bull due to fusariotoxicosis

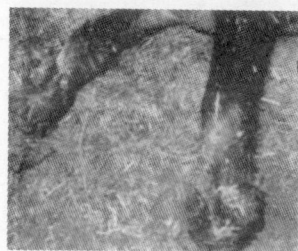

Fig.12.24. Photograph showing sloughing of hoofs in buffalo due to fusariotoxicosis

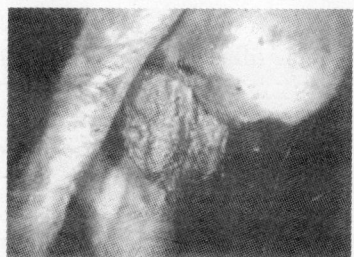

Fig.12.25. Photograph showing sloughing of skin from udder due to fusariotoxicosis

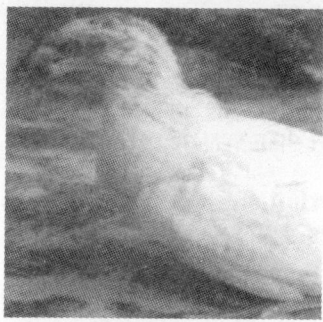

Fig.12.26. Photograph showing papule on beak and around eyes

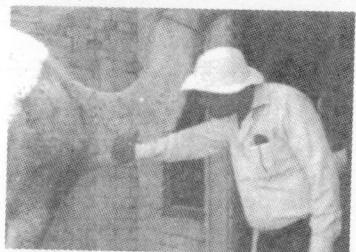

Fig.12.27. Photograph showing presence of scab and scar on skin of camel.

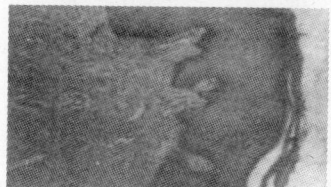

Fig.12.28. Photomicrograph of skin showing Acanthosis

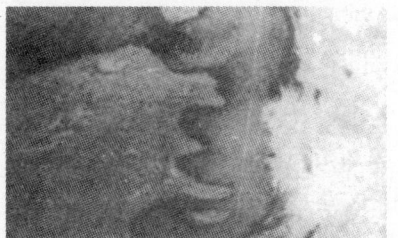

Fig.12.29 Photomicrograph of skin showing erosion

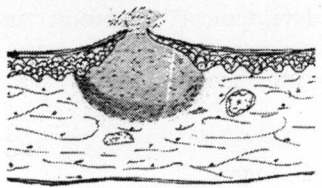

Fig.12.30. Diagram of abscess

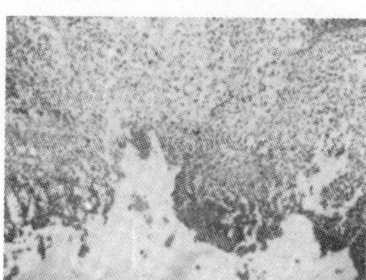

Fig.12.31. Photomicrograph of ulcer

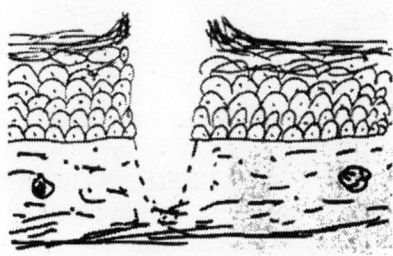

Fig.12.32. Diagram of ulcer

- Sloughing of skin leaving raw surface.
- Sloughing of hoofs with haemorrhage.

Microscopic features
- Inflammation of skin and invasion by saprophytes causing dissolution of cells/tissue.
- Infiltration of mononuclear cells at the periphery of the lesion.

EQUINE CUTANEOUS GRANULOMA
There is development of chronic, ulcerated and bloody granuloma on limb of horses due to wire cuts or other cutaneous injury.

Etiology
- Skin cuts/injury.
- Habronemiasis.
- Phycomycosis.
  o *Hyphomyces destruens*
  o *Entomorphthora coronata*

Macroscopic features
- Granulation of tissue in wound.
- Presence of yellowish/white specks.
- Summer sores/Bursatti.

Microscopic features
- Tissue composed of newly formed fibrous tissue, with large number of capillaries, infiltration of eosinophils.
- Presence of necrotic masses, stains deep red with H&E.
- Presence of helminths in section – cutaneous habronemiasis.
- Presence of septate hyphae of fungus.

MISCELLANEOUS LESIONS OF SKIN
Papule: Focal hyperplasia of stratum spinosum epithelium leading to hard nodular eruption on skin (Fig. 12.26).

Vesicle: A cavity in epidermis containing fluid and covered by a thin layer of epidermis elevated from the surface (Figs. 12.6 & 12.7).

Pustule: A vesicle filled with pus (Fig. 12.14).

Acanthosis: Thickening of epidermis due to hyperplasia of stratum spinosum/prickle cell layer (Fig. 12.28).

Hyperkeratosis: Thickening of keratin layer stratum corneum.

Parakeratosis: The retention of nucleus in keratin layer.

Bulla/bleb: Cavitations in epidermis filled with fluid and larger than vesicle.

Erosion/Excoriation: Superficial loss of epithelium (Fig. 12.29).

Fissure: Linear defect in epidermis, which may be crusted at mucocutaneous junctions.

Abscess: A circumscribed cavity filled with pus (Fig. 12.30).

Ulcer: A break in the continuity of the epidermis exposing dermis (Fig. 12.31 & 12.32).

Urticaria: A circumscribed area of swelling/oedema involving dermis.

Folliculitis: Inflammation of hair follicles.

Acne: Enlargement of sealed off hair follicles or sebaceous glands and rupture through the epidermis. It leaves a rounded hole in the epidermis and a canal down to the dermis.

Eczema: Eczema is a form of allergic dermatitis of obscure etiology and characterized by erythema, vesicular rash, serus exudate and pruritus.

MODEL QUESTIONS

Q. 1. **Fill in the blanks with appropriate word(s).**
1. .... is a cavity in epidermis containing fluid and covered by a thin layer of ...... elevated from the surface. If it is filled with pus, then it is known as...............
2. Superficial loss of epithelium in skin is known as .... or .... while the discontinuity of epidermis is termed as ....
3. In congenital icthyosis, the skin looks like .... as of fish.
4. Congenital discontinuity of epithelium of skin leaving patches without squamous epithelium is known as ....
5. Acanthosis nigricans is increased amount of...........caused by...........or tumors of ....and.............

Q. 2. **Write true or false against each statement and correct the false statement.**
1. ......Urticaria is a circumscribed area of swelling in dermis.
2. ......Ulcer is filled with fluid in epidermis.
3. ......Parakeratosis is thickening of keratin layer.
4. ......Bulla is a large cavity in epidermis filled with fluid.
5. ......Albinism is absence of melanin in skin.
6. ......Cutaneous asthenia occurs due to deficiency of procollagen peptidase.
7. ......Proliferation of melanocytes occurs in Acanthosis nigricans.
8. ......Sunlight may cause dermatitis.
9. ......Mange is caused by mites in animals.
10. ......Phycomycosis may lead to cutaneous granuloma in horses.

Q. 3. **Define the following.**
1. Scaly skin
2. Alopecia
3. Dermatitis
4. Papule
5. Pustule
6. Bleb
7. Parakeratosis
8. Erosion
9. Abscess
10. Urticaria

Q. 4. **Write short notes on.**
1. Epitheliogenesis imperfecta.
2. Acanthosis nigricans.
3. Allergic dermatitis.
4. Equine cutaneous granuloma.
5. Eczema.

Q. 5. **Select an appropriate word(s) from the four options given with each question.**
1. In congenital icthyosis, the skin of calves resembles the skin of ....
   (a) Toad   (b) Fish   (c)Tortoise   (d) Zebra
2. Acanthosis is .... of skin epithelium.
   (a) Hypoplasia   (b) Aplasia   (c) Hyperplasia   (d) Anaplasia
3. Vesicle formation occurs in skin as a result of ....
   (a) Cloudy swelling (b) Hydropic degeneration (c) Glycogen storage (d) Fatty change

4.   Acariasis is caused by ……..
     (a) Bacteria   (b) Virus   (c) Chlamydia   (d) Mite
5.   Enlargement of sealed off hair follicle or sebaceous gland is known as …….
     (a) Acne   (b) Folliculitis   (c) Fissure   (d) Bleb
6.   A break in the continuity of the epidermis exposing dermis is known as …….
     (a) Erosion   (b) Ulcer   (c) Fissure   (d) Vesicle
7.   Hyperkeratosis is the thickening of ………………..
     (a) Prickle cell layer   (b) Stratum lucidum   (c) Stratum corneum   (d) Dermis
8.   Superficial loss of epithelium on skin or mucous membrane is known as ………
     (a) Erosion   (b) Abrasion   (c) Ulcer   (d) Fissure
9.   Papule is hyperplasia of ………. Epithelium.
     (a) Stratum corneum   (b) Stratum lucidum   (c) Stratum spinosum   (d) Dermis
10. Retention of nucleus in keratin layer of skin is known as ………
     (a) Hyperkeratosis   (b) Parakeratosis   (c) Urticaria   (d) Acanthosis

13
PATHOLOGY OF MUSCULOSKELETAL SYSTEM

- **Pathology of muscles**
    - **Equine rhabdomyolysis**
    - **White muscle disease**
    - **Acute myositis**
    - **Haemorrhagic myositis**
    - **Chronic myositis**
- **Pathology of Bones**
    - **Fibrous osteodystrophy**
    - **Rickets**
    - **Osteomalacia**
    - **Osteoporosis**
    - **Osteopetrosis**
    - **Osteomyelitis**
    - **Bone fracture and repair**
    - **Pulmonary osteoarthropathy**
    - **Spondylitis**
- **Pathology of joints**
    - **Arthritis**
- **Model Questions**

PATHOLOGY OF MUSCLES
EQUINE RHABDOMYOLYSIS

It is also known as *Azoturia* or *Monday Morning Disease*. The disease occurs in well fed horse after a spell of inactivity. Suddenly after walking a few steps, the horse is unable to move further and feels pain with intense sweating and hardening of muscles.

Etiology

- Accumulation of lactic acid in muscles.
- High glycogen storage.
- Lack of oxygen supply.

Macroscopic features

- Hardening of muscle just like wood.
- Urine is dark brown with myoglobin – *myoglobinuria.*
- Tonic spasms in muscles.
- Atrophy of affected muscles in chronic cases.

Microscopic features

- Necrosis of muscle fibres
- Oedema.
- Hyaline degeneration (Fig. 13.1).
- Invasion of sarcolemma by macrophages and lymphocytes.
- Degeneration and necrosis of tubular epithelium in kidneys.

WHITE MUSCLE DISEASE

Extensive coagulative necrosis of muscles is observed in calves possibly due to deficiency of vitamin E during 6 months of age (Fig. 13.2).

Etiology

- Vitamin E deficiency.
- Selenium deficiency.
- Stress.

Macroscopic features

- Colour of muscle becomes pale pink, yellowish red, grey or white (Fig. 13.3).
- Muscle becomes dry, inelastic and firm.
- Urine is brown/red or chocolate brown in colour because of myoglobin.

Microscopic features

- Coagulative necrosis of muscles.
- In some muscle cells, cloudy swelling can be observed.
- Neutrophils, macrophages, lymphocytes and eosinophils may be present.
- Calcium may be deposited in necrosed areas.

ACUTE MYOSITIS

Acute myositis is the acute inflammation of skeletal muscles characterized by the presence of serous, fibrinous or haemorrhagic exudate (Figs. 13.4 & 13.5).

Etiology

- Trauma.
- Vitamin E/Selenium deficiency.
- *Clostridium chauvei,* the cause of black leg in cattle.

Macroscopic features

- Muscles become extremely moist.
- Colour becomes red, consistency is firm and tense.
- Swelling and accumulation of gas in muscles, crepitating sound on palpation.
- Muscle dark red/ black with gas mixed exudate (Figs. 13.6 & 13.7) (gangrenous myositis).

Microscopic features

- Presence of serous, fibrinous and/or haemorrhagic exudate.
- Infiltration of neutrophils, macrophages, lymphocytes, etc.
- Degenerative and necrotic changes in muscles.
- Presence of Gram positive rods in exudate.

HAEMORRHAGIC MYOSITIS

Haemorrhagic myositis is characterized by the presence of large amount of blood and inflammation in muscles. It may occur due to trauma and muscle rupture (Fig. 13.8).

Etiology

- Trauma.
- Clostridial infections.

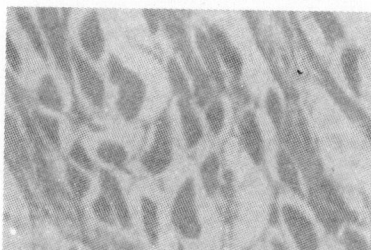

Fig.13.1. Photomicrograph showing hyaline
degeneration in muscle

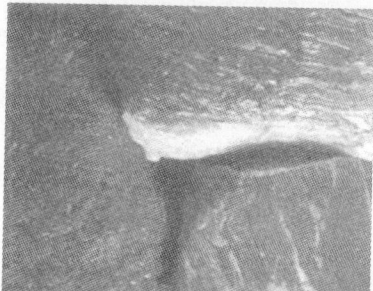

Fig.13.2. Photograph of white muscle
disease (ARS/USDA)

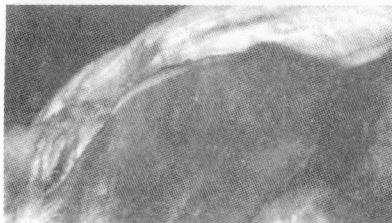

Fig.13.3. Photograph showing muscular
distrophy

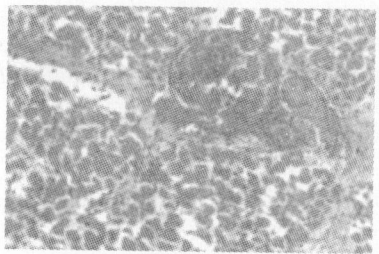

Fig.13.4. Photomicrograph *showing acute
myositis*

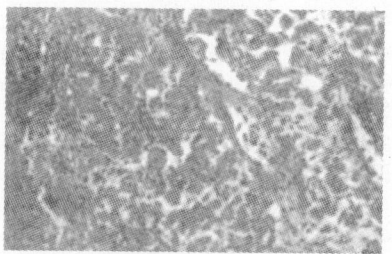

Fig.13.5. Photomicrograph showing acute
myositis due to clostridia

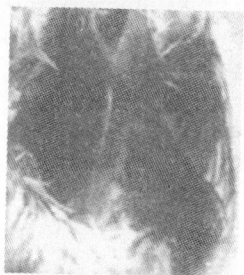

Fig.13.6. Photograph showing
gangrenous myositis in poultry

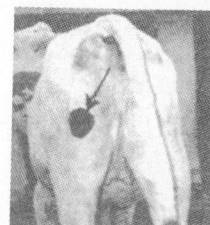

Fig.13.7. Photograph showing
gangrenous myositis in heifer

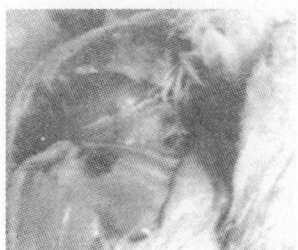

Fig.13.8. Photograph showing
haemorrhagic myositis

Macroscopic features
- Area becomes red/cyanotic.
- On cut, large amount of blood comes out from muscles.
- The affected area is hard and painful to touch.
- Regional lymphnodes may become enlarged and swollen.

Microscopic features
- Extravasation of blood in between the myofibrils.
- Infiltration of neutrophils, macrophages and lymphocytes in connective tissue between the muscle cells.

CHRONIC MYOSITIS

Chronic inflammation of muscle is characterized by necrosis, calcification and proliferation of fibrous connective tissue. In case of tuberculosis and pseudotuberculosis, there are multiple focal nodules containing caseation and fibrous capsule.

Etiology
- *Mycobacterium tuberculosis.*
- *Corynebacterium pseudotuberculosis.*
- *Trichinella* spp. infection.
- *Sarcosporidia* spp. infection.

Macroscopic features
- Muscles become hard to touch.
- Nodules can be seen (Fig. 13.9).
- On cut the lesions of caseation and calcification observed.

Microscopic features
- Caseative necrosis, infiltration of macrophages, lymphocytes and proliferation of fibrous tissue.
- Calcification can also be observed.
- In cases of pseudotuberculosis infiltration of neutrophils is seen.
- Extensive infiltration of eosinophils in sarcoporidia infection.

PATHOLOGY OF BONES
FIBROUS OSTEODYSTROPHY

Fibrous osteodystrophy occurs as excessive action of parathyroid hormone on bones and characterized by bone resorption with replacement by fibrous tissue, increased osteoid formation which does not get sufficient minerals for deposition and formation of cysts.

Etiology
- Hyperparathyroidism
- Dietary deficiency of calcium or excess of phosphorus
- Vitamin-D deficiency
- Excessive bran feeding (Disease in horses of flour millers).

Macroscopic features
- Lack of calcification in bone
- Resorption of calcium from bone, fibrosis
- Bone becomes shoft, flexible and deformed
- Rubbery jaw due to involvement of facial bones

Microscopic features
- Fibrous tissue hyperplasia in bones.
- Enlargement of Haversian canals.
- Boney tissue is replaced by fibroblasts, with osteoclastic giant cells lining the remaining bone tissue.

RICKETS

Rickets is failure of adequate deposition of calcium in bones of growing animals caused by deficiency of calcium and vitamin D and is characterized by bending of limbs, enlargement of ends of long bones and skeletal deformities (Fig. 13.10).

Etiology
- Vitamin D deficiency.
- Calcium deficiency.
- Deficiency of phosphorus.

Macroscopic features
- Bending of legs, bow legs.
- Pot belly.

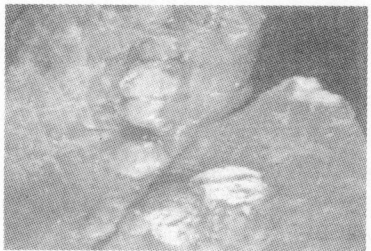

Fig.13.9. Photograph showing chronic myositis (ARS/USDA)

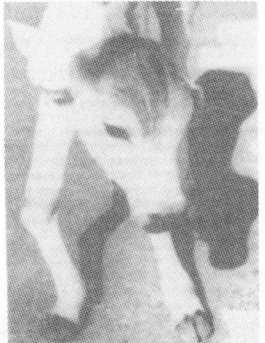

Fig.13.10. Photograph of calf showing rickets

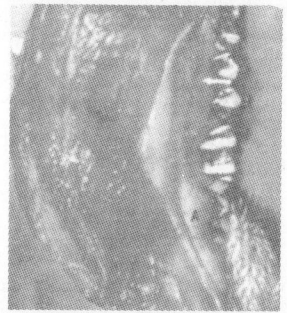

Fig.13.11. Photograph showing osteomyelitis in mandible (Actinomycosis) (ARS/USDA)

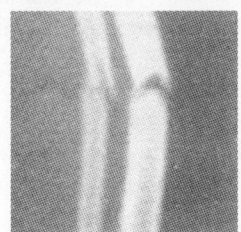

Fig.13.12. Photograph showing fracture

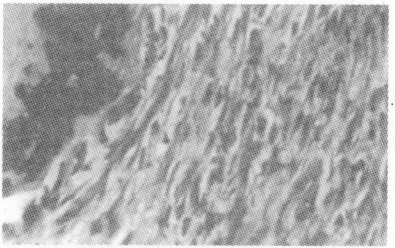

Fig.13.13. Photomicrograph of fracture healing

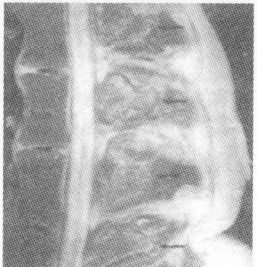

Fig.13.14. Photograph showing spondylitis(ARS/USDA)

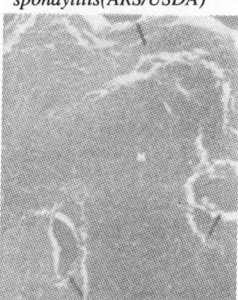

Fig. 13.15. Photomicrograph showing spondylitis (ARS/USDA)

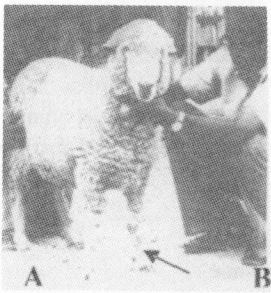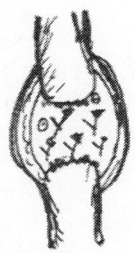

Fig. 13.16. A. Photograph showing arthritis B. Diagram showing immune complex deposition in joint

151

- Enlarged costochondral articulation.
- Softening of bones.

Microscopic features
- Increase in proliferating cartilage adjacent to the area of ossification and its disorderly arrangement.
- Disorderly penetration of cartilage by blood vessels.
- Increased area of uncalcified osteoid tissue
- Fibrosis of marrow.

OSTEOMALACIA

Osteomalacia is also known as *adult rickets*. It occurs in bone of adults and is caused by deficiency of vitamin D and calcium and characterized by softening of bones.

Etiology
- Vitamin D deficiency.
- Calcium-phosphorus ratio disturbance.

Macroscopic features
- Softening of bones.
- Irregular diffuse thickening of bones.
- Bone deformities.

Microscopic features
- Increase in osteoid tissue with failure of calcification.
- Increase in osteoclastic activity.

OSTEOPOROSIS

Osteoporosis is atrophy of bones caused by possibly hormonal imbalance and is characterized by inadequate deposition of calcium, brittleness of bones due to its increased porosity.

Etiology
- Hormonal imbalance.
- Vitamin C deficiency.
- Copper deficiency.

Macroscopic features
- Inadequate calcium deposition.

- Bone becomes brittle and porous.
- Increased fragility of bones.

Microscopic features
- Widening of Haversian canals.
- Increased activity of osteoclasts.
- Decrease in zona compacta and thickness of bone trabeculae.

OSTEOPETROSIS

Osteopetrosis is enlargement of bone caused by fluorosis or avian leukosis virus and is characterized by increase in bony tissue. It is also known as *marble bone disease*.

Etiology
- Avian leukosis virus of retroviridae family.
- Fluorosis.

Macroscopic features
- Enlargement of bone towards outside and inside.
- Reduced marrow cavity.
- Bone becomes brittle, marbelling of bones.

Microscopic features
- Cartilage is also calcified, surrounded by osteoid tissue.

OSTEOMYELITIS

Osteomyelitis is the inflammation of bone with bone marrow caused by trauma and pyogenic bacteria and is characterized by destruction, replacement and excessive growth of new bone adjacent to the infected part (Fig. 13.11).

Etiology
- Hematogenous infection.
- Direct infection through trauma/fracture.
- *Actinomyces pyogenes, A. bovis.*
- *Staphylococcus aureus.*
- *Pseudomonas aeruginosa.*

Macroscopic features
- Metastatic abscess in bone marrow.

- Excessive growth of bone in adjacent area.
- Exostosis or endostosis.

Microscopic features
- Infiltration of neutrophils.
- Proliferation of osteoid tissue.
- Demonstration of bacteria in pus.

BONE FRACTURE AND REPAIR

Fracture is the break in the continuity of bone due to trauma. A fracture may be simple or compound depending on the severity of trauma. Healing of fracture occurs by reunion of the broken ends of bone through development and proliferation of fibroblasts, angioblasts, osteoid tissue and infiltration of calcium salts (Figs. 13.12 & 13.13).

Etiology
- Trauma.
- Accidents – automobile accidents.

Macroscopic features
- Fracture can be identified by break in bones.
- Healing of fracture is characterized by development of callus at the site of reunion of break ends of bone.
- Callus may be soft or hard.

Microscopic features
- Proliferation of fibroblasts, angioblasts and metaplasia of connective tissue to osteoid tissue.
- Areas of calcification in osteoid tissue

PULMONARY OSTEOARTHROPATHY

Pulmonary osteoarthropathy is a rare disease of dog, sheep, cat, horse, and lion caused by prolonged anoxia and is characterized by cough, dyspnea, respiratory disturbances and formation of new bone leading to thickening and deformity of limbs.

Etiology
- Prolonged anoxia.
- Toxaemia.

Macroscopic features
- Pneumonia.
- New bone formation due to hyperplasia just beneath the periosteum in long bones.
- The proliferation of bone is irregular leading to development of rough surface on bone.
- Bone becomes enlarged twice to its normal size.
- Heart worms were also seen in case of dogs.

Microscopic features
- Bronchogenic carcinoma.
- Granulomatous lesions of tuberculosis.
- Chronic bronchiectasis.
- Hyperplasia of osteoid tissue with no indication of any kind of neoplastic growth in bones.

SPONDYLITIS

Spondylitis is the inflammation of vertebrae caused by bacteria/fungi and characterized by caseation, intraosseous abscess formation granulomatous lesions and fibrosis (Figs. 13.14 & 13.15).

Etiology
- *Brucella abortus, Br. ovis, Br. melitensis.*
- *Actinomyces bovis.*
- *Coccidioidomyces* sp.

Macroscopic features
- Intraosseous abscess.
- Granuloma encapsulated by fibrous tissue involving one or two adjacent vertebrae.
- Local enlargement of bone.

Microscopic features
- Granulomatous lesions with caseation.
- Proliferation of osteoid tissue.
- Infitration of neutrophils in intraosseous abscess.

PATHOLOGY OF JOINTS
ARTHRITIS

Arthritis is the inflammation of joint caused by bacteria, virus, chlamydia, mycoplasma and immune complexes and characterized by serus, fibrinous, purulent or ankylosing lesions in joints.

Etiology
- Bacteria – *E. coli, Erysipelas rhusiopathae, Streptococus* sp., *Shigella* sp. *Corynebacterium ovis, Brucella* sp.
- Mycoplasma – *Mycoplasma mycoides, Mycoplasma sinoviae.*
- Virus – Reovirus (Tenosynovitis in birds).
- Antigen antibody complexes.
- Trauma.

Macroscopic features
- Swelling of joints with increase in synovial fluid (Fig. 13.16).

- Difficulty in movement.
- In chronic cases fusion of two bony processes leaving no joint (ankylosing).
- Synovial fluid diminishes, becomes dirty, thick in chronic illness.

Microscopic features
- Presence of increased number of leucocytes in synovial fluid.
- Serus, fibrinous or purulent exudate in joints.
- Thickening of synovial membrane.
- Presence of plasma cells and immune complexes in synovial fluid.

MODEL QUESTIONS

Q. 1. *Fill in the blanks with suitable word(s).*
1. Gas gangrene is produced by.................... in thigh muscles of heifer which is manifested by ....sound on palpation due to accumulation of.................... and....................
2. Equine rhabdomyolysis occurs in horses on.................... after a day's rest and is characterized by...................,...................,.................... and.................... of muscles.
3. Osteomalacia is also known as.................... which is caused by deficiency of.................... and disturbances in ratio of.................... and.................... characterized by....................
4. ....,.................... and.................... may led to osteoporosis in animals characterized by.................... of bones.
5. Avian leucosis virus may cause........................ in birds characterized by........................ of bone.
6. Osteomyelitis is inflammation of.................... and.................... caused by .... and.................... and characterized by...................,.................... and................ of new bone adjacent to the infected part.
7. Healing fracture is characterized by the development of.................... at the site of reunion of break ends of bone.
8. Arthritis is inflammation of.................... characterized by.................... of joints.

Q. 2. *Write true and false and correct the false statement.*
1. ....In white muscle disease the colour of urine becomes redish brown due to presence of hemoglobin.
2. ....Sarcosporidia causes eosinophilic myositis.
3. ....In rickets, the deficiency of calcium may lead to softening of bones.
4. ....Osteopetrosis is enlargement of bones.
5. ....Osteoporosis is atrophy of bones.
6. ....Metastatic abscess are formed in bone marrow due to osteomyelitis.
7. ....Fracture is break in continuity of bones due to trauma.

8.   ....Prolonged anoxia may lead to pulmonary osteoarthropathy in dogs.
9.   ....Spondylitis is the inflammation of intervertebral disc.
10. ....Rheumatoid arthritis is caused by reovirus infection.

Q. 3.   Define the following

1. Myoglobinurea
2. Millers disease
3. Osteitis
4. Osteomyelitis
5. Exostosis
6. Enostosis
7. Callous
8. Spondylitis
9. Tenosynovitis
10. Ankylosis

Q.4.   Write short notes on the following

1. Azoturia
2. Osteoporosis
3. Gas gangrene
4. Rickets
5. Arthritis
6. White muscle disease
7. Osteopetrosis
8. Fibrous osteodystrophy
9. Pulmonary osteoarthropathy
10. Fracture healing

Q. 5.   Select most appropriate word(s) from the four options given against each statement.

1. Equine rhabdomyolysis is also known as .... morning disease
   (a) Sunday   (b) Monday   (c) Tuesday   (d) Wednesday
2. Accumulation of .... is responsible for hardening of muscles in azoturia.
   (a) Lactic acid   (b) Myoglobin   (d) Hemoglobin   (d) Glycogen
3. White muscle disease is caused by .... deficiency.
   (a) Vit-A   (b) Vit- D   (c) Vit-C   (d) Vit-E
4. Rickets is caused by deficiency of vitamin...............
   (a) A   (b) D   (c) C   (d) E
5. Osteoporosis is caused by deficiency of ....
   (a) Copper   (b) Zinc   (c) Iron   (d) Calcium
6. Osteopetrosis is also known as .... disease
   (a) Brittle bone (b) Marble bone   (c) Both a & b   (d) None
7. Fibrous osteodystrophy is characterized by .... condition.
   (a) Lock jaw   (b) Rubbery jaw   (c) Bottle jaw   (d) None
8. Osteomyelitis is inflammation of ....
   (a) Bone   (b) Bone marrow   (c) Both a & b   (d) None
9. *Brucella* sp may cause .... in animals and man.
   (a) Pulmonary osteoarthropathy (b) Spondylitis (c) Rickets   (d) Osteopetrosis
10. Rheumatoid arthritis is caused by ....
   (a) Antigen-antibody complex (b) *E. coli*   (c) Reovirus   (d) *Brucella* sp.

14
PATHOLOGY OF CARDIOVASCULAR SYSTEM

- **Developmental anomalies**
- **Cardiac failure**
    - **Acute cardiac failure**
    - **Chronic cardiac failure**
- **Pericarditis**
- **Myocarditis**
- **Endocarditis**
- **Brisket disease**
- **Mulberry heart disease**
- **Arteriosclerosis**
    - **Atherosclerosis**
    - **Medial sclerosis**
    - **Arteriolosclerosis**
- **Arteritis**
- **Aneurysm**
- **Phlebitis**
- **Lymphangitis**
- **Model Questions**

DEVELOPMENTAL ANOMALIES
Persistent right aortic arch
This is a developmental anomaly of aorta in which the aorta develops from right arch present on right side of trachea and oesophagus. The ductus arteriosus forms a ring around trachea and oesophagus by connecting aorta and pulmonary artery. This ring causes partial obstruction of trachea and/or oesophagus.

Patent ductus arteriosus
The ductus arteriosus is a short blood vessel which connects pulmonary artery to aorta in foetal life for diversion of blood. Normally, soon after birth this duct is sealed and remains in the form of a ligamentum arteriosum. But sometimes this ductus arteriosus remains open and blood is continuously shunted between aorta and pulmonary artery, after leading to congestive heart failure, pulmonary hypertension and cyanosis due to mixing of venous and arterial blood (Fig. 14.1).

Interventricular septal defects
In foetal life, there is no partition in ventricles and there is only one chamber which is divided into two – right and left – by inter-ventricular septum. But when interventricular septum does not develop completely, or there is defect in formation of complete partition, there is mixing of blood from both chambers. It is responsible for thickening of myocardium, roughening of endocardium and cyanosis (Fig. 14.2).

Transposition of aorta
THis condition develops if there is a shift in position of aorta and pulmonary artery i.e. the aorta arises from right ventricle and pulmonary artery from left ventricle. This results in arterial blood in right and venous blood in left side and has no clinical significance. However, it may create problems when aorta arises from venous ventricle and pulmonary artery from arterial side.

Tetrad of Fallot
Tetrad of Fallot includes four developmental defects of cardiovascular system and is also known as *tetralogy of Fallot* (Fig. 14.3).

1. Inter-ventricular septal defect.
2. Pulmonary stenosis is characterized by narrowing of lumen of pulmonary artery at its origin due to fibrous tissue causing 'jet' effect.
3. Hypertrophy of right ventricle.
4. Transposition of aorta.

Ectopia cordis
When heart lies outside the thorax under the subcutaneous tissue of lower cervical region.

Interatrial septal defect
There is a developmental defect in interatrial septa which remains as incomplete partition of atrium. It produces continuous overload on the right side of heart leading to pulmonary hypertension and hypertrophy of right side myocardium. However, a small defect in septum may persist throughout the life of animal without causing any clinical illness (Fig. 14.4).

CARDIAC FAILURE
Cardiac failure is the inability of heart to maintain adequate blood supply leading to death. It can be divided into two types: Acute and chronic heart failure.

Acute cardiac failure
Acute cardiac failure is sudden failure of contraction of heart leading to death within minutes.

Etiology
- Anoxia.
- Drugs/poisons.
- Shock.
- Cardiac temponade.
- Myocardial necrosis.
- Sudden occlusion of aorta and/or pulmonary artery.

Macroscopic features
- Cardiac temponade.
- Occlusive thrombus.
- Pulmonary congestion.
- Dialation of heart particularly of right ventricle

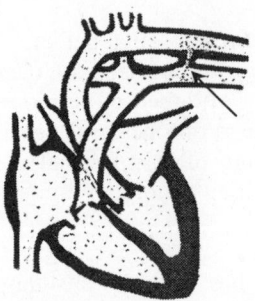

Fig.14.1 Diagram of heart showing developmental anomaly patent ductus arteriosus

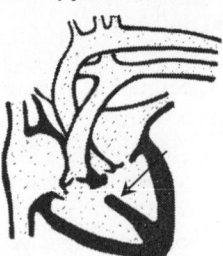

Fig.14.2. Diagram of heart showing developmental anomaly interventricular septal defect

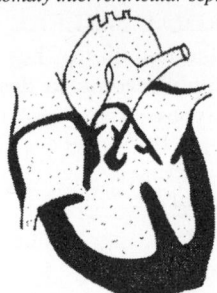

Fig.14.3. Diagram of heart showing developmental anamalies tetralogy of fallot

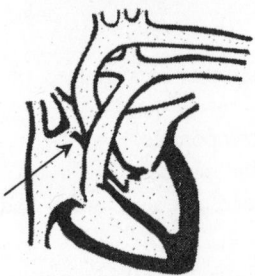

Fig.14.4. Diagram of heart showing developmental anomaly interatrial septal defect

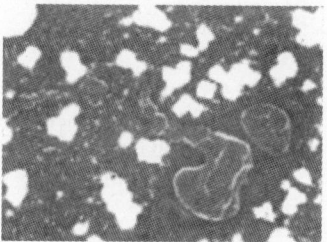

Fig.14.5. Photomicrograph of lung showing lesions of heart failure

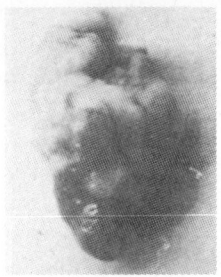

Fig.14.6. Photograph of heart showing necrotic lesions due to Salmonella gallinarum in poultry.

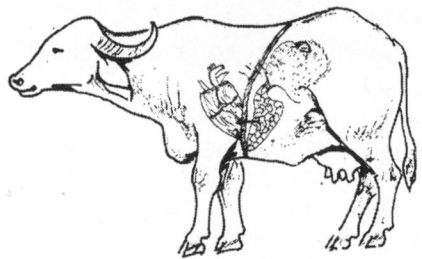

Fig. 14.7.Diagram showing traumatic reticulo pericarditis

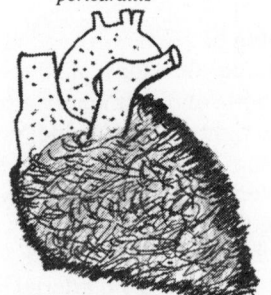

Fig.14.8. Diagram showing fibrinous pericarditis

Microscopic features
- Myocardial necrosis.
- Centrilobular necrosis in liver "nut meg liver".
- In prolonged cases, congestion and oedema in visceral organs.

Chronic Cardiac Failure

Chronic cardiac failure is the inability of heart to maintain balance between its output and venous return of blood. It can be further divided into two – left and right sided heart failure.

Left Sided Heart Failure

Left sided heart failure is caused by myocardial damage and is characterized by congestion and oedema in lungs with hypertrophy of alveolar lining cells (Fig. 14.5).

Etiology
- Myocardial degeneration/ necrosis
- Aortic and mitral valve disease
- Hypertension

Macroscopic features
- Congestion and oedema in lungs.
- Chronic dialation of heart.

Microscopic features
- Congestion of alveolar vessels.
- Oedema in lungs.
- Hypertrophy of alveolar lining cells.
- Alveolar macrophages contain hemosiderin pigment also called " heart failure cells".

Right Sided Heart Failure

Right sided heart failure is caused by a disease of lungs or pulmonary vasculature and mostly occurs after a left sided heart failure.

Etiology
- Left sided heart failure.
- Pulmonary lesions, congestion.

Macroscopic features
- Congestion of visceral organs.

- Subcutis oedema and ascites.
- Pulse in jugular vein.

Microscopic features
- "Nutmeg appearance" in liver due to centrilobular necrosis.
- Atrophy, necrosis and fibrosis in liver.
- Congestion in visceral organs.

PERICARDITIS

Pericarditis is the inflammation of pericardium, the upper layer of heart. It may be serus, fibrinous or suppurative depending on the type of exudate.

Etiology/Occurrence
- Pasteurellosis .
- Salmonellosis in poultry (Fig. 14.6).
- Hydropericardium syndrome in poultry.
- Gout in poultry.
- Trauma/foreign body *e.g.* traumatic reticulo pericarditis (TRP) (Fig. 14.7).

Macroscopic features
- Deposition of fibrin in between pericardium and heart gives an appearance of "bread and butter" (Fig. 14.8).
- In chronic cases, pericardium becomes thick due to excessive fibrosis.
- Accumulation of fluid (clear, serus) in pericardial sac is called *Hydropericardium* (Figs. 14.9 & 14.10).
- Presence of blood in pericardial sac is known as *hemopericardium* and the excessive accumulation of blood leading to heart failure is termed as *cardiac temponade* (Fig. 14.11).
- Accumulation of pus in pericardial sac is known as *pyopericardium*.
- Presence of gas in pericardial sac in known as *pneumopericardium*.

Microscopic features
- Hyperemia and haemorrhage in pericardium.
- Deposition of fibrin, formation of fibrin network, infiltration of neutrophils, macrophages and lymphocytes.

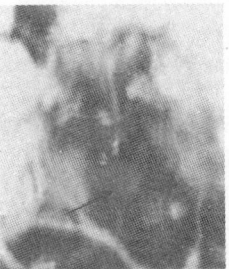

Fig.14.9. Photograph of hydropericardium in poultry

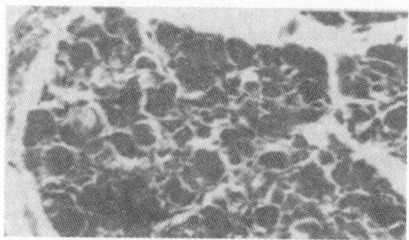

Fig.14.13. Photomicrograph showing myocarditis

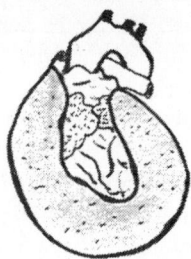

Fig.14.10. Diagram showing hydropericardium

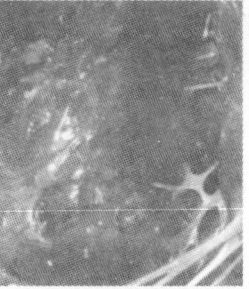

Fig.14.14. Photograph showing endocarditis (ARS/USDA)

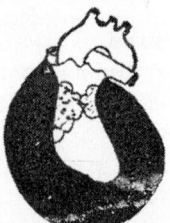

Fig.14.11. Diagram showing *hemopericardium (cardiac temponade)*

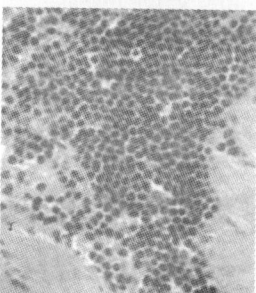

Fig.14.15. Photomicrograph showing eosinophilic endocarditis (ARS/USDA)

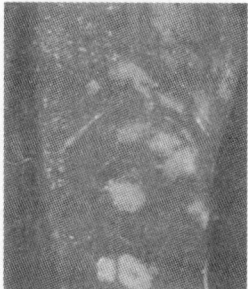

Fig.14.12. Photograph showing myocarditis (ARS/USDA)

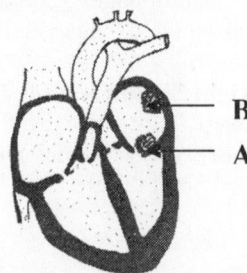

Fig.14.16. Diagram showing (A) valvular and (B) mural vegetative endocarditis

MYOCARDITIS

Myocarditis is the inflammation of myocardium, the middle layer of heart. It may be suppurative, eosinophlic or lymphocytic depending on the type of the exudate (Figs. 14.12 & 14.13).

Etiology

- Toxins/ Poisons.
- Bacteria / Virus.
- Parasites.
- Drugs / Chemicals.

Macroscopic features

- Colour of myocardium may become dark red or cyanotic due to accumulation of blood.
- In suppurative myocarditis, one can find abscesses in myocardium from where yellow/ green pus oozes out.
- Yellowish white streaks of necrosis in myocardium.
- Presence of cyst encapsulated by fibroplasia due to cysticercosis.

Microscopic features

- Hyperemia and haemorrhages in myocardium.
- Infiltration of neutrophils, eosinophils or lymphocytes.
- Coagulative necrosis of muscle fibres.
- In chronic cases, proliferation of fibrous connective tissue.

ENDOCARDITIS

Endocarditis is the inflammation of the endocardium, the inner layer of heart (Figs. 14.14 to 14.19).

Etiology/ Occurrence

- Chronic septicemic diseases like caused by *Actinomyces pyogenes*, *Erysipelothrix rhusiopathiae*.
- Staphylococci.
- Streptococci.
- *Pseudomonas aeruginosa*.
- Clostridial infections.

Macroscopic features

- Lesions in heart valves or wall of atrium/ ventricles.
- Presence of thrombi on endocardium.
- Vegetative/cauliflower like growth on endocardium either in valves (*Valvular vegetative endocarditis* e.g. swine erysepalas) or in wall (*Mural vegetative endocarditis*).
- Dilation of heart chambers.

Microscopic features

- Infiltration of thrombocytes, neutophils, macrophages and lymphocytes.
- Masses of bacterial organisms can be seen.
- Underlying endocardium and myocardium shows the presence of fibrin network and infiltration of RBC, neutrophils and macrophages.

BRISKET DISEASE/HIGH ALTITUDE DISEASE

Brisket disease is a condition of slow cardiac failure, which occurs at 2500 metres above sea level or higher where pressure of air is low (Fig. 14.20).

Etiology

- Low oxygen in environment.
- Decreased atmospheric pressure of air.
- In native cattle morbidity rate is only 2% and in imported cattle at hills it is upto 40%.

Macroscopic feature

- Dilation of heart.
- Hypertrophy of ventricular wall.
- Chronic passive congestion in visceral organs.
- Oedema in sternal region in between forelegs.

Microscopic feature

- Nutmeg liver due to chronic passive congestion.
- Polycythemia.
- Hypertrophy of muscle fibres in myocardium.

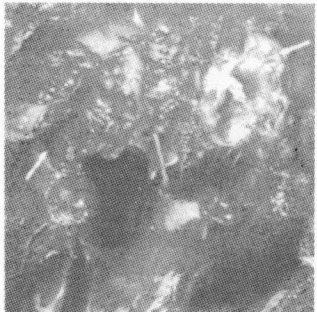

Fig.14.17 Photograph showing vegetative
endocarditis (ARS/USDA)

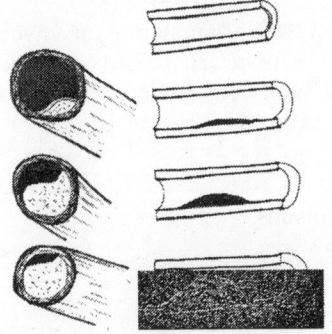

Fig.14.21. Diagram showing atherosclerosis
leading to obstruction of vessel

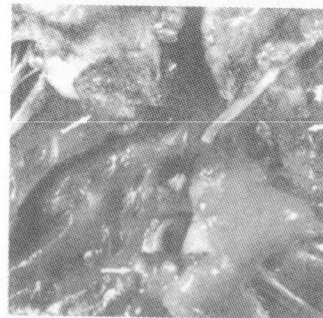

Fig.14.18. Photograph showing vegetative
endocarditis (ARS/USDA)

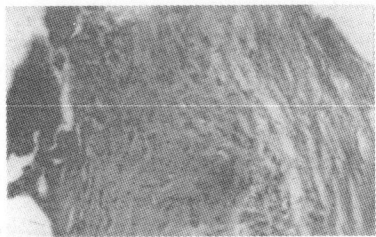

Fig.14.22. Photomicrograph showing arteriosclerosis

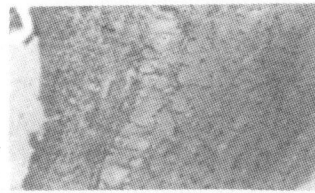

Fig.14.19 Photomicrograph showing endocarditis

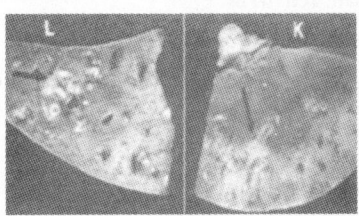

Fig.14.23. Photograph showing arteritis (L) Liver (K)
Kidney (ARS/USDA)

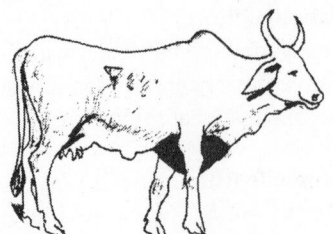

Fig.14.20. Diagram showing Brisket disease in cow

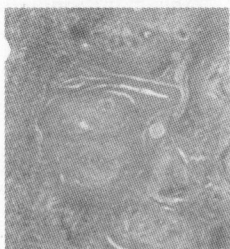

Fig.14.24 Photomicrograph showing arteritis
(ARS/USDA)

MULBERRY HEART DISEASE

It is characterized by firm contraction of heart and petechial haemorrhage on pericardium giving the appearance of mulberry.

Etiology
- Not known
- May be enterotoxaemia/poisoning

Macroscopic features
- Contraction of heart with petechial haemorrhage on pericardium looking like mulberry "Mulbery heart disease"
- Hydropericardium, hydroperitoneum and pulmonary oedema
- Oedema fluid has high protein content resulting in clot formation
- Congestion of fundic portion of stomach.

Microscopic features
- Congestion on serosa of visceral organs.

ARTERIOSCLEROSIS

Arteriosclerosis is hardening of arteries causing 3 types of diseases in arteries depending on their size and etiological factors viz., Atherosclerosis, medial sclerosis and arteriolosclerosis.

ATHEROSCLEROSIS

Atherosclerosis is characterized by hardening and thickening of intimal layer of large arteries and aorta due to proliferation of connective tissue, hyaline degeneration, infilteration of fat/ lipids and calcification. These intimal changes may lead to loss of elasticity of artery (*Athere* means mushy substance) (Fig. 14.21 & Fig. 14.22).

Etiology
- Exact cause is not clear
- Hypercholesterolemia and hyperlipidemia
- Hypertension

Macroscopic features
- Fatty streaks running parallel in the direction of the artery.

- Intimal layer of aorta/ coronary arteries is elevated due to plaques which are white/ yellow, fibrous and occluding the lumen of vessel.
- Occlusion of artery may lead to ischemia and infarction.

Microscopic features
- Macrophages are filled with lipid droplets including cholesterol, fatty acids, triglycerides and phospholipids.
- Fragmented internal elastic lamina in the intimal layer of artery
- Proliferation of altered smooth muscles may become metaplastic to macrophages.
- Deposition of mucoid ground substance and collagen fibers
- Hyalinization of connective tissue " Fibrous plaques".
- Presence of some fat droplets in between the lesion

MEDIAL SCLEROSIS

Medial sclerosis involve medium sized muscular arteries and characterized by fatty degeneration and hyalinization of muscular tissue of medial arteries leading to necrosis. This is also known as *Monckeberg medial sclerosis*.

Etiology
- Old age.
- Excessive administration of epinephrine (adrenaline).
- Nicotine.
- Vitamin D toxicity.
- Hyperparathyroidism.

Macroscopic features
- Hardening of medium sized arteries.
- Hyaline, fatty changes and calcification of arterial wall.

Microscopic features
- Fatty changes, hyalinization of muscular layer of medium sized arteries.
- Necrosis of myofibrils.
- Calcification.

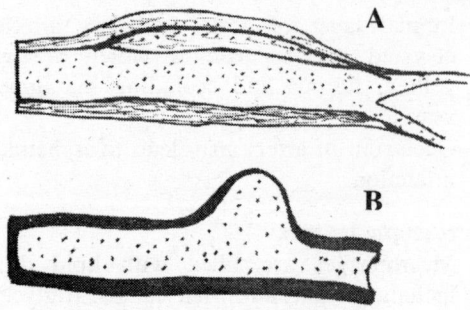

Fig.14.25. Diagram showing aneurysm
(a) dissecting (b) sacular

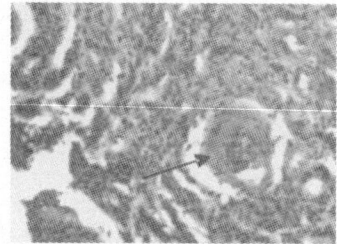

Fig.14.26. Photomicrograph showing phlebitis

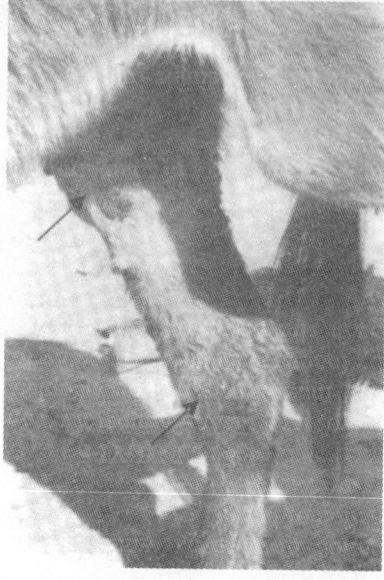

Fig.14.27. Photograph showing of lymphangitis

ARTERIOLOSCLEROSIS

Arteriolosclerosis affects arterioles in kidneys, spleen and pancreas and is characterized by hyperplasia of intimal cells of arterioles producing concentric lamellations occluding their lumen.

Etiology
- Hypertension.

Macroscopic features
- No characteristic macroscopic lesion.
- Atrophy of organ, hardening.

Microscopic features
- Proliferation of cells present in intima of blood vessels.
- Swelling and necrosis of cells in medial layer leading to occlusion of lumen.
- Calcification in chronic cases.

ARTERITIS

Arteritis is the inflammation of arteries characterized by infiltration of neutrophils, lymphocytes and macrophages in the media and intima of arterial wall (Figs. 14. 23 & 14.24).

Etiology
- Chemicals.
- Thermal.
- Virus *e.g.* Equine viral arteritis.
- Pyogenic bacteria.
- Parasite *e.g. Strongylus vulgaris.*

Macroscopic features
- Hyperemia.
- Conjunctivitis, oedema of eye.
- Presence of thrombi in artery.

164

Microscopic features

- Presence of thrombi in artery involving intimal layer.
- Equine viral arteritis virus causes infiltration of lymphocytes and macrophages in media.
- Occlusion of lumen of arteries due to thickening of wall.
- In parasitic arteritis, parasitic thrombi may present along with inflammatory reaction in intimal layer.

ANEURYSM

Aneurysm is dilation of an artery or cardiac chamber leading to formation of sac (Fig. 14.25).

Etiology

- Aflatoxin.
- Infectious emboli.
- Weak vessel wall due to rupture.
- Fracture or necrosis of medial layer of large blood vessel.
- Arteriolosclerosis.

Macroscopic features

- Fracture or necrosis of medial layer of large blood vessels permitting parallel blood circulation till the next division of blood vessel is called as *Dissecting aneurysm* or *false aneurysm*.
- Formation of sac in artery due to dilation, also known as *True aneurysm*.

Microscopic features

- Rough intimal layer.
- Wall of blood vessel damaged with inflammatory exudate.

PHLEBITIS

Phlebitis is the inflammation of veins characterized by presence of inflammatory exudate, thickening of the wall and dilation of the lumen (Fig. 14.26).

Etiology/Occurrence

- Naval infection in calves.

- Uterine infections.
- In jugular vein due to improper intravenous infection.
- *Varicose veins* are dilated and elongated veins following irregular and tortuous course.
- *Telangiectasis* is marked dilation of veins particularly of sinusoidal capillaries in one or more lobules in liver.

Macroscopic feature

- Wall of vein is thickened.
- Vein contain large thick necrotic material
- Lumen dialated
- Inner surface of vein is rough and hyperemic.

Microscopic feature

- Infilteration of neutrophils in the wall of veins
- Sometimes calcification may also present.
- Wall of vein becomes thick due to inflammatory cells and/or proliferation of fibrous tissue.

LYMPHANGITIS

Lymphangitis is the inflammation of lymph vessels characterized by aggregation of lymphocytes around lymphatics, oedema of dependent parts and distension of lymphatics (Fig. 14.27).

Etiology/Occurrence

- *Corynebacterium ovis* causes caseous lymphangitis and lymphadenitis
- Equine epizootic lymphangitis

Macroscopic lesions

- Distension of subcutaneous lymph vessels, nodules of lymphoid aggregates.
- Oedema due to failure of lymphatic drainage.

Microscopic lesions

- Lymphoid aggregation around lymphatics.
- Lymphatics distended.
- Oedema of dependent tissue.

MODEL QUESTIONS

Q. 1. *Fill in the blanks with suitable word(s).*
1. Right sided heart failure is caused by a disease in...............and occurs after ....failure and is characterized by ....pulse.
2. Interventricular septal defects may lead to ....and ....
3. Brisket disease is caused by ....in environment and is characterized by ....,................and oedema in ....region.
4. Arteriosclerosis is ....of arteries including ....,...............and ....
5. ....,................and ....may lead to occurrence of atherosclerosis.
6. Caseous lymphangitis is caused by...........and is characterized by...............,...............and ....
7. Hypertension may cause ....characterized by ....producing ....occluding ....of blood vessels.
8. Macrophages are filled with ....including ....,...............,...............and ....in atherosclerosis of large blood vessels.

Q. 2. *Write true or false and correct the false statements.*
1. ....Transposition of aorta includes the origin of aorta from left ventricle.
2. ....Myocardial necrosis and nutmeg liver are feature of acute heart failure.
3. ....Eosinophilic myocarditis is caused by Sarcosporidia.
4. ....Hypocholesterolemia may cause atherosclerosis.
5. ....Oedema occurs due to lymphangitis.
6. ....Phlebitis is inflammation of veins.
7. ....Excessive administration of adrenaline may cause medial sclerosis.
8. ....Arteriolosclerosis may affect medium and large size arteries.
9. ....Altered smooth muscle fibres may act as macrophages loaded with lipid content.
10. ....Lymphangitis may not cause oedema.

Q. 3. *Define the following.*
1. Ectopia cordis
2. Heart failure cells
3. Hydropericardium
4. Cardiac temponade
5. Pneumopericardium
6. Arteriolosclerosis
7. Arteriosclerosis
8. Nutmeg liver
9. Varicose veins
10. Telangiectasis

Q. 4. *Write short notes on.*
1. Tetralogy of Fallot
2. Vegetative endocarditis
3. Brisket disease
4. Mulberry heart disease
5. Atherosclerosis
6. Cardiac failure

Q. 5. *Match the word(s) from four options given against each statement.*
1. Acute heart failure is not caused by ....
   (a) Anoxia   (b) Shock   (c) Cardiac temponade   (d) Fever
2. Left sided heart failure is characterized by ....
   (a) Heart failure cells (b) Pulse in jugular vein   (c) Shock   (d) Oedema

3. "Bread and butter" appearance of heart is due to deposition of ....
   (a) Fibrin   (b) Neutrophils   (c) Fibroblasts   (d) Collagen

4. Endocarditis is caused by ....
   (a) *Actinomyces pyogenes* (b) Erysepalas   (c) Staphylococci   (d) All of the above

5. Vegetative growth in heart is caused by ....
   (a) *Actinomyces pyogenes* (b) Staphylococci   (c) Clostridia   (d) Erysipalas

6. Arteriolosclerosis affects arterioles in ....
   (a) Kidneys   (b) Spleen   (c) Pancreas   (d) All of the above

7. Atherosclerosis is ....of blood vessels
   (a) Hardening   (b) Softening   (c) Aneurysm   (d) Thinning

8. Arteritis is inflammation of arteries caused by ....
   (a) Equine viral arteritis (b) *E.coli*   (c) Salmonella   (d) Rotavirus

9. Phlebitis is the inflammation of ....
   (a) Artery   (b) Vein   (c) Lymph vessel   (d) Capillary

10. Lymphangitis is inflammation of ....
    (a) Lymphnode   (b) Lymph gland   (c) Lymph vessel   (d) Lymphocytes

15
PATHOLOGY RESPIRATORY SYSTEM

- **Pathology of upper respiratory passage**
  - **Nasal polyps**
  - **Nasal granuloma**
  - **Tracheitis**
  - **Bronchitis**
- **Pathology of lungs**
  - **Atelectasis**
  - **Emphysema**
  - **Pulmonary oedema**
  - **Pneumonia**
  - **Pulmonary adenomatosis**
  - **Hypersensitivity pneumonitis**
  - **Pneumoconiasis**
- **Pathology of air sacs**
  - **Air sacculitis**
- **Pathology of pleura**
  - **Pleuritis**
- **Model Questions**

PATHOLOGY OF UPPER RESPIRATORY TRACT

In many infectious diseases, there is inflammation of mucosa of upper respiratory passage leading to nasal discharge which is catarrhal, purulent or fibrinous, depending on the type of infection. The infection may extend to lower parts of respiratory tract and reach the lungs causing pathological alterations. *Rhinitis* is the inflammation of nasal mucosa (Fig. 15.1). *Sinusitis* is the inflammation of sinuses *e.g.* frontal sinusitis in dehorned cattle. The larvae of botfly *Oestrus ovis* enter the nasal passage and migrate upto frontal sinuses and turbinate bones and cause mucopurulent inflammation. Similarly leeches (*Dinobdella ferox)* is known to cause nasal cavity inflammation in domestic animals and suck blood. Rhinitis is caused by *Bordetella bronchiseptica* in pigs and is characterized by mucopurulent exudate, disappearance of nasal septum, retarded growth of snout and plugging of passage by solidified exudate and dead tissue. This condition is known as *porcine atrophic rhinitis*. *Epistaxis* is bleeding from nasal passage due to trauma, neoplasm and ulcerative lesions as a result of infections. *Pharyngitis* is the inflammation of pharynx while *laryngitis* is the inflammation of larynx.

NASAL POLYPS

Nasal polyps are the inflammatory conditions of respiratory mucosa resembling neoplastic growth caused by fungus and characterized by formation of new growth simulating benign neoplasm in nasal passage.

Etiology

- *Rhinosporidium sceberi*, a fungus most commonly prevalent in southern India.

Macroscopic features

- Formation of a single polyp in respiratory mucosa, pedunculated, elongated, fills nasal cavity.
- Cauliflower like growth may cause bleeding.

Microscopic features

- Fibrous covering by mucous membrane and heavily infiltrated by neutrophils, lymphocytes, eosinophils, macrophages around fungus.

NASAL GRANULOMA

Nasal granuloma is the granulomatus inflammation of respiratory mucosa in nasal cavity caused by blood flukes and characterized by the presence of granulomatous growth filling the nasal passage causing obstruction (Figs. 15.2 & 15.3).

Etiology

- *Schistosoma nasalis,* a blood fluke.
- Type II hypersensitivity reaction of nasal mucosa to plant pollens, fungi, mites etc (Fig. 15.4).

Macroscopic Features

- Nasal pruritus.
- Small tiny nodules on nasal mucosa later becomes cauliflower-like growth filling the cavity and causing obstruction.

Microscopic features

- Oedema in lamina propria.
- Infiltration of eosinophils, mast cells, lymphocytes and plasma cells and absence of epithelioid cells.
- Proliferation of fibroblasts.
- The lesion is covered by squamous epithelium.
- Mucous glands may have metaplastic pseudostratified columnar epithelium.

TRACHEITIS

Tracheitis is the inflammation of trachea. In canines, it is tracheobronchitis while in poultry it is manifested by laryngotracheitis (Fig. 15.5).

Etiology

- Canine tracheobronchitis caused by adenovirus, influenza virus and herpes virus.
- Avian infectious laryngotracheitis (ILT) is caused by herpes virus.

169

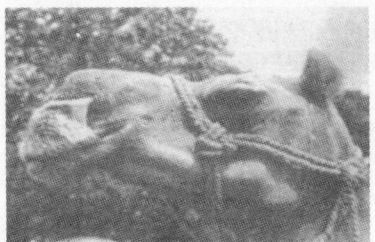

Fig.15.1. Photograph showing rhinitis in a camel and catarrhal nasal discharge

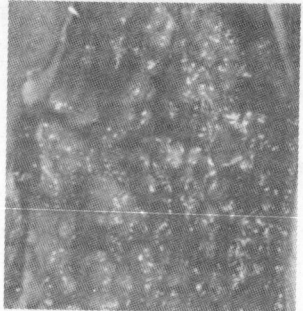

Fig.15.2. Photograph showing nasal granuloma (ARS/USDA)

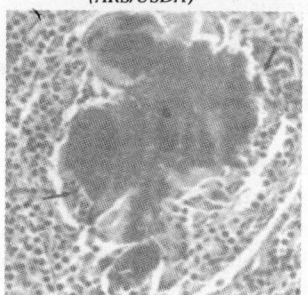

Fig.15.3. Photomicrograph showing nasal granuloma (ARS/USDA)

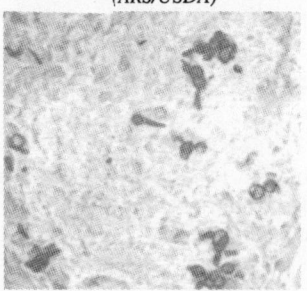

Fig.15.4. Photomicrograph showing causative fungus in nasal granuloma (ARS/USDA)

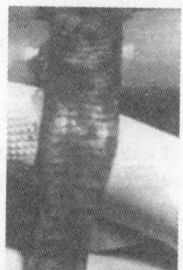

Fig.15.5. Photograph showing haemorrhagic tracheitis in poultry

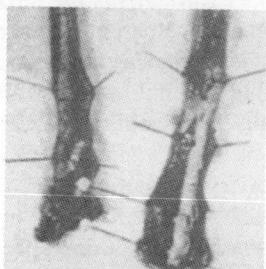

Fig.15.6. Photograph showing presence of caseous exudate in larynx and trachea.

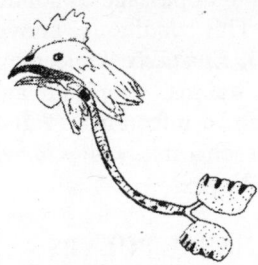

Fig.15.7. Diagram showing presence of caseous exudates in larynx and trachea.

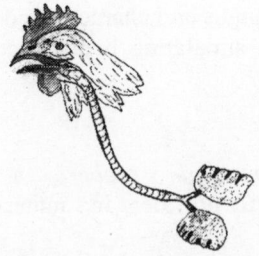

Fig.15.8. Diagram showing lesions of infectious bronchitis in poultry

Macroscopic features
- Canine tracheobronchitis or *kennel cough* includes congestion of trachea and presence of catarrhal exudate.
- In poultry, haemorrhage in trachea and caseous plug in trachea towards larynx causing obstruction (Figs. 15.6 & 15.7).

Microscopic features
- Inclusion bodies in tracheal and bronchial epithelium in canines.
- Haemorrhagic tracheitis, presence of intra nuclear basophilic inclusions in tracheal epithelial cells in infectious laryngotracheitis.

BRONCHITIS

Bronchitis is the inflammation of bronchi, characterized by catarrhal, suppurative, fibrinous or haemorrhagic exudate.

Etiology
- Bacteria *e.g.* Pasteurella.
- Virus *e.g.* infectious bronchitis in poultry.
- Parasites.
- Allergy/ Inhalation of pollens etc.

Macroscopic features
- Coughing, dyspnoea.
- Mucous exudate in lumen.
- Congestion and/or haemorrhages in bronchi.
- Presence of caseous plugs at the point where bronchi enters in lungs in infectious bronchitis of poultry (Fig. 15.8).

Microscopic features
- Mucous exudate along with inflammatory cells in the lumen of bronchi.
- Hyperplasia and/or necrosis of bronchiolar epithelium.
- Accumulation of mononuclear cells in the bronchial mucosa and in peribronchiolar area.

PATHOLOGY OF LUNGS
ATELECTASIS

Atelectasis is the failure of alveoli to open or the alveoli are collapsed and thus do not have air.

Etiology
- Obstruction in bronchi/ bronchiole.
- Pleuritis.
- Atelectasis neonatorum in new born animals. In the absence of respiration, lung alveoli remain closed and thus sink in water indicating still birth.

Macroscopic features
- Dull red in colour, hard area of lung like liver in consistency.
- Atelectic lung sinks in water.

Microscopic features
- Compressed alveoli (Fig. 15.9).
- Absence of air spaces.
- Collapsed bronchioles.
- In inflammatory condition, exudate compresses alveoli.

EMPHYSEMA

Emphysema is the increase in amount of air in lungs characterized by dilation of the alveoli. It may be acute or chronic and focal or generalized.

Etiology
- Bronchitis.
- Atelectasis in adjoining area of lung.
- Pneumonia.
- Allergy to dust, pollens etc.
- Pulmonary adenomatosis.

Macroscopic features
- Lungs are enlarged and flabby.
- Imprints of ribs can be seen. Colour of lungs becomes pale.
- Cut surface is smooth and dry.

Microscopic features
- Alveoli are distended (Fig. 15.10).
- Some alveoli may rupture and form giant alveoli.
- Alveolar wall becomes thin due to stretching.
- Mild bronchitis.
- Hyperplasia of lymphoid tissue.

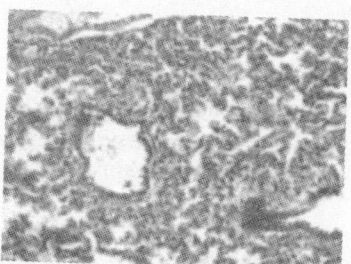

Fig.15.9. Photomicrograph of lung showing
atelectasis.

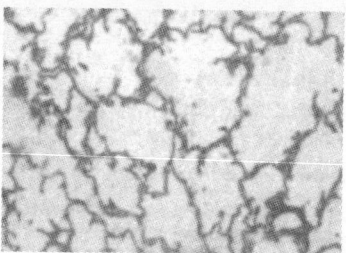

Fig.15.10. Photomicrograph of lung
showing emphysema

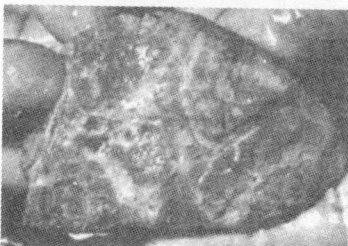

Fig.15.11. Photograph of lung showing
odema

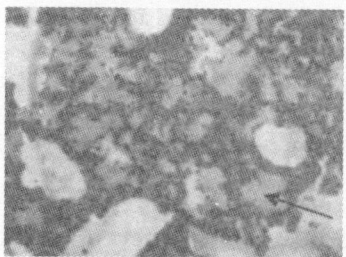

Fig.15.12. Photomicrograph of lung showing
oedematous fluid in alveoli

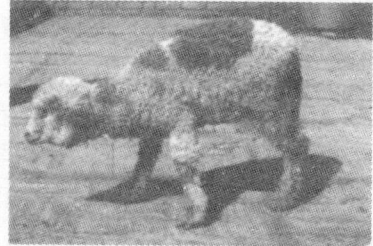

Fig.15.13. Photograph of lamb showing signs of
pneumonia

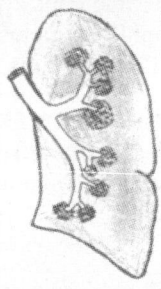

Fig-15.14. Diagram showing bronchogenous
spread of causal agent in lung

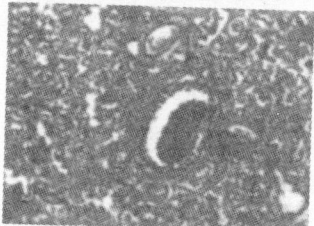

Fig.15.15. Photomicrograph showing
bronchopneumonia

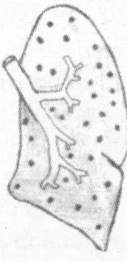

Fig.15.16. Diagram showing hematogenous
spread of causal agent in lung

PULMONARY OEDEMA

In pulmonary oedema, there is accumulation of serous fluid in alveoli of lungs (Figs. 15.11 & 15.12).

Etiology

- Bacteria.
- Virus.
- Allergy.

Macroscopic features

- Lungs become enlarged.
- Weight of lungs increases.
- Cut surface releases fluid and frothy exudate in trachea and/or bronchi.

Microscopic features

- Serous fluid accumulation in alveoli of lungs
- Fluid may also be seen in some bronchi/ bronchioles.
- Infiltration of inflammatory cells.
- Congestion of lungs.

PNEUMONIA

Pneumonia is the inflammation of lungs characterized by congestion and consolidation of lungs. Clinically, it is menifested by dyspnoea, coughing, weakness and nasal discharge (Fig. 15.13). The pathological lesions in lungs are produced in a similar way irrespective of the type of etiological agent and includes various stages like congestion, red hepatization, grey hepatization and resolution.

Stage of congestion: This stage of lung is characterized by active hyperemia and pulmonary oedema. The capillaries are distended with engorged blood and alveoli are filled with watery serous exudate. This requires 2 minutes to few hours to initiate the congestion.

Stage of red hepatization: This stage of lung is characterized by the consolidation of lungs due to accumulation of blood in blood vessels (congestion). The consolidated lungs are firm and look like liver and hence the name "red hepatization". Such affected lung always sinks in water. Alveoli are filled with serous or serofibrinous exudate giving hardness to lungs. In inflammatory condition, the neutrophils, macrophages and lymphocytes along with erythrocytes infiltrate the affected area of lungs. This stage of red hepatization takes 2 days for development of firmness of lung.

Stage of grey hepatization: The lung remains hard but due to lysis and removal of erythrocytes, it becomes grey or less red in colour. Firmness/ hardness of lung remains same and thus, the name grey hepatization. There is increase in infiltration of inflammatory cells like macrophages, lymphocytes, epithelioid cells depending on the virulence of etiological agents.

Stage of resolution: After a week, the recovery starts in the form of resorption of fluid; autolized cells and debris is removed by phagocytic cells. The causative organism is neutralized or removed from the lungs through immunity of body. After a few days the lung parenchyma becomes normal and starts functioning. If the causative agent is more virulent, it may cause death of animal due to respiratory failure or may cause permanent lesions like formation of scar, carnification, granuloma etc. There are various types of pneumonia caused by bacteria, virus, fungi, parasites, allergens, chemicals and all such affections of lungs are classified as under.

BRONCHOPNEUMONIA

Bronchopneumonia is the inflammation of lungs involving bronchi or bronchioles along with alveoli. It is thought to be spread through bronchogenous route and is the common type of pneumonia in animals (Figs. 15.14 & 15.15).

Etiology

- Virus.
- Bacteria.
- Chemicals.
- Mycoplasma.
- Chlamydia.
- Parasites.
- Fungus.
- Mainly through bronchogenous route.

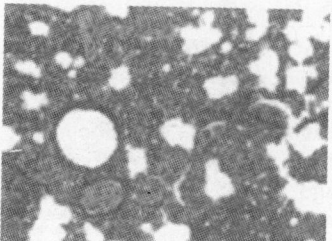

Fig.15.17. Photomicrograph showing interstitial pneumonia

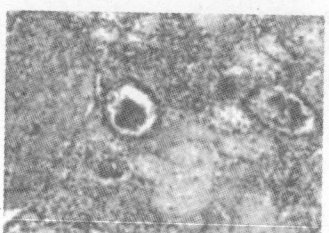

Fig.15.18. Photomicrograph of fibrinous pneumonia

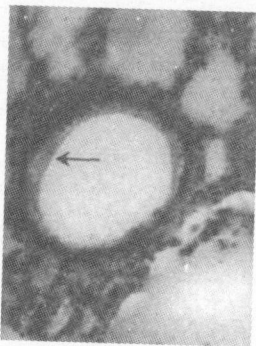

Fig.15.19. Photomicrograph showing hyaline membrane pneumonia

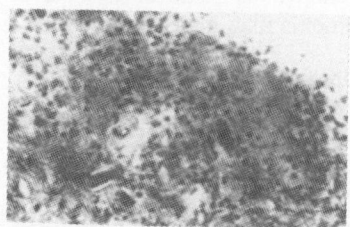

Fig.15.20. Photomicrograph showing verminous pneumonia

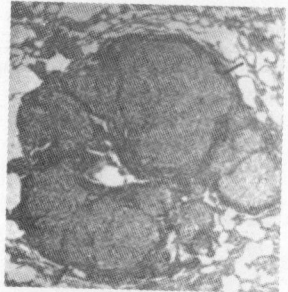

Fig.15.21. Photomicrograph showing aspiration pneumonia (ARS/USDA)

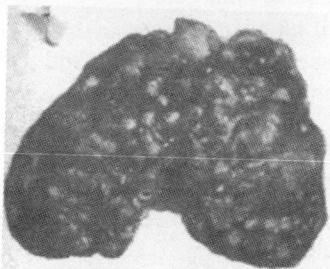

Fig.15.22. Photograph showing mycotic pneumonia

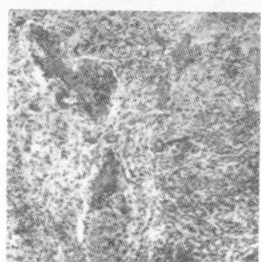

Fig.15.23. Photomicrograph showing mycotic pneumonia.

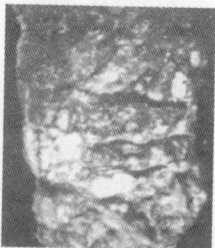

Fig.15.24. Photograph of lung showing tubercle/granulomatous lesion (ARS/USDA)

Macroscopic features

- Congestion and consolidation of anterior and ventral parts of lungs (lobular pneumonia).
- Patchy lesions on one or several lobes and adjacent area showing emphysema.
- Mediastinal lymphnodes are swollen.

Microscopic features

- Congestion, oedema or haemorrhage in lung.
- Infiltration of neutrophils, mononuclear cells in and around bronchioles/ bronchi.
- Catarrhal inflammation of bronchi.
- Proliferation of bronchiolar epithelium.

Interstitial Pneumonia

Interstitial pneumonia is the inflammation of the lungs characterized by thickening of alveolar septa due to serous/fibrinous exudate along with infiltration of neutrophils and/or mononuclear cells and proliferation of fibroblasts. It is also known as lobar pneumonia (Figs. 15.16 & 15.17).

Etiology

- Bacteria.
- Virus.
- Chlamydia.
- Parasites.
- Mainly through hematogenous route.

Macroscopic features

- Lungs are pale or dark red in colour.
- Oedema, dripping of fluid from cut surface.

Microscopic features

- Alveoli may have serous or fibrinous exudate.
- Thickening of alveolar septa due to accumulation of exudate, inflammatory cells and in chronic cases, proliferation of fibrous tissue.
- Infiltration of mononuclear cells in alveolar septa.

Fibrinous Pneumonia

Fibrinous pneumonia is the inflammation of lungs characterized by the presence of fibrin in alveoli or bronchioles and may give rise to hyaline membrane formation over the surface of alveoli or bronchiole.

Etiology

- Bacteria.
- Virus.
- Parasites.
- Toxin/poisons.

Macroscopic features

- Antero-ventral portion of lung is congested and consolidation.
- Colour of lungs become deep red due to congestion.
- Surface of lungs is covered by fibrin sheet.
- Interlobular septa are prominent due to accumulation of plasma and fibrin.

Microscopic features

- Principal exudate is fibrin, fills alveoli, bronchioles and bronchi (Fig. 15.18).
- Congestion and/or haemorrhages.
- Infiltration of neutrophils, macrophages and giant cells.
- Formation of eosinophilic false membrane of fibrin over the surface of alveoli and bronchiole known as *"hyaline membrane pneumonia"* (Fig. 15.19).

Verminous Pneumonia

Verminous pneumonia is caused by parasites and is characterized by the presence of lesions of bronchopneumonia along with parasites or their larva (Fig. 15.20).

Etiology

- *Metastrongylus apri* in pig.
- *Dictyocaulus filariae* in sheep and goat.
- *D. viviparus* in cattle and buffaloes.
- *D. arnfieldi* in horse and donkeys.
- *Capillaria aerophila* in dogs and cats.

Macroscopic features

- Multiple petechial haemorrhage in lungs at the site of parasite penetration.

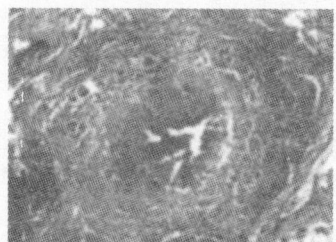

Fig.15.25. Photomicrograph of lung showing tubercle

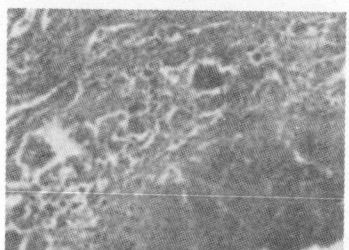

Fig.15.26. Photomicrograph.of lung showing granulomatous lesions

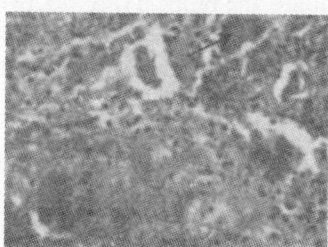

Fig.15.27. Photomicrograph of lung showing granulomatous lesions and giant cells

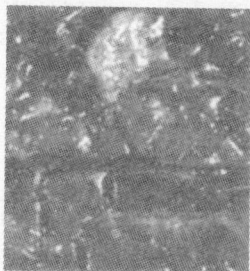

Fig.15.28. Photograph showing pulmonary adenomatosis (ARS/USDA)

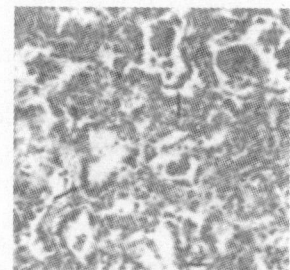

Fig.15.29. Photomicrograph showing pulmonary adenomatosis (ARS/USDA)

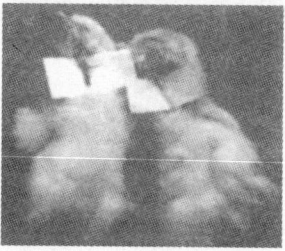

Fig.15.30. Photograph showing deposition of carbon particles in trachea in chicks

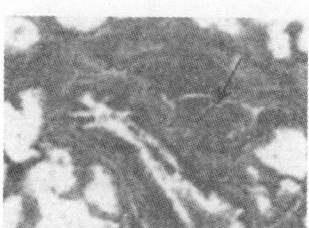

Fig.15.31. Photomicrograph showing pneumoconiasis

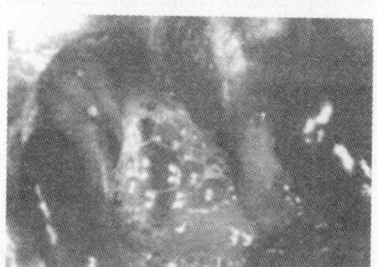

Fig.15.32. Photograph showing air sacculitis in poultry

- Mature worms in alveoli, bronchioles and bronchi.
- Mucopurulent exudate in alveoli/bronchi.
- Pulmonary oedema, emphysema.

Microscopic features
- Dilation of bronchiole/ bronchi
- Lesions of chronic suppurative bronchiolitis
- Focal areas of inflammation in the vicinity of parasites and around bronchioles.
- Hyperplasia of bronchiolar epithelium.
- Infiltration of eosinophils and lymphocytes.

Aspiration Pneumonia

Aspiration pneumonia is caused by faulty medication through drenching which reaches lungs instead of targetted place (digestive tract) and characterized by necrosis and gangrene of lung paranchyma.

Etiology
- Drugs, food, foreign body and oil drench which reaches in lungs through trachea.
- Paresis of throat predisposes the animal for aspiration pneumonia.

Macroscopic features
- Congestion and consolidation of anterior and ventral portion of lung.
- Affected part becomes green/ black in colour, moist gangrene.
- Affected lungs are often foul smelling.
- Presence of foreign body like heads of wheats, parts of corn, oil, milk etc.

Microscopic features
- Thrombosis of blood vessels.
- Necrosis in lungs.
- Presence of saprophytes, leucocytes and bacteria cause liquefaction and gangrene.
- Gangrenous lesions surrounded by intense inflammation (Fig. 15.21).
- Congestion.

Mycotic Pneumonia

Mycotic pneumonia is caused by a variety of fungi and characterized by the presence of chronic granulomatous lesions in lungs (Figs. 15.22 & 15.23).

Etiology
- *Aspergillus fumigatus.*
- *Blastomyces* sp.
- *Cryptococcus* sp.
- *Coccidioidomyces immitis.*

Macroscopic features
- Nodules in lungs.
- On cut, cheese-like caseative mass comes out from nodules.
- Caseation involves both bronchiole and alveoli.
- Such lesions may also be present in trachea, bronchi and air sacs.

Microscopic features
- Presence of granulomatus lesions *i.e.* caseative necrosis, macrophages, epithelioid cells, lymphocytes, giant cells, fibroblasts etc.
- Presence of branched hyphae of fungi in the necrosed area.

Tuberculous Pneumonia

Tuberculous pneumonia is caused by *Mycobacterium* sp. and is characterized by the presence of chronic granulomatous lesions in the lungs (Figs. 15.24 to 15.27).

Etiology
- *Mycobacterium tuberculosis.*
- *M. bovis.*

Macroscopic features
- Grey, white or light yellowish nodules in lungs.
- Nodules are hard, painful and/or calcified.
- Animal carcass is cachectic, weak or emaciated.

Table 15.1 Differential features of various types of Pneumonia

	Bronchopneumonia	Interstitial	Fibrinous	Verminous	Aspiration	Mycotic	Tuberculous
Macroscopic features	1. Congestion and consolidation of anterior and ventral parts of lungs (Lobular pneumonia). 2. Patchy lesions on one or several lobes and adjacent area shows emphysema. 3. Mediastinal lymphnodes are swollen.	1. Lungs are pale or dark red in colour. 2. Oedema, dripping of fluid from cut surface	1. Antero-ventral portion of lung is congested and consolidated. 2. Colour of lungs become deep red due to congestion 3. Surface of lungs is covered by fibrin sheet. 4. Interlobular septa are prominent due to accumulation of plasma and fibrin.	1. Multiple petechial haemorrhage in lungs at the site of parasite penetration. 2. Mature worms in alveoli, bronchioles and bronchi. 3. Mucopurulent exudate in alveoli/bronchi. 4. Pulmonary oedema, emphysema.	1. Congestion and consolidation of anterior and ventral portion of lung. 2. Affected part becomes green/ black in colour, moist gangrene. 3. Affected lungs are often foul smelling. 4. Presence of foreign body like heads of wheats, parts of corn, oil, milk etc.	1. Nodules in lungs 2. On cut, cheese like caseative mass comes out from nodules. 3. Caseation involves both bronchiole and alveoli. 4. Such lesions may also present in trachea, bronchi and air sacs.	1. Grey, white or light yellowish nodules in lungs. 2. Nodules are hard, painful and/or calcified. 3. Animal carcass is cachectic, weak or emaciated. 4. On cut, the cheesy material comes out from the nodules.
Microscopic features	1. Congestion, oedema or haemorrhage in lung. 2. Infiltration of neutrophils, mononuclear cells in and around bronchioles/ bronchi. 3. Catarrhal inflammation of bronchi. 4. Proliferation of bronchiolar epithelium	1. Alveoli may have serous or fibrinous exudate. 2. Thickening of alveolar septa due to accumulation of exudate, inflammatory cells and in chronic cases, proliferation of fibrous tissue. 3. Infiltration of mononuclear cells in alveolar septa.	1. Principal exudate is fibrin, fills alveoli, bronchioles and bronchi. 2. Congestion and/or haemorrhages 3. Infiltration of neutrophils, macrophages and giant cells 4. Formation of eosinophilic false membrane of fibrin over the surface of alveoli and bronchiole and then known as "hyaline membrane pneumonia".	1. Dilation of bronchiole/ bronchi 2. Lesions of chronic suppurative bronchiolitis 3. Focal areas of inflammation in the vicinity of parasites and around bronchioles. 4. Hyperplasia of bronchiolar epithelium. 5. Infiltration of eosinophils and lymphocytes.	1. Thrombosis of blood vessels. 2. Necrosis in lungs. 3. Presence of saprophytes, leucocytes and bacteria cause liquefaction and gangrene. 4. Gangrenous lesions surrounded by intense inflammation 5. Congestion	1. Presence of granulomatus lesions i.e. caseative necrosis, macrophages, epithelioid cells, lymphocytes, giant cells, fibroblasts etc. 2. Presence of branched hyphae of fungi in the necrosed area.	1. Presence of tubercle/granuloma in lungs which comprises a central necrosed area surrounded by macrophages, epithelioid cells, lymphocytes, Langhan's giant cells and covered by fibrous covering. 2. Acid-fast rod shaped bacteria may present in necrosed area. 3. Central area may be calcified.

178

On cut, the cheesy material comes out from the nodules.

Microscopic features

- Presence of tubercle/granuloma in lungs which comprises a central necrosed area surrounded by macrophages, epithelioid cells, lymphocytes, Langhan's giant cells and covered by fibrous covering.
- Acid-fast rod shaped bacteria may be present in necrosed area.
- Central area may be calcified.

PULMONARY ADENOMATOSIS

Pulmonary adenomatosis is a slow viral disease of sheep and is characterized by metaplasia of alveolar squamous epithelium to cuboidal and /or columnar epithelium leading to glandular appearance of alveoli (Figs. 15.28 & 15.29).

Etiology

- Retrovirus.
  - Pulmonary adenomatosis virus.

Macroscopic features

- Multiple focal areas of consolidation in lungs.
- Imprint of ribs on lungs.
- Congestion and hardening of mediastinal lymphnodes.

Microscopic features

- Metaplasia of alveolar epithelium leading to formation of glandular structures in alveoli.
- Metaplasia of simple squamous epithelium to cuboidal or columnar epithelium which gives alveoli a gland like look.
- Mild inflammatory reaction.
- Proliferation of fibrous tissue.

HYPERSENSITIVITY PNEUMONITIS

Hypersensitivity pneumonitis is the inflammation of lung caused by an allergic reaction of antigen (allergen) and characterized by interstitial pneumonia, emphysema, hyaline membrane formation and hyperplasia of alveolar epithelium.

Etiology

- Allergens.
- Parasites – *Dictyocaulus viviparous.*
- Moldy hay.
- Fungus – *Aspergillus* sp.

Macroscopic features

- Lobes may contain small grey foci.
- Presence of yellow and dense mucus in lumen of bronchi.
- Excessive accumulation of air in lungs due to emphysema.
- Presence of worms/larvae.

Microscopic features

- Extensive infiltration of lymphocytes, monocytes and eosinophils around the bronchi and bronchioles.
- Accumulation of catarrhal exudate in bronchi/bronchiole.
- Emphysema as a result of widening of alveoli.
- Hyperplasia of bronchiolar musculature.
- Inflammatory cells in interalveolar septa may form small granulomas.
- Formation of hyaline membrane over alveolar and bronchiolar epithelium.

PNEUMOCONIASIS

Pneumoconiasis is the granulomatous inflammation of lungs caused by aerogenous dust particles of sand, silica, beryllium, carbon or asbestos. It is also known as anthracosis (Figs. 15.30 & 15.31).

Etiology

- Silica.
- Asbestos.
- Beryllium.
- Bauxite.
- Graphite.
- Carbon.
- Bronchogenous/aerogenous administration of particles inhaled with air, mostly around mines/factories.
- Generator smoke.

Macroscopic features

- Dense fibrous nodules in lungs.
- Presence of carbon particles in trachea/bronchi mixed with mucous exudate.

Microscopic features

- Granuloma formation around the particles of silica/asbestos infiltrated by macrophages, lymphocytes and giant cells
- Silica produces cellular reaction *'Silicosis'*.
- *Beryllium granuloma* looks like tubercule without caseation.
- *Asbestosis* is characterized by the presence of club shaped filaments bearing cells in lesion.

PATHOLOGY OF AIR SACS
AIR SACCULITIS

Air sacculitis is inflammation of air sacs caused by *E. coli*, Mycoplasma, reovirus etc. and characterized by thickening of the wall of air sacs and presence of cheesy exudate (Fig. 15.32).

Etiology

- *Escherichia coli.*
- *Mycoplasma gallisepticum.*
- Avian reovirus.

Macroscopic features

- Thickening of the air sac wall, which becomes dirty and cloudy.
- Presence of cheesy exudate in air sacs, congestion of lungs.
- Fibrinous pericarditis.
- Liver is covered with thin fibrinous membrane.

Microscopic features

- Oedema and infiltration of neutrophils and lymphocytes in air sacs.
- Caseous exudate in lungs and air sacs.

PATHOLOGY OF PLEURA
PLEURITIS

Pleuritis is the inflammation of pleura character--ized by serous, fibrinous or purulent exudate. It is also known as *pleurisy*.

Etiology

- *Mycobacterium tuberculosis.*
- *Mycoplasma mycoides.*
- *Haemophilus suis.*
- Organisms responsible for pneumonia/traumatic pericarditis may also cause pleuritis.

Macroscopic features

- Congestion of pleura.
- Serous, fibrinous or purulent exudate.
- Accumulation of clear fluid in pleura/thoracic cavity is called as *hydrothorax*.
- Presence of blood in thoracic cavity is known as *Hemothorax*.
- Suppurative exudate in thoracic cavity is known as *pyothorax*.
- Presence of air in pleural cavity is termed as *pneumothorax*, while presence of lymph in pleural cavity is called as *chylothorax*.
- Tuberculous pleuritis is characterized by small nodules on pleura and is known as *"pearly disease"*.
- In chronic cases, development of fibrous tissue causes adhesions and is known as *adhesive pleuritis*.

Microscopic features

- Congestion of blood vessels.
- Infiltration of neutrophils and lymphocytes.
- Thickening of pleura due to oedema.
- Proliferation of fibroblasts producing adhesive lesions.

MODEL QUESTIONS

Q. 1. **Fill in the gaps with suitable word(s).**
1. .... is the inflammation of lungs characterized by .... and .... of lungs.
2. Lobar pneumonia is characterized by .... of interalveolar septa.
3. Fibrinous pneumonia is characterized by the presence of .... exudate in alveoli and may give rise to.............formation which is............of fibrin over the surface of............and ....
4. Aspiration pneumonia is caused by .... of drugs/ milk and is characterized by .... and .... formation in the lungs.
5. *Mycobacterium tuberculosis* produces .... pneumonia in lungs characterized by .... formation consisting of .... central area surrounded by ...., ..., ..., ..., and covered by .... capsule.
6. Pulmonary adenomatosis is caused by .... and is characterized by .... of alveolar squamous epithelium to .... or .... leading to .... appearance of alveoli.
7. Allergic reaction due to .... may cause .... characterized by ...., ..., ... and .... of alveolar epithelium.
8. Pneumoconiasis is .... inflammation of lungs caused by aerogenous................. of ...., ... or .... and it is also known as ....
9. Inflammation of air sacs in poultry is known as.................and is caused by ...., ... and................. and characterized by................. and ....
10. .... pleuritis is also known as................. while the presence of lymph in pleural cavity is termed as.................

Q. 2. **Write true or false against each statement and correct the false statements.**
1. ....Bronchopneumonia is the inflammation of lungs characterized by thickening of interalveolar septa.
2. ....Verminous pneumonia is caused by *Bordetella bronchiseptica*.
3. ....Gangrenous pneumonia occurs due to faulty drenching of medicines.
4. ....Mycotic pneumonia is caused by *E. coli*.
5. ....Granulomatous pneumonia is produced by *Blastomyces* sp.
6. ....Pearly disease is caused by *Mycoplasma myoides*.
7. ....Atelectic lung floats in water.
8. ....*Oestrus ovis* is the cause of nasal granuloma is sheep.
9. ....Metaplasia of alveolar epithelium occurs in hypersensitivity pneumonitis.
10. ....Air sacculitis is caused by *E. coli*.

Q.3. **Define the followings.**
1. Rhinitis
2. Sinusitis
3. Laryngitis
4. Pharyngitis
5. Hydrothorax
6. Pyothorax
7. Epistaxis
8. Hyaline membrane
9. Silicosis
14. Tracheobronchitis
15. Pneumothorax
16. Red hepatization
17. Carnification
18. Lung worms
19. Atelectasis neonatorum
20. Bronchiolitis
21. Beryllium granuloma
22. Peribronchitis

10. Asbestosis
11. Pleurisy
12. Chylothorax
13. Adhesive pleuritis

23. Hemothorax
24. Alveolitis
25. Pearly disease

Q. 4.   *Write short notes on.*
1. Porcine atrophic rhinitis
2. Nasal polyps
3. Nasal granuloma
4. Atelectasis
5. Pathogenesis of pneumonia
6. Lobar pneumonia
7. Hyaline membrane pneumonia
8. Gangrenous pneumonia
9. Infectious laryngotracheitis
10. Emphysema
11. Pulmonary adenomatosis
12. Bronchopneumonia
13. Mycotic pneumonia
14. Granulomatous pneumonia
15. Air sacculitis

Q. 5.   *Match the word(s) from four options given against each statement.*
1. Nasal polyps are caused by ....
   (a) *Schistosoma nasalis* (b) *Rhinosporidium sceberi* (c) *E. coli* (d) *Mycoplasma mycoides*
2. Canine tracheobronchitis is caused by...........
   (a) Adenovirus   (b) Influenza virus   (c) Herpes virus   (d)All of the above
3. Presence of caseous plugs in bronchi at the point of entrance in lungs in characteristic lesions of ....
   (a) Infectious bronchitis (b) Infectious laryngotracheitis (c) Air sacculitis   (d) Pleuritis
4. This is not the pathologic lesion of pneumonia...........
   (a) Congestion   (b) Red hepatization   (c) Yellow hepatization   (d) Resolution
5. Infection through aerogenous route may cause ....pneumonia
   (a) Lobar   (b) Lobular   (c) Hypersensitivity   (d) Fibrinous
6. Verminous pneumonia is caused by ....
   (a) Mycoplasma   (b) Chlamydia   (c) *Dictayocaulus* sp.   (d) *E. coli*
7. Langhan's type giant cell is characteristic feature of ....pneumonia
   (a) Tuberculous   (b) Verminous   (c) Broncho   (d) Pulmonary adenomatosis
8. Atelectasis neonatorum is characteristic features of ....
   (a) Premature birth   (b) Aborted foetus   (c) Still birth   (d) None
9. Hypersensitivity pneumonitis is caused by ....
   (a) Allergens   (b) Parasites   (c) Moldy hay   (d)All of the above
10. Pneumoconiasis is characterized by ....lesions in lungs
    (a) Serus   (b) Fibrinous   (c) Haemorrhagic   (d) Granulomatous

16

PATHOLOGY OF DIGESTIVE SYSTEM

- **Developmental anomalies**
- **Pathology of Mouth cavity**
- **Pathology of Esophagus and crop**
- **Pathology of Stomach**
- **Pathology of Intestines**
- **Pathology of liver and pancreas**
- **Pathology of peritoneum**
- **Model Questions**

DEVELOPMENTAL ANOMALIES

Epitheliogenesis imperfecta of tongue
Abnormal smooth surface of tongue due to small filiform papillae. It occurs as a defect in autosomal recessive gene and occurs in Holstein-Friesian cattle. This is also known as smooth tongue.

Cleft palate
This is most common congenital abnormality that occurs due to failure of oral-nasal cavity to divide leaving cleft. It may also extend towards lips producing 'harelip' condition.

Mega colon
There is distention of colon which abruptly terminates in rectum due to mutant gene in dogs.

Duplication of colon
In dog, the colon is duplicated from caecum to rectum and this defect is associated with malformation in the body of vertebrae T_4 and T_5.

Atresia coli
In calf, the absence of colon occurs and the intestine terminates in blind caecum.

Atresia ani
This is absence of anal opening.

PATHOLOGY OF MOUTH CAVITY STOMATITIS
Stomatitis in the inflammation of mucosa of oral cavity (Figs. 16.1 to 16.6). It includes:
Gingivitis: Inflammation of gums.
Glossitis: Inflammation of tongue.
Cheilitis: Inflammation of lips.
Tonsilitis: Inflammation of tonsil.
Palatitis/Lampas: Inflammation of palates.

Etiology
- Trauma due to nails, wire, or any sharp object like needle.
- Physical due to hot milk, medicines etc.
- Chemical – Alkali / acids.
- Microorganisms – Bacteria, virus, fungi.

Macroscopic features
- Catarrhal stomatitis: Mucous exudation in oral cavity.
- Vesicular stomatitis: Vesicles in oral mucosal *e.g.* FMD.
- Erosive stomatitis: Erosions in oral mucosa *e.g.* Rinderpest.
- Fibrinous stomatitis: False membrane in oral mucosa.
- Ulcerative stomatitis: Presence of ulcers in oral mucosa *e.g.* mucosal disease.

Microscopic features
- Congestion of oral mucosa.
- Presence of erosions, vesicles or ulcers.
- Infiltration of neutrophils, lymphocytes and macrophages.
- Presence of fibrinous exudate in the form of diphtheritic membrane.

PATHOLOGY OF OESOPHAGUS AND CROP CHOKE
Choke is complete or partial obstruction of oesophagus either due to any foreign material or pressure from adjoining areas (Fig. 16.7).

Etiology
- Beets, turnip, carrots, bone.
- Abscess, tumor of neck area.

Macroscopic features
- Tympany.
- Gangrene, sapremia and toxaemia.
- Sac-like dilatation "Oesophageal diverticulum"
- Perforation due to sharp bone ends.

Microscopic features
- Necrosis gangrene at a point of obstruction.
- Congestion haemorrhage in perforated cases.

OESOPHAGITIS
Oesophagitis is the inflammation of oesophagus caused by trauma, parasites etc. and is characterized by catarrhal inflammation, ulceration or stenosis due to fibrosis.

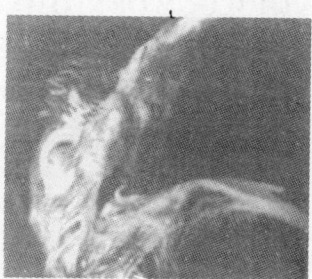

Fig. 16.1. Photograph of mouth cavity of a bird showing stomatitis due to avian pox

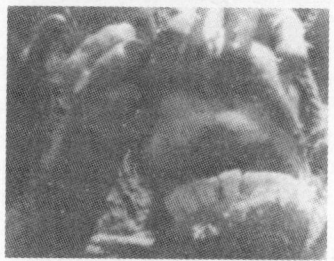

Fig 16.2. Photograph of mouth cavity of a buffalo having erosive palatitis

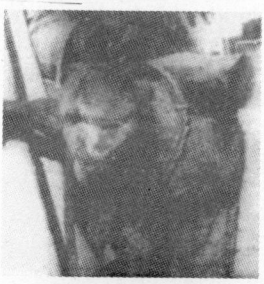

Fig. 16.3. Photograph of mouth of a camel showing cheilitis

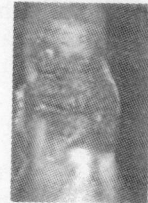

Fig 16.4. Photograph of tongue showing granulomatous lesions (ARS/USDA)

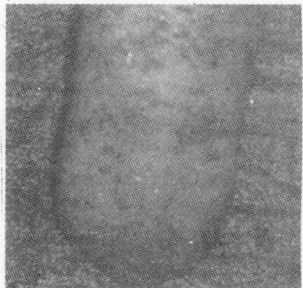

Fig 16.5. Photograph of tongue showing ulcerative glossitis (ARS/USDA)

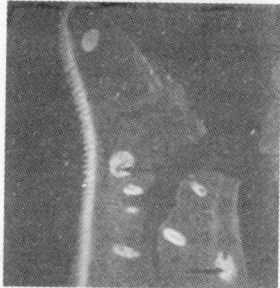

Fig 16.6. Photograph of tongue showing glossitis due to cysticercosis.(ARS/USDA)

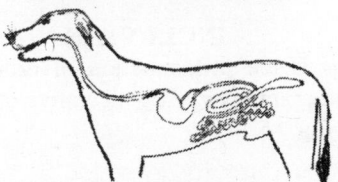

Fig 16.7. Diagram of alimentary tract of dog showing choke in oesophagus due to bone

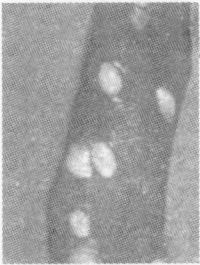

Fig 16.8. Photograph of oesophagus showing presence of cysts due to sarcosporidiosis (ARS/USDA)

Etiology

- Trauma due to foreign bodies.
- Chemicals – Acids, alkalies.
- Infection – Mucosal disease virus.
- Parasite – *Spirocerca lupi, sarcosporidiosis (Fig. 16.8)*.
- Nutritional – Vit. A deficiency.

Macroscopic features

- Congestion.
- Ulcer formation (Fig. 16.9).
- Red streaks of catarrhal inflammation.
- Stenosis due to fibrous nodules or inflammatory exudate.
- Enlargement of glands due to Vit A. defi. (Fig. 16.10).

Microscopic features

- Congestion, haemorrhage.
- Ulceration.
- Infilteration of neutrophils, lymphocytes.
- Sub-epithelial fibrosis/nodules by *Spirocerea lupi*.

INGLUVITIS

Ingluvitis is the inflammation of crop caused by fungi and characterized by ulcerative or diphtheritic lesions (Fig. 16.11).

Etiology

- *Candida albicans.*
- *Monilia albicans.*

Macroscopic features

- Turkis towl-like appearance in crop mucosa.
- Round and raised ulcers.
- In moniliasis, formation of diphtheritic membrane.

Microscopic features

- Necrotic and ulcerative lesions.
- Fibrinous inflammation with infiltration of mononuclear cells.

PATHOLOGY OF STOMACH
TYMPANY

Tympany is accumulation of gases in rumen due to failure of eructation as a result of obstruction or due to excessive production of gases characterized by distended rumen and dyspnoea. It is also known as *bloat* (Fig. 16.12).

Etiology

- Choke of oesophagus.
- Sudden change in animal feed with high content of legumes.
- Excessive lush green fodder.

Macroscopic features

- Rumen is distended due to excessive accumulation of gases (CO_2, H_2S, CO).
- Distended rumen compresses diaphragm to hinder respiration.
- Tarry colour blood, pale liver and rupture of diaphragm.
- On rupture of rumen gas comes out (dry tympany).
- The gas is trapped in small bubbles in the ruminal fluid forming foams and is not easily removed. This is known as *"frothy bloat"*, which is produced by saponin and water soluble proteins and due to reduction in surface tension in the absence of fatty acids that favours froth formation.

Microscopic features

- Haemorrhage in lungs, pericardium, trachea and lymphnodes.
- Atelectasis in lungs.

RUMENITIS

Rumenitis is the inflammation of rumen in ruminant animals caused by change in diet, chemicals or drugs and characterized by seropurulent exudate or ulcer formation with or without parakeratosis.

Etiology

- Change in diet, corn or alfaalfa hay.
- Chemicals/drugs *e.g.* potassium antimony tarterate.
- *Spherophorus necrophorus* infection

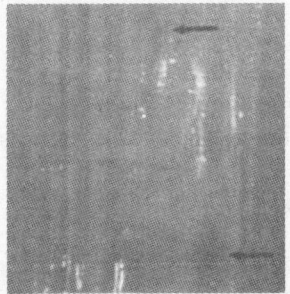

Fig. 16.9. Photograph showing ulcerative esophagitis due to bovine viral diarrhoea.virus

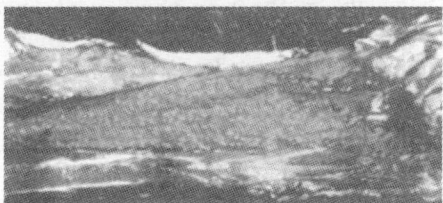

Fig. 16.10. Photograph of oesophagus showing nutritional roup

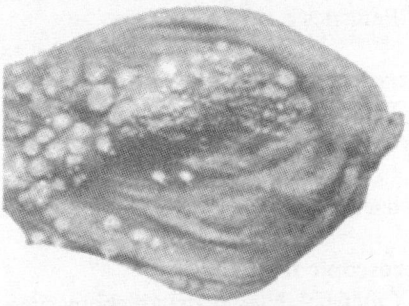

Fig. 16.11. Photograph of crop showing ingluvitis

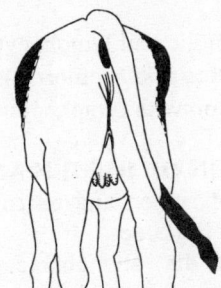

Fig. 16.12. Diagram showing tympauy in a cow

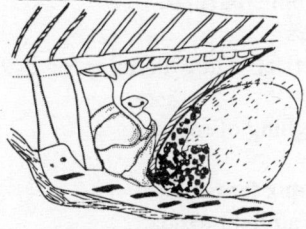

Fig. 16.13. Diagram showing penetration of needle from reticulum (Traumatic reticulitis)

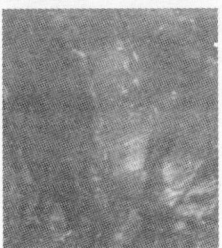

Fig. 16.14. Photograph showing ulcerative abomasitis

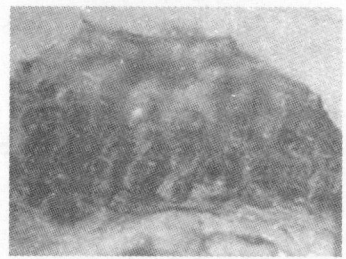

Fig 16.15. Photograph showing proventriculitis

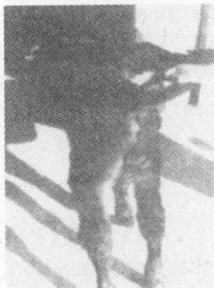

Fig 16.16. Photograph of calf showing diarrhoea

Macroscopic features
- Ulcers.
- Spherical white nodules of 1-2 cm diameter size.
- Sloughing of mucosa.

Microscopic features
- Seropurulent exudate.
- Ulcers
- Infiltration of lymphocytes and neutrophils.
- Fibrous nodules due to hyperplasia of fibroblasts.
- Parakeratosis.

RETICULITIS

Reticulitis is the inflammation of reticulum in ruminant animals caused by trauma/perforation by foreign body including sharp object like needles, wires, etc. and characterized by abscess formation, adhesions, peritonitis and pericarditis (Fig. 16.13).

Etiology
- Foreign body – sharp objects like needles, wires etc.

Macroscopic features
- Perforation of reticulum by foreign body.
- Abscessation/suppuration.
- Peritonitis, adhesions of reticulum with diaphragm.
- Pericarditis due to foreign body (traumatic reticulo pericarditis).

Microscopic features
- Infiltration of neutrophils, macrophages, lymphocytes.
- Proliferation of fibroblasts producing adhesions.
- Liquifactive necrosis.

OMASITIS

Omasitis is the inflammation of omasum in ruminant animals caused by *Actinobacillus* sp. and characterized by granulomatous inflammatory reaction.

Etiology
- *Actinobacillus ligneiresi*.

Macroscopic features
- Granulomatous nodules in omasum.

Microscopic features
- Typical granuloma formation.
- Sulphur granules of Actinobacillus in the centre of lesion.

ABOMASITIS

Abomasitis is the inflammation of abomasum in ruminants caused by chemicals/drugs, bacteria, virus or parasites and characterized by congestion, oedema and/or haemorrhagic ulcers (Fig. 16.14).

Etiology
- Chemicals/drugs.
- Bacteria *e.g. Clostridium septicum* cause of braxy.
- Virus *e.g.* Hog cholera, mucosal disease.
- Parasites *e.g. Theileria* sp.

Macroscopic features
- Presence of ulcers (button ulcers in Hog cholera).
- Congestion, oedema of abomasal folds, haemorrhage in braxy.

Microscopic features
- Catarrhal, haemorrhagic abomasits.
- Presence of Gram positive rods in case of braxy.
- Neutrophilic and lymphocytic infiltration.
- Congestion and haemorrhages.
- Ulceration with lymphocytic infiltration.

IMPACTION OF RUMEN AND RETICULUM

Impaction of rumen and reticulum is common in cattle and buffaloes. It is caused by heavy carbohydrate diet and characterized by atony of rumen, indigestion, acidosis and haemorrhage on serous membranes.

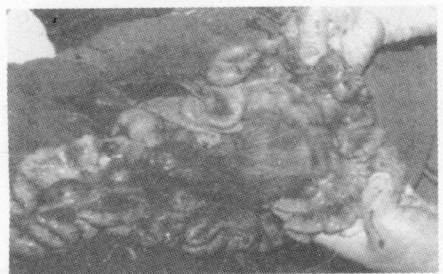

Fig. 16.17. Photograph showing enteritis

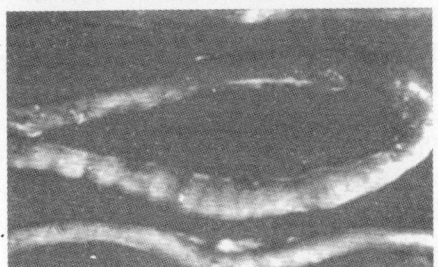

Fig. 16.18. Photograph showing catarrhal enteritis

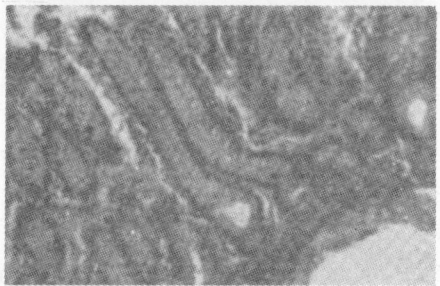

Fig. 16.19. Photomicrograph showing catarrhal enteritis

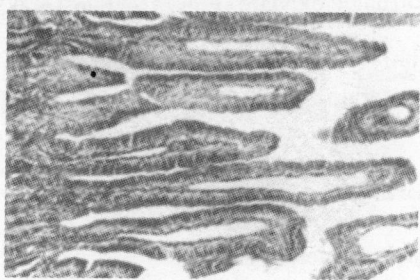

Fig. 16.20. Photomicrograph showing normal length of villi in intestine

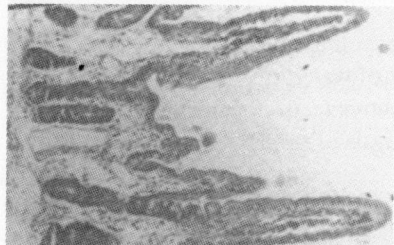

Fig. 16.21. Photomicrograph showing reduced length of villi due to rotavirus

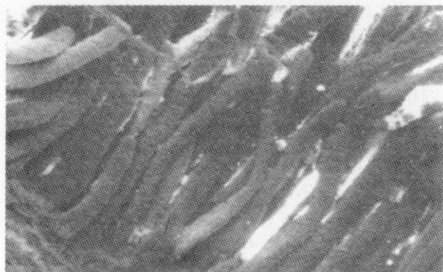

Fig. 16.22. Scanning electron microphotograph showing normal length of villi

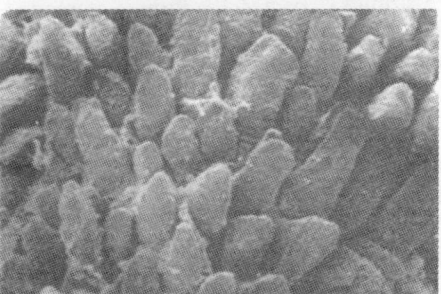

Fig. 16.23. Scanning electron microphotograph showing reduced length of villi with rough surface

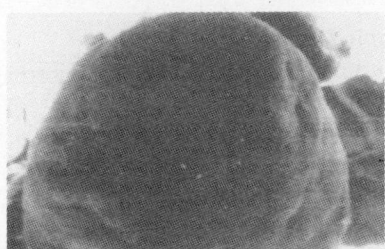

Fig. 16.24. Scanning electron microphotograph showing smooth surface of villi

Etiology

- Overfeeding of carbohydrate feed.
- Lack of water.
- Defective teeth or damaged tongue.
- Paralysis of rumen.

Macroscopic features

- Atony of rumen due to lactic acid production.
- Rumen is filled with hard, caked undigested food with foul odour.
- Hemoconcentration, anuria, blood becomes dark in colour.

Microscopic features

- Haemorrhage in lungs.
- Desquamation of ruminal epithelium.
- Lesions of acidosis/toxicosis.

GASTRITIS

Gastritis is the inflammation of stomach in non-ruminant animals having simple stomach caused by chemicals/drugs, bacteria, virus, parasite and characterized by congestion, oedema, haemorrhage and ulceration. Inflammation of proventriculus in poultry is termed as proventriculitis (Fig. 16.15).

Etiology

- Physical – overfeeding, trauma.
- Chemicals – Acid/alkali.
- Microorganisms such as bacteria, virus, fungi.
- Parasites *e.g. Trichostrongyles* sp., *Hemonchus* sp.
- Uremia.

Macroscopic features

- Congestion, oedema and haemorrhage of mucosal surface.
- Thick mucous exudate in stomach.
- Presence of vesicles/ulcers on gastric mucosa.

Microscopic features

- Congestion and haemorrhage of gastric mucosa.
- Presence of ulcers/necrosis.
- Infiltration of mononuclear cells.
- Lymphoid hyperplasia.

PATHOLOGY OF INTESTINES
CATARRHAL ENTERITIS

Catarrhal enteritis is characterized by increased number of goblet cells, congestion and infiltration of neutrophils and mononuclear cells in mucosa of intestine (Figs. 16.16 to 16.25).

Etiology

- Physical – Foreign bodies and corase feed
- Chemical – drugs
- Microorganisms – *E.coli, Salmonella* sp., viruses
- Parasites – Coccidia

Macroscopic features

- Presence of catarrhal exudate in lumen of intestine and congestion.
- Thickening of the wall of intestine.
- Diarrhoea.
- Presence of parasites in lumen of intestine.

Microscopic features

- Increased number of goblet cells in intestinal villi, reduced length of villi.
- Congestion.
- Infiltration of polymorphonuclear and mononuclear cells.

HAEMORRHAGIC ENTERITIS

Haemorrhagic enteritis is characterized by inflammation of the intestines along with haemorrhagic exudate (Figs. 16.26 to 16.28).

Etiology

- Bacteria – *E. coli, Bacillus anthracis, Salmonella* sp.
- Virus – Coronavirus, BVD, MD, RP.
- Parasites – Coccidia.

Macroscopic features

- Haemorrhagic exudate in intestines; blood mixed intestinal contents.
- Petechial or echymotic haemorrhage in mucosa and submucosa of intestine.
- Presence of erosions/ulcers in mucosa.

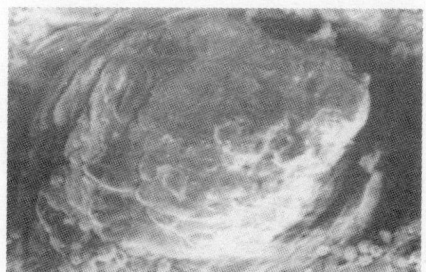

Fig. 16.25. Scanning electron microphotograph
showing rough surface of villi

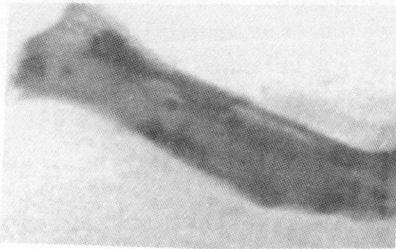

Fig. 16.26. Photograph showing haemorrhagic
enteritis

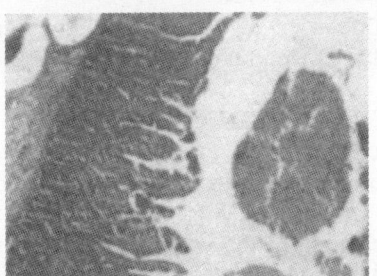

Fig. 16.27. Photomicrograph showing haemorrhagic
enteritis

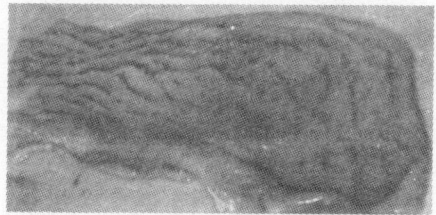

Fig. 16.28. Photograph showing linear
haemorrhage (Zebra marking) in large intestine

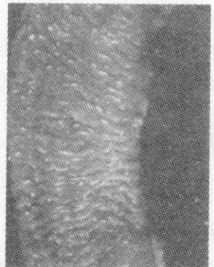

Fig. 16.29. Photograph showing corrugations in
large intistine indicative of chronic enteritis

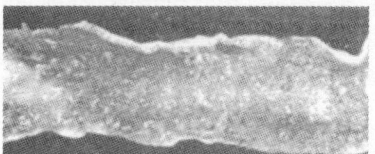

Fig. 16.30. Photograph showing necrotic enteritis
in birds due to clostridia

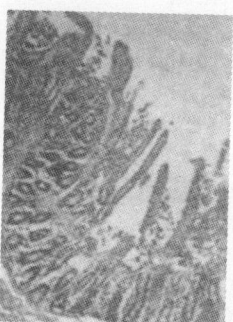

Fig. 16.31. Photomicrograph showing
necrotic enteritis

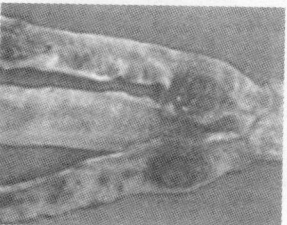

Fig. 16.32. Photograph showing
necrotic enteritis

Microscopic features
- Haemorrhage in the mucosa of intestine.
- Infiltration of neutrophils and mononuclear cells.
- Erosion or ulcers in intestinal mucosa.
- Presence of coccidia in the mucosa.

CHRONIC ENTERITIS

Chronic enteritis is the chronic inflammation of intestine characterized by proliferative changes like proliferation of fibrous tissue, infiltration of mononuclear cells and plasma cells in lamina propria leading to hardening of intestinal wall.

Etiology
- *Mycobacterium paratuberculosis* in bovines
- Intestinal helminths
- *E. coli* in poultry (Hjarre's disease)

Macroscopic features
- Thickening of the wall of intestine (corrugations in Johne's disease) (Fig. 16.29).
- Thick mucous cover over mucosa of intestine
- Transverse corrugations in the large intestine.
- Granulomatous nodules in duodenum.
- Small, round, raised necrotic foci on serosal surface of intestine covering whole length of intestine.

Microscopic features
- Proliferation of fibrous tissue in lamina propria.
- Infiltration of macrophages, lymphocytes, plasma cells.
- Atrophy of intestinal glands.

NECROTIC ENTERITIS

Necrotic enteritis is characterized by necrosis of mucosal epithelium of intestine leading to erosions/ulcer formation and exposition of underlying tissues (Figs. 16.30 to 16.32).

Etiology
- Salmonella.

- Rinderpest, rotavirus, cornovirus, Hog cholera virus.
- Coccidia, Histoplasma.
- Niacin deficiency.
- *Clostridium* sp. after coccidial infection in birds.

Macroscopic features
- Necrotic patches in intestines.
- Fibrinous deposits over necrotic patches like bran deposits.
- Swelling of mesenteric lymphnodes.
- Ulcers in intestine.

Microscopic features
- Congestion and infiltration of mononuclear cells.
- Necrosis and desquamation of intestinal villus epithelium, leading to exposed underlying tissue.
- Ulcers in mucosa.
- Proliferation of crypt epithelium, presence of abnormal epithelium over villus surface.

PARASITIC ENTERITIS

Parasitic enteritis is caused by parasites and is characterized by catarrhal and/or haemorrhagic exudate in intestine, presence of ova/adult parasite and thickening of the wall of intestine (Figs. 16.33 & 16.34).

Etiology
- Helminths :
  - Roundworms
  - Tapeworms
- Protozoa :
  - Coccidia
  - Histoplasma

Macroscopic features
- Presence of parasite helminths in the lumen of intestine.
- Thickening of the wall of intestine.
- Catarrhal or haemorrhagic exudate in intestine.

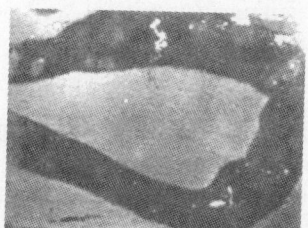

Fig.16.33.Photograph showing parasitic
enteritis (Coccidiosis)

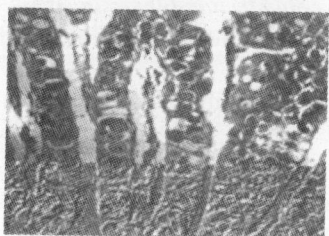

Fig.16.34.Photomicrograph showing
parasitic enteritis (Coccidiosis)

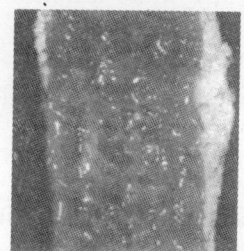

Fig.16.35.Photograph showing
fibrinous enteritis

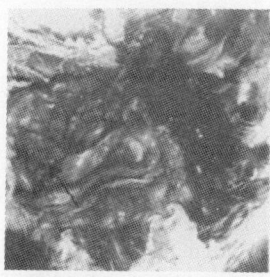

Fig.16.36.Photograph showing granulomatous
lesion in duodenum of poultry

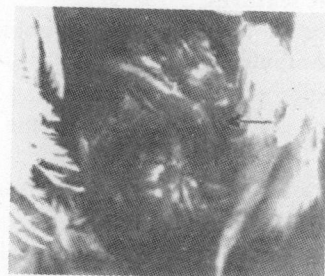

Fig.16.37. Photograph showing small tiny
necrotic granulomatous lesion on intestine

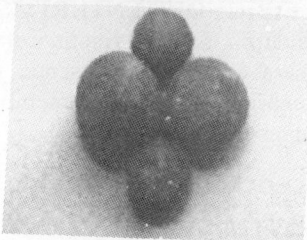

Fig.16.38. Photograph showing piliconcretions
(hair balls) recovered from stomach of calves

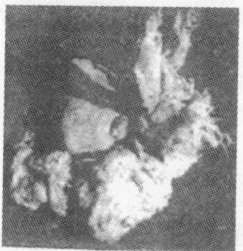

Fig.16.39.Photograph showing polybezoars
recovered from stomach of a barking deer

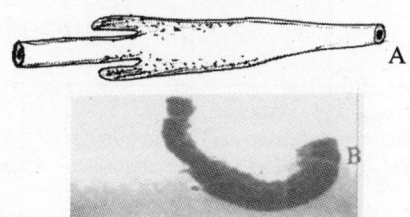

Fig.16.40.Diagram (A) and photograph (B)
showing intussusception in intestine

Microscopic features
- Presence of large number of goblet cells in mucosa of intestine.
- Congestion and/or haemorrhage.
- Presence of parasite/ova in the intestinal lumen.
- Infiltration of eosinophils in mucosa and submucosa of the intestines.
- Coccidia can be seen on mucosal scrapings under microscope.

FIBRINOUS ENTERITIS

Fibrinous enteritis is the fibrinous inflammation of intestine characterized by presence of fibrinous exudate comprising of pseudomembrane in the mucosa of intestine (Fig. 16.35).

Etiology
- *Salmonella choleraesuis.*
- *Spherophorus necrophorus.*

Macroscopic features
- Presence of diphtheritic membrane over mucosa of intestine.
- Button ulcers.
- Sometimes, diphtheritic membrane covers the faeces.

Microscopic features
- Congestion and haemorrhage in intestine.

- Thickening of intestinal wall due to fibrinous exudate.
- Fibrin network in mucosa.

GRANULOMATOUS ENTERITIS

Granulomatous enteritis is caused by bacteria or fungi and is characterized by granuloma formation in the intestines (Figs. 16.36 & 16.37).

Etiology
- *Mycobacterium tuberculosis.*
- Coli granuloma – *E. coli* in poultry (Hjarre's disease).
- Coccidioidomycosis / candidiasis.

Macroscopic features
- Granulomatous about cm diameter elevated/ raised areas on the serus surface of intestine.
- Thickening of the wall of intestine.
- Small, tiny, white necrotic nodules on serosa.

Microscopic features
- Granuloma formation consisting of central necrosed area covered by lymphocytes, macrophages, epithelioid cells, giant cells and fibrous connective tissue.
- Extensive proliferation of fibrous tissue.
- Presence of bacteria / fungus in the lesion.

Table 16.1 Differential features of various types of Enteritis

	Catarrhal	Haemorrhagic	Chronic	Necrotic	Parasitic	Fibrinous	Granulomatous
Macroscopic features	1. Presence of catarrhal exudate in lumen of intestine and congestion. 2. Thickening of the wall of intestine.	1. Haemorrhagic exudate in intestines; blood mixed intestinal contents. 2. Petechial or echymotic haemorrhage	1. Thickening of the wall of intestine (Corrugations in Johne's disease). 2. Thick mucous cover over	1. Necrotic patches in intestines. 2. Fibrinous deposits over necrotic patches like bran deposits 3. Swelling of mesenteric	1. Presence of parasite helminths in the lumen of intestine. 2. Thickening of the wall of intestine. 3. Catarrhal or	1. Presence of diphtheritic membrane over mucosa of intestine. 2. Button ulcers 3. Sometimes,	1. Granulomatous about one cm diameter elevated/ raised areas on the serus surface of intestine. 2. Thickening

	3. Presence of parasites in lumen of intestine.	in mucosa and submucosa of intestine. 3. Presence of erosions/ ulcers in mucosa.	mucosa of intestine 3. Transverse corrugations in the large intestine. 4. Granulomatous nodules in duodenum. 5. Small, round, raised necrotic foci on serosal surface of intestine covering whole length of intestine.	lymphnodes 4. Ulcers in intestine.	haemorrhagic exudate in intestine.	diphtheritic membrane covers the faeces.	of the wall of intestine. 3. Small, tiny, white necrotic nodules on serosa.
Microscopic features	1. Increased number of goblet cells in intestinal villi, reduced length of villi. 2. Congestion. 3. Infiltration of polymorpho nuclear and mononuclear cells.	1. Haemorrhage in the mucosa of intestine 2. Infiltration of neutrophils and mononuclear cells. 3. Erosion or ulcers in intestinal mucosa	1. Proliferation of fibrous tissue in lamina propria. 2. Infiltration of macrophages, lymphocytes, plasma cells. 3. Atrophy of intestinal glands.	1. Congestion and infiltration of mononuclear cells. 2. Necrosis and desquamation of intestinal villus epithelium, leading to exposed underlying tissue. 3. Ulcers in mucosa. 4. Proliferation of crypt epithelium, presence of abnormal epithelium over villus surface.	1. Presence of large number of goblet cells in mucosa of intestine. 2. Congestion and/ or haemorrhage. 3. Presence of parasite/ova in the intestinal lumen 4. Infiltration of eosinophils in mucosa and submucosa of the intestines. 5. Coccidia can be seen on mucosal scrapings under microscope.	1. Congestion and haemorrhage in intestine. 2. Thickening of intestinal wall due to fibrinous exudate. 3. Fibrin network in mucosa.	1. Granuloma formation consisting of central necrosed area covered by lymphocytes, macrophages, epithelioid cells, giant cells and fibrous connective tissue 2. Extensive proliferation of fibrus tissue. 3. Presence of bacteria/ fungus in the lesion.

INTESTINAL OBSTRUCTION

Obstruction of intestines may occur as a result of foreign body, enterolith, piliconcretions, phytobezoars, polybezoars or due to hypermotility of intestines leading to intussusception, volvulus or torsion.

Piliconcretions

Piliconcretions are hair balls mostly found in stomach/intestines of animals having habit of licking. This vice is more common in suckling calves and in animals with pica related to phosphorus deficiency. The hairs are accumulated in stomach which become in rounded shape due to movements of stomach and look like balls. Such hair balls are not degradable in gastrointestinal tract and may cause obstruction (Fig. 16.38).

Phytobezoars/Polybezoars

Concretions formed in gastrointestinal tract as a result of deposition of salts around a nidus of undigested plants or polythenes. They may cause obstruction in gastrointestinal tract (Fig. 16.39).

Foreign bodies

Foreign bodies like rubber balls, nuts, bones, stones, plastic and rubber materials, polythenes may obstruct the intestinal tract as they are not degradable in the gastrointestinal tract.

Hernia

Hernia is presence of intestinal loop in umbilical area, scrotum or inguinal cavity which causes passive congestion, oedema and obstruction in intestines.

Intussusception

Intussusception is telescoping of intestine means a portion of intestine enters in caudal segment due to violent peristaltic movement. It causes obstruction, passive congestion and oedema (Fig. 16.40).

Volvulus

In volvulus, the loop of intestine passes through a tear in mesentry. It causes obstruction at both ends of loop (Fig. 16.41).

Torsion

Torsion is twisting of intestine upon itself causing obstruction (Fig. 16.42).

Enterolith

Concretions in intestines particularly in horses are responsible for obstruction of intestinal tract and cause "colic in horse" and enterocolitis (Fig. 16.43).

TYPHLITIS

Typhlitis is the inflammation of caecum. It is particularly important in poultry, caused by protozoan parasites and characterized by haemorrhage, thickening of the wall, presence of cheesy exudates and/or necrotic ulcers (Fig. 16.44).

Etiology

- *Eimeria tennella.*
- *Histomonas meleagridis.*

Macroscopic features

- Haemorrhage in caecum, blood mixed contents.
- Thickening of the wall, with congestion and cheesy exudates.

Presence of necrotic ulcers in caecum in case of histomoniasis which is further supported by round, depressed, yellowish-green areas of necrosis in liver.

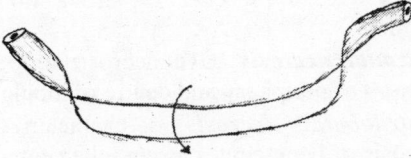

Fig.16.41. Diagram showing volvulus in intestine

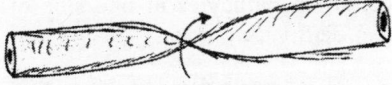

Fig.16.42.Diagram showing torsion in intestine

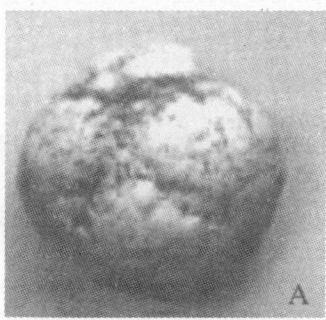

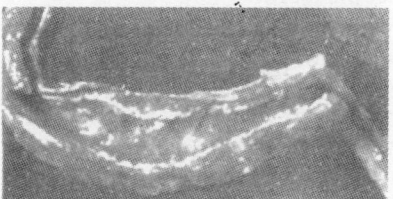

Fig.16.44.Photograph showing typhlitis in poultry

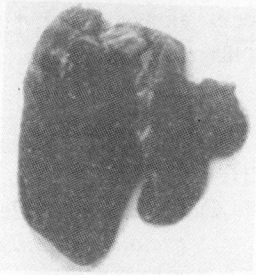

Fig.16.45.Photograph of liver showing hepatitis with focal necrosis

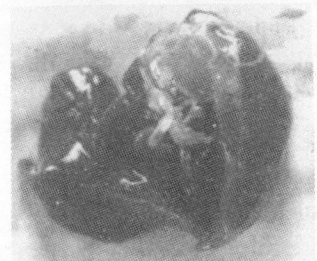

Fig.16.46.Photograph showing presence of fibrinous membrane on liver (Colisepticemia.)

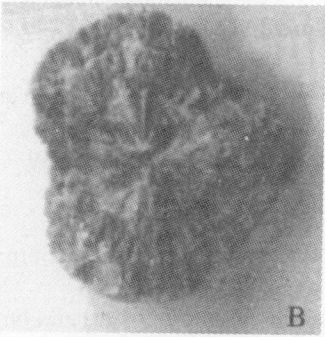

Fig.16.43.Photograph showing A. enterolith recovered from colon of a horse B. cross section of enterolith showing lamillated deposition of salts

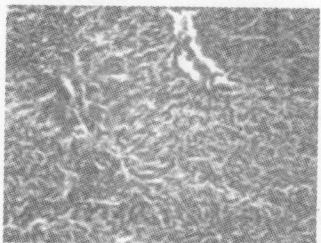

Fig.16.47.Photomicrograph showing focal necrosis

Microscopic features

- Congestion, haemorrhage, necrosis.
- Presence of protozoan parasites.
- Necrotic hepatic lesions.

HEPATITIS

Hepatitis is the inflammation of liver. It may be acute or chronic. Acute hepatitis is characterized by the presence of degeneration and necrosis of hepatocytes and infiltration of neutrophils and mononuclear cells along with hyperemia and/or haemorrhage (Figs. 16.45 to 16.48).

Etiology

- Bacteria – Necrobacillosis, *Salmonella, E. coli.*
- Virus – ICH.
- Chemicals – Carbon tetrachloride.
- Parasites – *Fasciola gigantica, Fasciola hepatica.*

Macroscopic features

- Enlargement of liver.
- Congestion and/or haemorrhage.
- Presence of necrotic patches in liver.
- Presence of fibrinous diphtheritic membrane on liver.

Microscopic features

- Cloudy swelling and/or fatty changes in liver.
- Congestion in blood vessels and in sinusoidal area.
- Infiltration of neutrophils, macrophages and lymphocytes.
- Necrosis of hepatic parenchyma.

In acute toxic hepatitis there is necrosis of hepatocytes. According to location it can be classified as under which is helpful in making diagnosis.

- *Diffused necrosis* covers a considerable area crossing over the lobular boundaries.
- *Focal necrosis* occupying only a part of lobule *e.g.* EHV induced aborted foetal liver.
- *Peripheral necrosis* is characterized by necrosis at the periphery of lobule which

occurs due to presence of strong toxins in blood.

- *Midzonal necrosis* have necrosis of cells in midway of periphery and centre of lobule.
- *Centrilobular necrosis* is characterized by necrosis of hepatocytes around the central vein and occurs due to stagnation of blood with toxaemia.
- *Paracentral necrosis* is characterized by necrosis of hepatocytes at one side of central vein *e.g.* Rift valley fever.

CIRRHOSIS

Cirrhosis is the chronic inflammation of liver characterized by extensive fibrosis, hepatic degeneration and necrosis (Fig. 16.49 to 16.51).

Etiology

- Bacteria – Salmonella, *Spherophorus necrophorous.*
- Virus – Infectious canine hepatitis.
- Chemicals – Carbon tetrachloride.
- Parasites – *Fasciola hepatica, F. giantica.*
- Poisons/toxins – Aflatoxins.
- Once cirrhosis of liver starts, it is not checked even after removal of the cause as the newly formed fibrous tissue itself acts as an irritant to cause further proliferation of fibroblasts.

Macroscopic features

- Liver becomes hard and firm.
- Surface of liver becomes uneven and nodular.
- Size of liver becomes reduced due to atrophy.
- Colour becomes yellowish, grey.

Microscopic features

- Increase in fibrous tissue within and around lobules.
- Infiltration of macrophages and lymphocytes.
- Central vein is either absent or placed eccentrically.
- Hepatocytes show degenerative and necrotic changes.

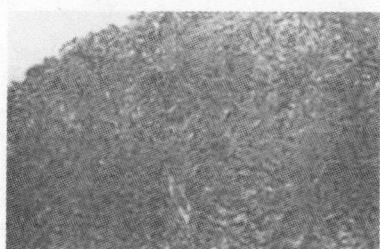

Fig.16.48.Photomicrograph of liver showing
diffuse necrosis

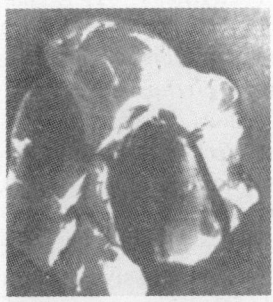

Fig.16.52.Photograph showing cholecystitis in birds

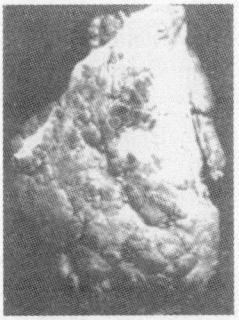

Fig.16.49.Photograph showing cirrhosis in liver

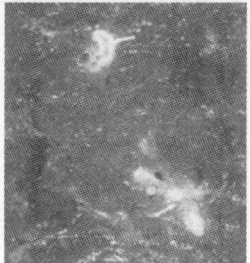

Fig.16.53.Photograph showing cholangitis
(ARS/USDA)

Fig.16.50.Photomicrograph showing
cirrhosis in liver

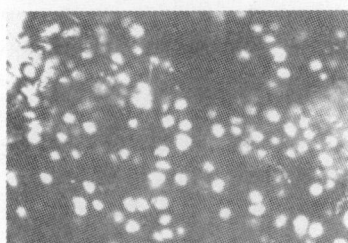

Fig.16.54.Photograph showing pearly
disease

Fig.16.51.Photomicrograph showing
cirrhosis in liver

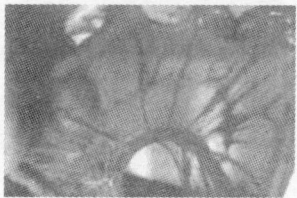

Fig.16.55.Photograph showing
haemorrhage in mesentry due to peritonitis

Biliary cirrhosis is characterized by proliferation of fibrous tissue around the bile ducts encircling them *e.g. Fasciola giantica.*

- ***Glissonian cirrhosis*** is mostly confined to areas at a short distance beneath the capsule.
- ***Pigment cirrhosis*** is associated with yellow discolouration.
- ***Central or cardiac cirrhosis*** is increase in fibrous tissue around the central vein as a result of chronic passive congestion.
- ***Parasitic cirrhosis*** occurs due to damage caused by migration of parasites *e.g. Ascaris lumbricoides, Schistosoma* sp.

CHOLECYSTITIS

Cholecystitis is the inflammation of gall bladder characterized by congestion, thickening of wall and infiltration of mononuclear cells. Cholangitis is the inflammation of bile duct (Figs. 16.52 & 16.53).

Etiology
- Parasites – *Fasciola* sp.
- Foreign body – Stones
- Bacteria – *E. coli.*

Macroscopic features
- Thickening of the wall of gall bladder.
- On opening of gall bladder, there may be parasites/stones/foreign body.
- Contents of gall bladder may be watery or thick oily.

Microscopic features
- Congestion.
- Proliferation of fibrous tissue in the wall of gall bladder.
- Infiltration of mononuclear cells.
- Increased number of mucus secreting cells.

PANCREATITIS

Pancreatitis is the inflammation of pancreas characterized by necrosis of pancreatic tissue, infiltration of neutrophils and mononuclear cells and fibrous tissue proliferation.

Etiology
- Bacteria.
- Virus- Reovirus in poultry.
- Parasites.

Macroscopic features
- Pancreas becomes pale, swollen, oedematous.
- In chronic cases, atrophy of pancreas.
- Pancreas becomes hard, firm, and fibrous.

Microscopic features
- Necrosis of pancreatic cells.
- Oedema, infiltration of leucocytes, haemorrhage.
- Fibrosis characterized by proliferation of fibroblasts.

PATHOLOGY OF PERITONIUM

Peritonitis is the inflammation of peritoneum characterized by hemorrhagic suppurative, serofibrinous or nodular lesions (FIg. 16.54 & 16.55).

Etiology
- Bacteria – Staphylococci, *Mycobacterium* sp.
- Virus.
- Neoplasia.
- Parasites .

Macroscopic features
- Serofibrinous, fibrinous, haemorrhagic, suppurative or granulomatous lesions.
- Accumulation of clear fluid is known as ***Hydroperitoneum*** or ***Ascites***.
- Presence of nodules in tuberculosis is also termed as *"**Pearly disease**"*.

Microscopic features
- Serofibrinous, suppurative or granulomatous lesions.
- Thickening of peritoneum, adhesions due to fibrosis.

MODEL QUESTIONS

Q. 1.   Fill in the blanks with suitable word(s).
1.   In esophagus sub-epithelial fibrous nodules are produced by ....
2.   Esophageal choke may lead to .... in ruminants characterized by .... rumen.
3.   Omasitis is the inflammation of..........caused by...............and characterized by...........nodules.
4.   *Clostridium septicum* may cause .... in sheep characterized by ...., ... and .... of abomasal folds.
5.   Haemorrhagic enteritis is the inflammation of .... along with .... exudates caused by ...., ... and .... bacteria and characterized by .... or .... haemorrhage in the intestinal wall.
6.   Chronic enteritis is the..............inflammation of intestine characterized by...............changes like ...., ...and .... in lamina propria leading to .... of intestinal wall.
7.   In poultry necrotic enteritis is caused by ....after the primary damage caused by ....
8.   Coligranuloma is also known as .... in poultry and is caused by ....
9.   .... is the cause of ingluvitis in poultry which produce .... like lesions.
10. In acute toxic hepatitis, necrosis occupying a considerable area in lobule is known as ....

Q. 2.   Write true or false, correct the false statements.
1.   ....Ulcerative stomatitis is a feature of mucosal disease in cattle.
2.   ....Impaction of rumen may lead to alkalosis.
3.   ....Hog cholera virus produces punched out ulcers in abomasum.
4.   ....Actinobacillosis in omasum is characterized by haemorrhagic lesions.
5.   ....Focal necrosis of liver covers a considerable area of lobules.
6.   ....Cirrhosis is the extensive fibrosis of liver.
7.   ....Once cirrhosis starts it can't be checked in spite of removal of causative agent.
8.   ....Parasitic cirrhosis is caused by *Fasciola gigantica*.
9.   ....Cholangitis is the inflammation of gall bladder.
10. ....Midzonal necrosis occurs in rift valley fever.

Q.3.   Define the followings.
1.   Necrotic enteritis
2.   Atresia ani
3.   Piliconcretions
4.   Glossitis
5.   Cleft palate
6.   Intussusception
7.   Phytobezoars
8.   Cardiac cirrhosis
9.   Cholangitis
10. Pearly disease
11. Ingluvitis
12. Polybezoars
13. Cheilitis
14. Volvulus
15. Gingivitis
16. Torsion of intestine
17. Atresia coli
18. Typhlitis
19. Glissonian cirrhosis
20. Parasitic cirrhosis

Q.4.   Write short notes on.
1.   Frothy blot
2.   Hjarre's disease
9.   Hernia
10. Necrosis in liver

3. Enteroliths
4. Cholecystitis
5. Traumatic reticulitis
6. Fibrinous enteritis
7. Impaction
8. Cirrhosis

11. Peritonitis
12. Chronic enteritis
13. Acute toxic hepatitis
14. Developmental anomalies of digestive system
15. Choke in esophagus

Q. 5. *Select appropriate word(s) from the four options given with each statement.*

1. Turkish towel like lesions are observed in ....
   (a) Candidiasis   (b) Histomoniasis   (c) Moniliasis   (d) Coccidiosis

2. Vesicular stomatitis is seen in cases of ....
   (a) Rinderpest   (b) Mucosal disease   (c) Hog cholera   (d) FMD

3. Choked oesophagus may cause .... in ruminants.
   (a) Impaction   (b) Vomition   (c) Tympany   (d) Gastritis

4. Rumen is distended due to accumulation of .... in bloat.
   (a) H_2S (b) CO_2 (c) CO   (d) All of the above

5. Traumatic reticulitis may lead to ....
   (a) Pericarditis   (b) Peritonitis   (c) Pleurisy   (d) All of the above

6. Increase in .... cells is observed in catarrhal enteritis.
   (a) Mast cells   (b) Eosinophils   (c) Goblet   (d) Neutrophils

7. Punched out ulcers are produced by ....
   (a) Theileria   (b) Babesia   (c) Hog cholera   (d) *Clostridium* sp.

8. Granulomatous lesions in intestine of poultry are observed in ....
   (a) Coli granuloma   (b) *E. coli* infection   (c) Hjarre's disease   (d) All of the above

9. Telescoping of intestine is also known as ....
   (a) Torsion   (b) Volvulus   (c) Intussusception   (d) None

10. *Eimeria tennella* causes .... in intestines.
   (a) Typhlitis   (b) Enteritis   (c) Colitis   (d) Proctitis

11. Necrosis of hepatocytes at one side of central vein in liver is known as .... necrosis.
   (a) Centrilobular   (b) Midzonal   (c) Paracentral   (d) Focal

12. Parasitic cirrhosis is caused by ....
   (a) *Hemonchus* sp.   (b) *Ascaris lumbricoides*   (c) *Fasciola* sp.   (d) Amphistomes

13. Cholecystitis is the inflammation of ....
   (a) Urinary bladder   (b) Bile duct   (c) Gall bladder   (d) Pancreas

14. Reovirus causes .... of pancreas.
   (a) Hypertrophy   (b) Atrophy   (c) Hyperplasia   (d) Hypoplasia

15. 'Pearly disease' is caused by ....
   (a) Streptococci   (b) Staphylococci   (c) *Mycobacterium* sp.   (d) None

16. Erosive stomatitis is seen in ....
   (a) Rinderpest   (b) Mucosal disease   (c) Pox   (d) FMD

17. Ingluvitis is the inflammation of ....
   (a) Colon   (b) Rectum   (c) Jejunum   (d) Crop

18. Sub-epithelial fibrous nodules are produced in .... esophagitis.
   (a) Traumatic   (b) Bacterial   (c) Viral   (d) Parasitic

19. Sudden change in feed with lush green fodder is the cause of ....
   (a) Impaction   (b) Tympany   (c) Reticulitis   (d) None

20. Acute abomasitis characterized by oedema, congestion and haemorrhage of abomasal folds is feature of ....
    (a) Enterotoxaemia   (b) Black disease   (c) Braxy   (d) Blue tongue

21. Corrugations in large intestines are observed in ....
    (a) Tuberculosis   (b) Paratuberculosis   (c) Pseudotuberculosis   (d)All of the above

22. Pica may lead to formation of ....
    (a) Piliconcretions   (b) Polybezoars   (c) Both a & b   (d) None

23. Enterolith may cause ....in horses.
    (a) Enterotoxaemia   (b) Colic   (c) Lameness   (d) Diarrhoea

24. Frothy bloat occurs in buffaloes due to ....
    (a) Saponin   (b) Fatty acids   (c) Carbohydrate   (d) None

25. Button ulcers are produced in abomasum due to ....
    (a) *Salmonella* sp.   (b) Staphylococci   (c) *E. coli*   (d) FMD

17
PATHOLOGY OF HEMOPOITIC AND IMMUNE SYSTEM

- **Developmental anomalies**
- **Anemia**
  - **Hemolytic**
  - **Haemorrhagic**
  - **Deficiency**
  - **Toxic/Aplastic**
  - **Autoimmune Hemolytic**
- **Polycythemia**
- **Leukocytosis**
- **Leukopenia**
- **Pathology of Spleen**
- **Pathology of Lymphnodes**
- **Pathology of Thymus**
- **Pathology of Bursa**
- **Model Questions**

DEVELOPMENTAL ANOMALIES

Hereditary anemia

Hereditary anemia has been reported in mice due to defects in erythropoiesis or reduced vitality of erythrocytes. Erythropenia along with leucopenia occurs in mouse foetus on 20th day of gestation due to defective autosomal chromosome 4. Sex linked anemia in mouse is hypochromic with deficient bone marrow and occurs in hemizygus males or homozygus females. This anemia occurs due to deficiency of iron as a result of poor absorption from gastrointestinal tract.

Autoimmune hemolytic anemia in foals

It occurs due to incompatible blood group antigens of male and female parents. The mare does not have that blood group antigen but foetus acquires it from father. The foetal blood exposed to dam through placental exchanges leads to induction of antibody production in mares against foetal blood group antigen. These antibodies accumulate in colustrum and when foal suck the milk from mares, they are readily absorbed through G.I. tract of foals in blood and cause destruction of erythrocytes leading to anemia.

Congenital defects in lymphocytes

Congenital defects in lymphocytes are classified under stem cell aplasia/agenesis leading to combined immunodeficiency with absence of both T- and B-lymphocytes in Arabian foals. It occurs either due to inherited gene defect or differentiation/maturation defects in lymphocytes. It is characterized by agammaglobulinemia, lymphopenia, hypoplasia of thymus, lymphnodes and spleen.

Chediak-Higashi Syndrome

This syndrome is related with defects in phagocytic cells such as defective neutrophils and monocytes. The defects are in chemotaxis, engulfment and killing of bacteria and associated with defective assembly of cytoplasmic microtubules responsible for degranulation and release of lysosomal enzymes, there is depression of superoxide anions leading to persistent bacterial infections.

ANEMIA

Anemia is the decrease in number of erythrocytes or hemoglobin concentration in erythrocytes per unit of blood and is characterized by pale mucus membrane, dyspnoea, cardiac hypertrophy and weakness. Anemia is classified according to morphological characteristics of erythrocytes and on the basis of causative factors. Morphologically, anemia is classified as macrocytic, normocytic and microcytic depending on the size of red blood cells and normochromic and hypochromic based on the presence of quantity of hemoglobin in RBC. *Macrocytic anemia* is characterized by increased size of RBC and occurs due to acute blood loss or hemolysis resulting in excessive production and availability of immature erythrocytes in blood. Such cells also have reduced amount of hemoglobin and are termed as hypochromic. *Macrocytic normochromic* anemia is increase size of RBC with normal hemoglobin and has been observed in deficiency of folic acid, niacin and vitamin B_{12}. *Normocytic anemia* is most common in animals occurs due to neoplasia, irradiation and is also known as *aplastic anemia* as a result of aplasia or agenesis of RBC. In Normocytic normochromic, normal size of RBC with normal hemoglobin occurs as a result of depression of erythrogenesis. *Microcytic anemia* is reduction in size of erythrocytes with decreased hemoglobin (Microcytic hypochromic) and occurs in deficiency of iron and pyridoxine or chronic blood loss.

In anemia, the size of RBC varies markedly, some being of large size and some of small size and is known as *anisocytosis*. The presence of abnormal shape (elongated, angular, ovoid, distorted) of RBC is termed as *poikilocytosis*. In some blood smears, there are nucleated RBC's which are immature due to increased production to meet the demand. Sometimes, the erythrocytes have minute dark spots known as *basophilic stippling* which occurs in acute blood loss. Some erythrocytes stain unevenly with some dark and light colour spots and are known as *polychromatophilia* which is an indication of active erythrogenesis. The denaturation and precipitation of hemoglobin leads to appearance of purplish granules in RBC near the

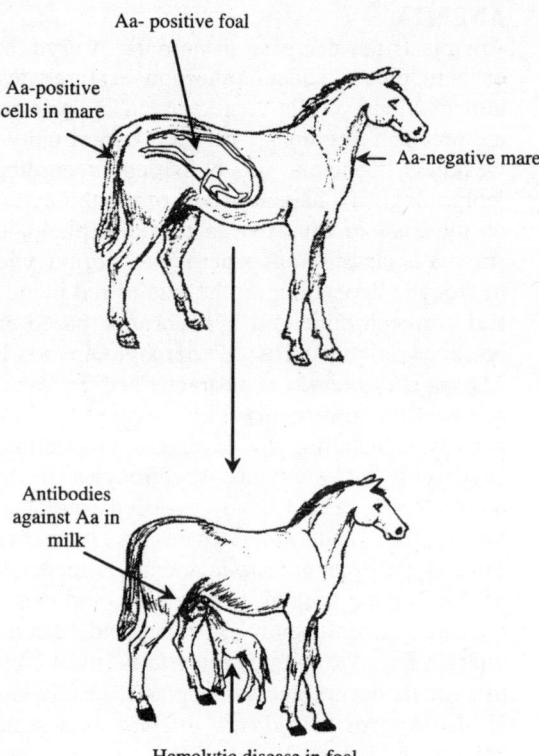

Aa- positive foal

Aa-positive cells in mare

Aa-negative mare

Antibodies against Aa in milk

Hemolytic disease in foal

Fig.17.1.Diagram showing autoimmune
hemolytic anemia in foal

RBC with surface Ag

Processing of Ag by APC

Generation of T-cytotoxic cells

Generation of plasma cells

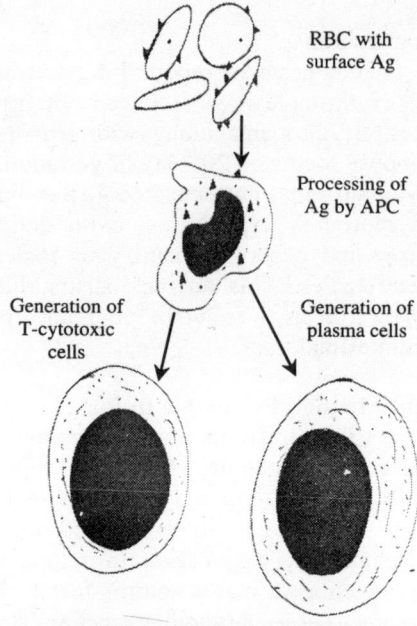

Fig.17.3. Diagram showing autoimmune
hemolytic anemia

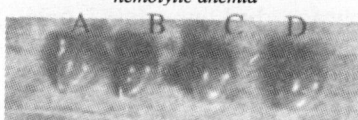

Fig.17.4. Photograph showing atrophy in spleen
(A. Normal, B, C and D Progressive atrophied of
spleen)

A

B

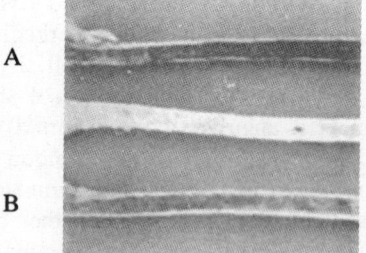

Fig.17.2. Photograph showing toxic aplastic
anemia A. Normal B. Yellow bone marrow

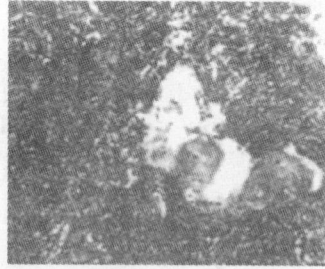

Fig.17.5. Photograph showing depletion
of lymphoid tissue

cytoplasmic membrane which are known as "Heinz bodies". According to etiological factors, anemia is classified as hemolytic, haemorrhagic or deficiency anemia.

HEMOLYTIC ANEMIA

Hemolytic anemia occurs due to excessive lysis of erythrocytes and is characterized by icterus, hemoglobinuria and presence of nucleated erythrocytes in blood and hemosiderosis in spleen.

Etiology
- Infections *e.g. Anaplasma* spp. *Babesia* spp., Equine infectious anemia virus.
- Toxins/ poisons *e.g.* snake venom, chronic lead poisoning.
- Immune mechanisms *e.g.* autoimmunity against erythrocytes (Fig. 17.1).

Macroscopic features
- Pale mucus membranes.
- Icterus.
- Blood is thin, watery.
- Hemoglobinurea.

Microscopic features
- Decreased number of erythrocytes.
- Presence of nucleated/immature RBC in blood.
- Hemosiderin laden cells in spleen.

HAEMORRHAGIC ANEMIA

Haemorrhagic anemia occurs due to severe haemorrhage, extravasation of blood and is characterized by pale mucus membrane and haemorrhage in body.

Etiology
- Infections *e.g.* Acute septicemic diseases.
- Toxins/poisons *e.g.* Bracken fern poisoning.
- Parasites *e.g. Hemonchus contortus.*
- Deficiency *e.g.* vitamin C deficiency.

Macroscopic features
- Petechiae or echymotic haemorrhage.
- Pale mucus membrane.
- Hematuria.

Microscopic features
- Haemorrhage in various tissues /organs.
- Macrocytic or normocytic characters of RBC.
- Poikilocytosis.
- Hyperplasia of bone marrow.

DEFICIENCY ANEMIA

Deficiency anemia occurs as a result of deficiency of iron, copper, cobalt and vitamins and is characterized by pale mucus membrane, weak and debilitated body and decreased number of erythrocytes with hypochromasia in blood.

Etiology
- Deficiency of iron.
- Deficiency of copper.
- Deficiency of cobalt.
- Deficiency of vitamin B_{12}, Pyridoxine, riboflavin and folic acid.
- Parasitic infestation may lead to deficiency.

Macroscopic features
- Pale mucus membrane.
- Thin watery blood with light red colour.
- Weak and debilitated carcass.
- Heavy parasitic load in gastrointestinal tract.

Microscopic features
- Microcytic hypochromic erythrocytes.
- Poikilocytosis.

TOXIC APLASTIC ANEMIA

Toxic aplastic anemia is agenesis or aplasia of hemopoietic tissues in bone marrow and there is lack of erythrocyte production. It is characterized by the absence of developmental stages of erythrocytes viz., normoblasts, megaloblasts etc.

Etiology
- Radiation *e.g.* X-rays, γ rays, or UV rays.
- Sulfonamides.
- Bracken fern toxicity.
- Uremia.
- Feline panleukopenia.

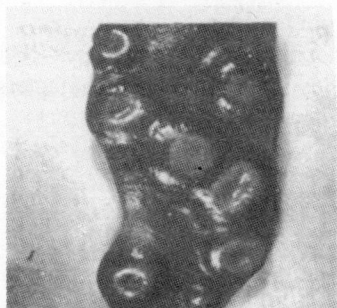

Fig.17.6. Photograph of spleen showing tubercles/granulomatous lesions (ARS/USDA)

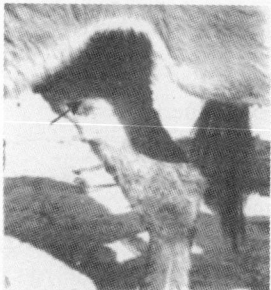

Fig.17.7. Photograph showing lymphadenitis in horse due to glanders

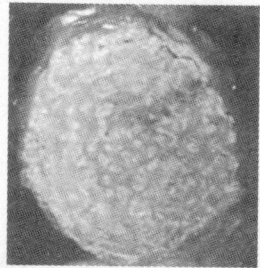

Fig.17.8. Photograph showing caseous lymphadenitis (ARS/USDA)

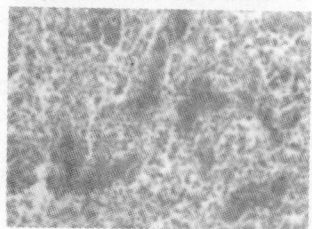

Fig.17.9. Photomicrograph of lymphnode showing acute lymphadenitis

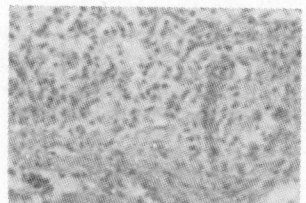

Fig.17.10. Photomicrograph of lymphnode showing chronic lymphadenitis

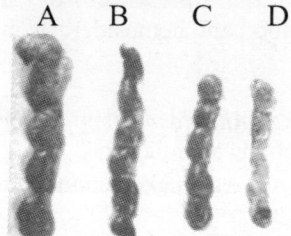

Fig.17.11. Photograph showing atrophy of thymus A. Normal B, C and D. progressive atrophy

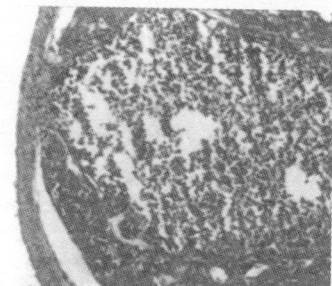

Fig.17.12. Photomicrograph of thymus showing depletion of lymphoid tissue.

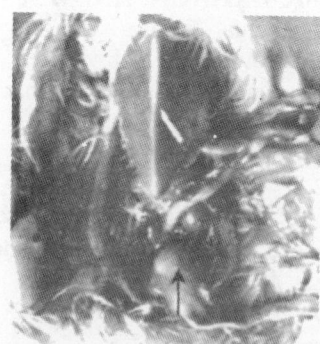

Fig.17.13. Photograph showing oedema in bursa of Fabricius due to Gumboro disease.

Macroscopic features

- Pale mucus membrane.
- Weak and debilitated animal.
- Dyspnoea.
- Bone marrow becomes yellow/fatty (Fig. 17.2).

Microscopic features

- Absence of developmental stages or RBC such as normoblasts, megaloblasts etc.
- Agranulocytosis i.e. reduction of WBC in circulating blood.
- Bone marrow becomes fatty.

AUTOIMMUNE HEMOLYTIC ANEMIA

Autoimmune hemolytic anemia occurs as a result of destruction of erythrocytes by immune mechanisms developed against erythrocytes.

Etiology

- Autoimmune hemolytic anemia in foals.
- Antibodies produced against own RBC of an animal (Fig. 17.3).
- Equine infectious anemia.
- Anaplasmosis.
- Systemic lupus erythematosus.

Table 17.1 Differential features of various types of Anaemia

	Hemolytic	Haemorrhagic	Deficiency	Toxic/ Aplastic	Autoimmune Hemolytic
Macroscopic features	1. Pale mucus membranes 2. Icterus 3. Blood is thin, watery. 4. Hemoglobinurea	1. Petechiae or Echymotic haemorrhage 2. Pale mucus membrane 3. Hematuria	1. Pale mucus membrane 2. Thin watery blood with light red colour 3. Weak and debilitated carcass 4. Heavy parasitic load in gastrointestinal tract.	1. Pale mucus membrane 2. Weak and debilitated animal 3. Dyspnoea 4. Bone marrow becomes yellow/fatty	1. Pale mucus membrane 2. Enlargement of liver, spleen and lymphnodes 3. Hemoglobinuria 4. Lameness due to rheumatoid arthritis
Microscopic features	1. Decreased number of erythrocytes 2. Presence of nucleated/immature RBC in blood 3. Hemosiderin laden cells in spleen	1. Haemorrhage in various tissues /organs 2. Macrocytic or normocytic characters of RBC 3. Poikilocytosis 4. Hyperplasia of bone marrow	1. Microcytic hypochromic erythrocytes. 2. Poikilocytosis	1. Absence of developmental stages or RBC such as normoblasts, megaloblasts etc. 2. Agranulocytosis i.e. Reduction of WBC in circulating blood. 3. Bone marrow becomes fatty.	1. Erythrophagocytosis 2. Demonstration of antibodies against own RBC in sera of animals. 3. Active erythropoiesis 4. Glomerulonephritis

Macroscopic features
- Pale mucus membrane.
- Enlargement of liver, spleen and lymphnodes.
- Hemoglobinuria.
- Lameness due to rheumatoid arthritis.

Microscopic features
- Erythrophagocytosis.
- Demonstration of antibodies against own RBC in sera of animals.
- Active erythropoiesis.
- Glomerulonephritis.

POLYCYTHEMIA

Polycythemia is increase in number of erythrocytes in circulating blood. It may be relative increase as a result of dehydration or decrease in plasma volume or absolute due to anoxia.

Etiology
- Dehydration due to diarrhoea, vomiting and loss of fluid in oedema/inflammation.
- Anoxia in high altitudes.
- Heart diseases *e.g.* patent ductus arteriosus.
- Severe pulmonary emphysema.

- Erythroid leukemia.

Macroscopic features
- Dehydration, mucus membrane dry, sticky.
- Pulmonary emphysema, fibrosis in lungs.
- Increase hemoglobin concentration.

Microscopic features
- Increased number of erythrocytes
- Severe damage in lungs, congestion, emphysema, fibrosis

LEUCOCYTOSIS

Leucocytosis is increase in number of leucocytes in circulating blood caused by various infections. There is also increase in white blood cells in blood due to neoplastic condition and is known as *Leukemia*. As the leucocytes consist of neutrophils, lymphocytes eosinophils, monocytes and basophils; the increase in number of neutrophils is termed as *neutrophilia*, eosinophils as *eosinophilia*, lymphocytes as *lymphocytosis*, basophils as *basophilia* and of monocytes as *monocytosis*.

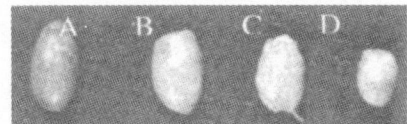

Fig.17.15. Photograph of bursa of Fabricius showing atrophy and fibrosis (A. Normal, B,C and D. progressive atrophic changes)

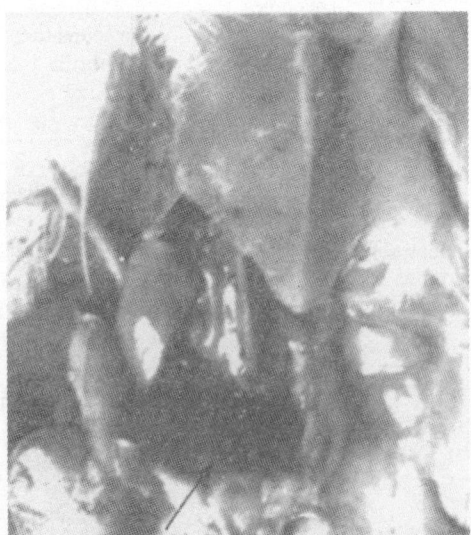

Fig.17.14. Photograph showing haemorrhage in bursa of Fabricius due to Gumboro disease

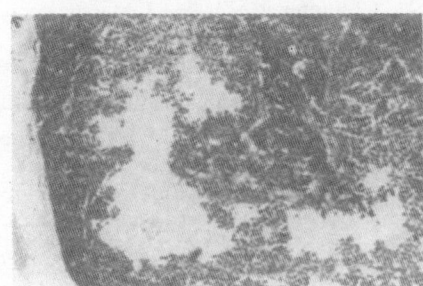

Fig.17.16. Photomicrograph of bursa of Fabricius showing depletion of lymphoid tissue

Etiology
- Infections.
- Bacterial infection – neutrophilia.
- Viral infections and chronic bacterial infections – lymphocytosis.
- Parasites – eosinophilia.
- Allergies – basophilia, lymphocytosis.

Macroscopic features
- No characteristic lesion.
- Reactive lymphnode hyperplasia.
- Enlargement of lymphoid organs such as spleen, thymus and bursa.

Microscopic features
- Increase in number of total leucocytes in blood.
- Increase in absolute lymphocyte, absolute neutrophil, absolute eosinophil counts.
- Hyperplastic lesions in lymphoid organs.

LEUCOPENIA

Leucopenia is decrease in number of white blood cells. The leucocytes are neutrophils, lymphocytes monocytes, eosinophils and basophils. If there is decrease in number of all 5 cells of leucocytes, it is known as *panleucopenia*. The decrease in number of neutrophils is termed as *neutropenia* and lymphocytes as *lymphopenia*.

Etiology
- Congenital *e.g.* Chediak-Higashi Syndrome.
- Infections *e.g.* Feline panleucopenia virus, infectious bursal disease virus.
- Chemicals *e.g.* Pesticides, heavy metals.
- Radiation *e.g.* X-rays.

Macroscopic features
- Atrophy of lymphoid organs.
- Recurrent infections, vaccination failures, pyogenic disorders.
- Oedema, haemorrhage in bursa, atrophy of bursa due to fibrosis in IBD infection.

Microscopic features
- Decrease in total leucocyte count and absolute neutrophil and absolute lymphocyte counts.
- Degeneration and necrosis of lymphoid cells in follicles of lymphoid organ.
- Oedema, necrosis, proliferation of fibrous tissue in bursa in IBD infection.

PATHOLOGY OF SPLEEN
SPLEENITIS

Spleenitis is the inflammation of spleen characterized by enlargement, infiltration of inflammatory cells, proliferation of lymphoid follicles, congestion and oedema followed by proliferation of fibrous tissue (Figs. 17.4 to 17.6).

Etiology
- Infections *e.g.* bacteria, virus.
- Deficiency of vitamins and minerals.
- Amyloidosis.
- Immunodeficiency *e.g.*environmental pollution

Macroscopic features
- Enlargement of spleen.
- Necrotic patches on spleen.
- In chronic cases or in immunological disorders.
- There is atrophy of spleen due to fibrosis.
- Necrotic patches and congestion leading to mottling.

Microscopic features
- Congestion in spleen.
- Proliferation of lymphoid follicles/cells.
- Oedema.
- In atrophied spleen, proliferation of fibrous tissue, depletion of lymphoid cells/follicles.

PATHOLOGY OF LYMPHNODES
LYMPHADENITIS

Lymphadenitis is the inflammation of lymphnodes characterized by enlargement/atrophy, congestion proliferation of lymphoid cells/depletion of lymphoid cells, oedema and fibrosis of lymphnodes (Figs. 17.7 to 17.10).

Etiology
- Infections *e.g.* Rinderpest.
- Immunological disorders *e.g.* immuno-deficiency.
- Deficiency *e.g.* deficiency of protein.
- Environmental pollution *e.g.* pesticides, heavy metals.
- Tumors/neoplasm *e.g.* lymphosarcoma.

Macroscopic features
- Enlargement of lymphnodes.
- Congestion.
- Oedema.
- In chronic cases- fibrosis.
- Atrophy.

Microscopic features
- Congestion, oedema, proliferation of lymphoid cells.
- In chronic cases, proliferation of fibrous tissue, depletion of lymphoid cells.

PATHOLOGY OF THYMUS
THYMOMA /THYMIC HYPERPLASIA
It is characterized by congestion and hyperplasia of lymphoid cells in thymus. The inflammation of thymus in chronic cases is characterized by atrophy and proliferation of fibrous tissue (Figs. 17.11 & 17.12).

Etiology
- Immunological disorders.
- Environmental pollution *e.g.* pesticide, heavy metals.
- Toxins/poisons.
- Aging *e.g.* in adult poultry thymus regresses.

Macroscopic features
- Congestion, reddening of thymus.
- Oedema.
- Increase in size.
- Atrophy, thinning like thread.

Microscopic features
- Congestion, oedema.
- Proliferation of lymphoid cells.
- Depletion of lymphoid cells.
- Proliferation of fibrous tissue.

PATHOLOGY OF BURSA
BURSITIS
Bursitis is the inflammation of bursa of Fabricius in poultry characterized by oedema, congestion, haemorrhage or atrophy and depletion of lymphoid cells (Figs. 17.13 to 17.16).

Etiology
- Infectious Bursal disease virus (Birnavirus).
- Environmental pollution *e.g.* Pesticides, heavy metals.

Macroscopic features
- Enlargement of bursa.
- Congestion and/or haemorrhage.
- Oedema.
- In chronic cases, atrophy and fibrosis.

Microscopic features
- Oedema.
- Depletion of lymphoid tissue.
- Degeneration and necrosis of lymphoid cells.
- Congestion and/or haemorrhage.
- Proliferation fibrous tissue.

MODEL QUESTIONS

Q. 1.   Fill in the blanks with suitable word(s).
1. Hereditary anemia occurs in mice due to defects in .... or .... of erythrocytes leading to............... and...............
2. Chediak-Higashi Syndrome is related with defects in........... including........... and............... . The defect are in..............., ... and............... of bacteria.

3. Morphologically, anemia is classified as.........., ... and......... while on the basis of presence of hemoglobin in RBC, it is divided into............ and...........
4. Hemolytic anemia occurs due to............... of erythrocytes in............... and is characterized by............... and...............
5. .... (parasitic infection) may cause haemorrhagic anemia.
6. Deficiency anemia occurs due to deficiency of..............., ..., ... and vitamin ...., ..., ..., ... and characterized by............,., ... and............
7. Leucocytosis is............... number of WBC in............... caused by............... and............... .

Q. 2.   *Write true or false against each statement, correct the false statement.*
1. ....Leukemia is increase in number of all leucocytes in blood.
2. ....Polycythemia is decrease in RBC in blood.
3. ....Inflammation of spleen may lead to immunosuppression.
4. ....Pesticides do not cause lymphadenitis.
5. ....Lymphopenia is a feature of congenital defects of stem cells.
6. ....Birna virus causes thymic hyperplasia
7. ....Atrophy of bursa occurs due to heavy metal toxicity
8. ....Chediak-Higashi Syndrome is decrease in WBC in blood
9. ....Sex linked anemia in mouse is hypochromic in nature due to iron deficiency.
10. ....Anisocytosis is variation in size of RBC

Q.3.   *Define the followings.*
1. Polycythemia
2. Poikitocytosis
3. Panleucopenia
4. Leukemia
5. Anisocytosis
6. Macrocytic normochronic
7. Neutropenia
8. Microcytic
9. Polychromatophilia
10. Lymphopenia

Q. 4.   *Write short notes on.*
1. Hemolytic anemia.
2. Anemia due to nutritional deficiency.
3. Impact of environmental pollution on lymphoid organs.
4. Leucopenia.
5. Chediak Higashi syndrome.

Q. 5.   *Select most appropriate word(s) from the four options given against each statement.*
1. Congenital defects in lymphocytes may result into ....
   (a) Lymphopenia   (b) Agammaglobulinemia (c) Hypoplasia of spleen   (d)All of the above
2. The size of RBC varies from small to large in peripheral blood and this condition is known as...
   (a) Poikilosytosis   (b) Anisocytosis   (c) Polychromatophilia   (d) Heinz bodies
3. Hemolytic anemia is caused by ....
   (a) *Anaplasma* spp.   (b) Coccidia   (c) Hemonchus   (d) *Proteus* sp.
4. Hematuria is an example of ....anemia
   (a) Hemolytic   (b) Autoimmune   (c) Haemorrhagic   (d) Deficiency
5. Eosinophilia occurs in ....infection
   (a) Bacterial   (b) Prion   (c) Viroid   (d) Parasitic

6. Decrease in number of all components of leucocytes is known as ....
   (a) Leucopoenia   (b) Panleucopenia   (c) Leucocytosis   (d) Leukemia
7. Pesticides may cause ....
   (a) Neutropenia   (b) Lymphopenia   (c) Hypogammaglobulimia   (d)All of the above
8. Depletion of lymphoid tissue from follicles of bursa ....
   (a) Gumboro disease   (b) Rinderpest   (c) Coccidiosis   (d) Salmonellosis
9. Macrocytic normochromic anemia is.........
   (a) Large size RBC   (b) Decreased Hb
   (c) Small size RBC   (d) Large size RBC & normal Hb
10. Erythrocytes having minute dark spots are known as ....
    (a) Heinz bodies   (b) Theleiria   (c) Basophilic stippling   (d) None

18
PATHOLOGY OF URINARY SYSTEM

- **Developmental anomalies**
- **Functional disturbances**
- **Pathology of kidneys**
  - **Glomerulonephritis**
  - **Interstitial nephritis**
  - **Pyelonephritis**
  - **Nephrosclerosis**
  - **Urolithiasis**
- **Pathology of ureter**
- **Pathology of urinary bladder**
  - **Cystitis**
- **Pathology of urethra**
  - **Urethritis**
- **Model Questions**

DEVELOPMENTAL ANOMALIES

Aplasia
Absence of one or both kidneys. Absence of one kidney is observed in animals with compensatory hypertrophy of another kidney and such animals may survive well.

Hypoplasia
The size of kidneys remain small as they don't grow properly due to defect in a single recessive autosomal gene.

Cyst in kidney
Single or multiple cysts in pig and dog kidney are reported with tinged yellow colour. They may arise from nephron due to its distension. Presence of multiple cysts is also termed as congenital polycystic kidney.
- *Type-I* cysts are formed due to dilation and hyperplasia of collecting tubules resulting in spongiform kidneys. In such neonates cystic bile ducts are also present.
- *Type-II* polycystic kidney is formed due to absence of collecting tubules and developmental failure of nephron. The cysts are thick walled with dense connective tissue and may involve one or both kidneys.
- *Type-III* cysts in kidneys occur due to multiple abnormalities during development. Cysts develop from tubules or Bowmen's capsule with part of glomeruli in cyst. This condition is bilateral and causes considerable enlargement of kidney due to clear fluid or blood mixed fluid containing cysts.

FUNCTIONAL DISTURBANCES

Proteinuria
Presence of protein particularly albumin in urine. Protein is found as smooth, homogenous, pink staining precipitate also called as 'cast'. The presence of albumin in urine is indicative of damage in glomeruli. It is also characterized by oedema due to protein deficiency.

Hematuria
Presence of blood in urine giving bright red colour. It may occur due to damage in glomeruli, tubule or haemorrhage anywhere from glomeruli to urethra. The most important cause of hematuria is bracken fern toxicity (Fig. 18.1).

Hemoglobinuria
When hemoglobin is present in urine without erythrocytes due to intravascular haemolysis. The urine becomes brownish red in colour. It must be differentiated from hematuria in which intact erythrocytes are present and settle down after some time leaving clear urine as supernatant. Hemoglobinuria is caused by various infections such as *Leptospira* sp., *Babesia* sp. or phosphorus deficiency in animals (Fig. 18.1).

Anuria
Absence of urine is known as anuria which may be due to:
- Absence of urinary secretion due to glomerulonephritis.
- Inelastic renal capsule unable to exert sufficient pressure required for glomerular filtration leading to nephrosis.
- Due to hydronephrosis or calculi urine already secreted puts back pressure to prevent further secretion.
- Low blood pressure.
- Dehydration.
- Necrosis of tubular epithelium.

Polyuria
Increased amount of urine leading to frequent urination caused due to diabetes insipedus, hormonal imbalance and polydipsia. In this condition, waste products are successfully eliminated.

Uremia
The presence of harmful waste products like uric acid, creatinine and urea in blood. Normally such waste products are removed by excretion through kidneys. But due to damage in kidneys or obstruction by inflammation, neoplasm, abscess

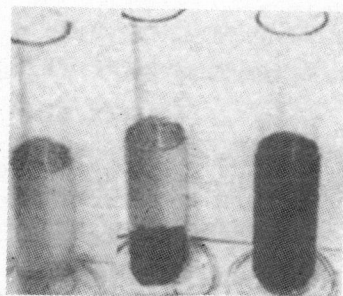

Fig. 18.1. Photograph showing (A) Normal (B) hematuria and (C) hemoglobinuria

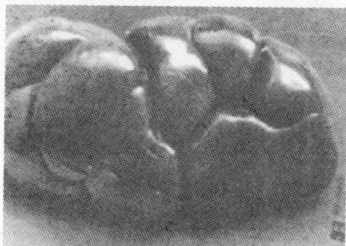

Fig. 18.2. Photograph showing nephrosis

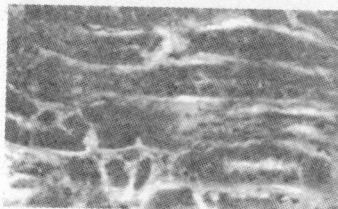

Fig. 18.3. Photomicrograph showing nephrosis (coagulative necrosis)

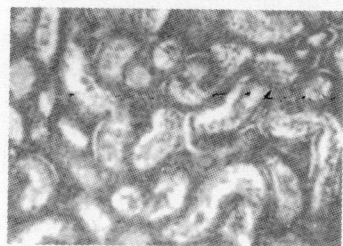

Fig. 184. Photomicrograph showing nephrosis

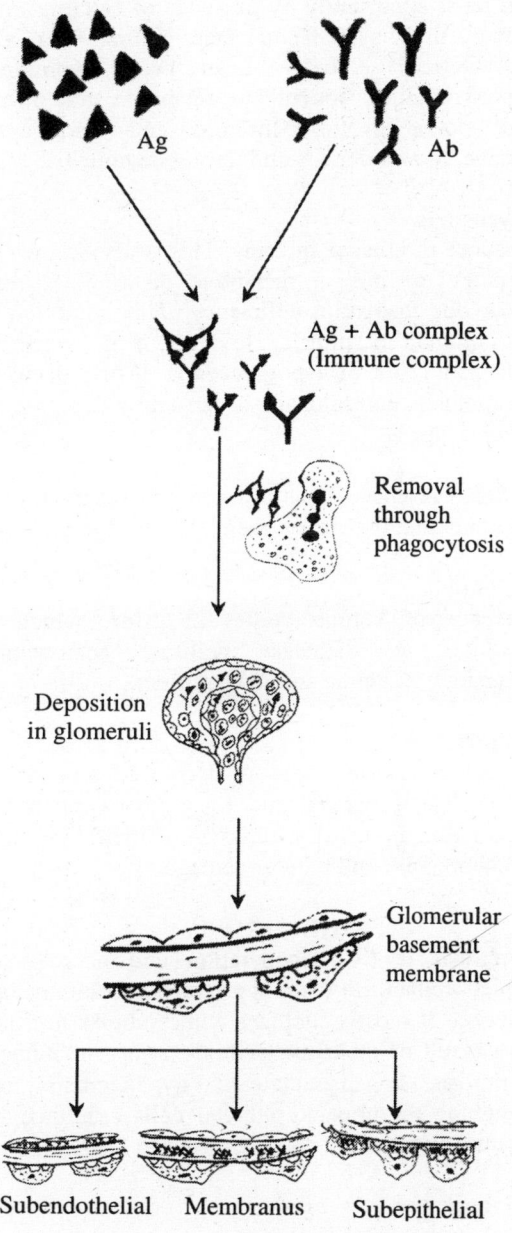

Fig. 18.5. Diagram of immune complex mediated glomerulonephritis

and most importantly by presence of calculi, urine remains in the system and causes uremia. Uremia is characterized by headache, vomiting, hyperirritability, convulsion, ulcers in oral cavity and stomach, normochromic and normocytic anemia, hemosiderosis and thrombocytopenia.

Glycosuria

Presence of glucose in urine. This is also known as diabetes mellitus, a metabolic disorder. It may occur due to insulin deficiency. This condition is not common in animals. However, it may occur in dogs as a result of hypoglyecemia. It may occur in sheep due to enterotoxaemia caused by *Clostridium welchii* type D.

Pyuria Presence of pus in urine due to suppurative inflammation in urinary tract.

Ketonuria

Presence of ketone bodies in urine, which is common in diabetes mellitus, acetonemia, pregnancy toxaemia and in starvation.

Oliguria

In this condition, there is decreased amount of urine, which occurs due to glomerulonephritis, obstruction in urinary passage, dehydration, low blood pressure and tubular damage.

NEPHROSIS

Nephrosis is the degeneration and necrosis of tubular epithelium without producing inflammatory reaction. It mostly includes acute tubular necrosis as a result of ischemia or toxic injury to kidney. Nephrosis is characterized by necrosis and sloughing of tubular epithelial cells exhibited by uremia, oliguria, anuria (Figs. 18.2 to 18.4).

Etiology
- Hypotension.
- Heavy metals.
- Mycotoxins *e.g.* Ochratoxin.
- Antibiotics *e.g.* Gentamicin.

Macroscopic features
- Swelling of kidneys.
- Capsular surface smooth, pale and translucent.

Microscopic features
- Vacuolation in tubular epithelium.
- Coagulative necrosis.
- Sloughing of tubular epithelium.

GLOMERULONEPHRITIS

Glomerulonephritis is the inflammation of glomeruli primarily characterized by pale and enlarged kidneys with potential haemorrhage, oedema of glomeruli, congestion and infiltration of inflammatory cells. Due to presence of mesangial proliferation, it is also called mesangio proliferative glomerulonephritis (MPGN) (Figs. 18.5 to 18.7).

Etiology
- Streptococci infection.
- Immune complexes.
- Environmental pollutants such as Organochlorine pesticides.

Macroscopic features
- Enlarged kidneys.
- Oedema, pale kidneys.
- Petechiae on kidneys.
- Proteinuria, uremia, hypercholesterolemia and increased creatinine level in blood.

Microscopic features
- Oedema of glomeruli leading to increase in size.
- Infiltration of neutrophils, macrophages.
- Compression of blood capillaries and absence of erythrocytes.
- Thrombosis and necrosis of glomerular capillaries.

Based on type of lesions, it can be divided into 5 subtypes.

1. Type-I MPGN
- Proliferation of mesangial cells.

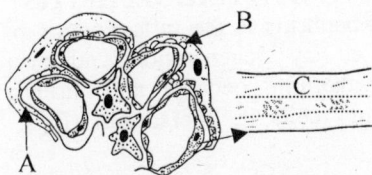

*Fig. 18.6. Diagram showing different locations
of deposits of immune complexes A.
subendothelial B. Membranous and C. Sub
epithelial deposits of immune complexes.*

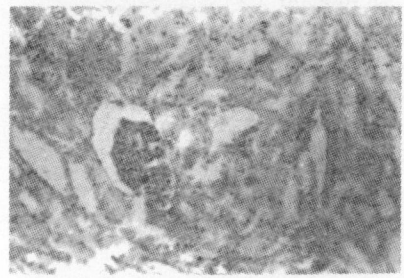

*Fig. 18.7. Photomicrograph showing immune
complexes in glomeruli (Immunoperoxidase staining)*

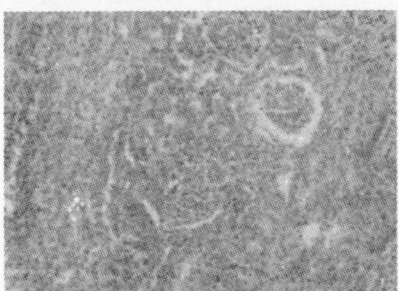

*Fig. 18.8. Photomicrograph showing
interstitial nephritis*

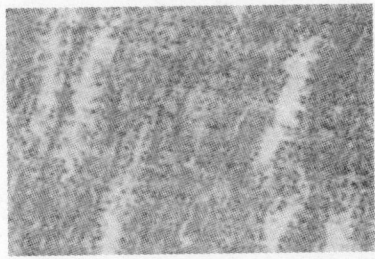

*Fig. 18.9. Photomicrograph showing interstitial
nephritis with severe haemorrhages in interstium.*

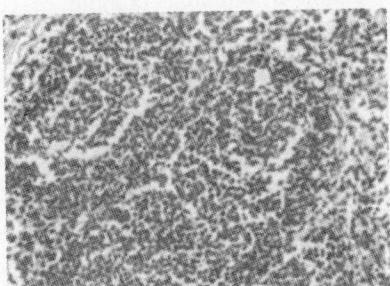

*Fig. 18.10. Photomicrograph showing
suppurative nephritis*

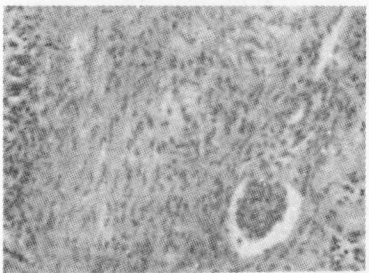

*Fig. 18.11. Photomicrograph of kidney showing
nephrosclerosis*

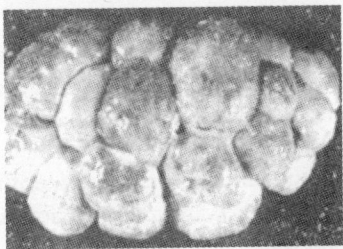

*Fig. 18.12. Photograph of kidney showing
nephrolithiasis*

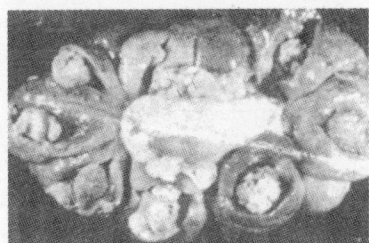

*Fig. 18.13. Photograph of kidney showing
nephrolithiasis*

- Deposition of immune complexes containing IgG, IgM, IgA and C_3.
- Immune complexes penetrate vascular endothelium but not the basement membrane and are deposited in subendothelial region.
- Proliferation and swelling of endothelial cells.
- Immune complexes induce production of transforming growth factor ($TGFB_1$) which increases production of fibrinolectin, collagen and proteoglycans leading to thickness of basement membrane; this is also known as "wire loop" lesions.

2. Type-II MPGN (Membranous)
- Deposition of immune complexes in basement membrane (lamina densa).
- Due to uncontrolled activation of complement.
- Proliferation of endothelium and mesangial cells.
- Demonstration of C_3 component, no immunoglobulin.

3. Type III MPGN (Acute Proliferative)
- Subepithelial deposits of immune complexes and disruption of basement membrane.
- Swelling of epithelium and its proliferation forming "Epithelial cresent".
- Demonstration of IgG in subepithelial region.
- Congestion and oedema of glomeruli.
- Infiltration of neutrophils, macrophages and lymphocytes.

4. Chronic glomerulonephritis
- Proliferation of epithelial and endothelial cells.
- Reduplication, thickening and disorganization of glomerular basement membrane.
- Lumen of capillaries occluded.
- Entire glomerulus is replaced by Hyaline connective tissue.

5. Focal embolic glomerulonephritis
- Focal zone of necrosis in glomeruli.
- Infiltration of neutrophils.
- Proliferation of epithelial cells and formation of crescent.

INTERSTITIAL NEPHRITIS
Interstitial nephritis is the inflammation of kidney characterized by degeneration and necrosis of tubular epithelium, oedema and infilteration of inflammatory cells in interstitium (Figs. 18.8 & 18.9).

Etiology
- Ochratoxins and atrinin.
- Leptospira.
- Toxins/ poisons *e.g.* pesticides.
- Herpes virus.
- Endogenous toxaemia *e.g.* ketosis.
- Immune complexes.

Macroscopic features
- Enlargement of kidneys.
- Necrosis, congestion and haemorrhage.

Microscopic features
- Oedema, congestion, haemorrhage.
- Necrosis and degeneration of tubular epithelium.
- Infiltration of inflammatory cells like neutrophils, macrophages and lymphocytes in interstitium.
- Loss of tubules, foci of mononuclear cells, fibrosis in chronic cases.
- Immune complexes are deposited in granular form causing degeneration of epithelial cells of tubules and mononuclear cell infiltration.

PYELONEPHRITIS
Pyelonephritis is the inflammation of renal pelvis and parenchyma i.e. tubules characterized by congestion, suppurative inflammation and fibrosis.

Etiology
- *Corynebacterium renale.*
- *Staphylococcus aureus.*
- *E. coli.*
- *Actinomyces pyogenes.*
- *Pseudomonas aeruginosa.*

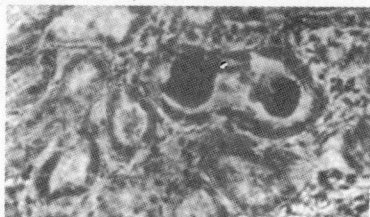

Fig. 18.14. Photomicrograph of kidney
showing nephrolithiasis

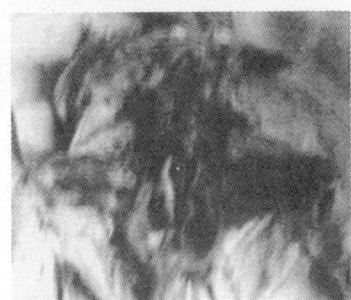

Fig. 18.15.Photograph showing ureteritis due
to deposition of salts

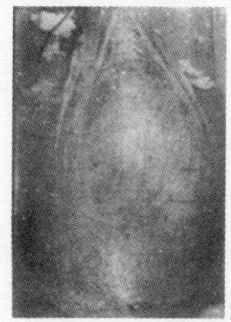

Fig. 18.16. Photograph showing cystitis

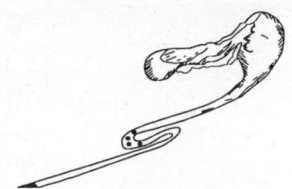

Fig. 18.17. Diagram showing retention of
calculi in urethra of bovines

Macroscopic features

- Congestion, haemorrhage and abscess formation in renal cortex, pelvis and ureters.
- Pyuria – pus mixed urine in bladder.
- Enlargement of kidneys.

Microscopic features

- Congestion, haemorrhage.

- Suppurative inflammation of pelvis and kidney parenchyma (Fig. 18.10).
- Necrosis of collecting ducts.
- Purulent exudate in pelvis.
- Infiltration of neutrophils, lymphocytes and plasma cells in interstitium.

Table 18.1 Differential features of various types of Nephritis

	Glomerulonephritis	Interstitial	*Pyelonephritis*
Macros copic features	1. Enlarged kidneys 2. Oedema, pale kidneys 3. Petechiae on kidneys 4. Proteinuria, uremia, hypercholesterolemia and increased creatinine level in blood.	1. Enlargement of kidneys 2. Necrosis, congestion and haemorrhage	1. Congestion, haemorrhage and abscess formation in renal cortex, pelvis and ureters. 2. Pyuria- Pus mixed urine in bladder. 3. Enlargement of kidneys

Microsc opic features	1. Oedema of glomeruli leading to increase in size. 2. Infiltration of neutrophils, macrophages. 3. Compression of blood capillaries and absence of erythrocytes. 4. Thrombosis and necrosis of glomerular capillaries.	1. Oedema, congestion, haemorrhage 2. Necrosis and degeneration of tubular epithelium 3. Infiltration of inflammatory cells like neutrophils, macrophages and lymphocytes in interstitium. 4. Loss of tubules, foci of mononuclear cells, fibrosis in chronic cases 5. Immune complexes are deposited in granular form causing degeneration of epithelial cells of tubules and mononuclear cell infiltration.	1. Congestion, haemorrhage 2. Suppurative inflammation of pelvis and kidney parenchyma. 3. Necrosis of collecting ducts. 4. Purulent exudate in pelvis. 5. Infiltration of neutrophils, lymphocytes and plasma cells in interstitium.

NEPHROSCLEROSIS

Nephrosclerosis is chronic fibrosis of kidney characterized by loss of glomeruli and tubules and extensive fibrosis (Fig. 18.11).

Etiology
- Glomerulonephritis.
- Interstitial nephritis.
- Arteriolosclerosis.

Macroscopic features
- Hard, atrophied kidneys.
- Fibrous nodules on kidneys.
- Thickening of capsule.
- Small white firm kidneys.

Microscopic features
- Ischemia, tubular atrophy.
- Loss of glomeruli and tubules.
- Extensive fibrosis.
- Deposition of hyaline mass.
- Infiltration of mononuclear cells.

UROLITHIASIS

Urolithiasis is the formation of stony precipitates anywhere in the urinary passage including kidneys, ureter, urinary bladder or urethra.

Etiology
- Bacterial infections.
- Metabolic defects.
- Vitamin A deficiency.
- Hyperparathyroidism.
- Mineral imbalance.

Macroscopic features
- Nephrosis, hydronephrosis.
- Distension of ureters.
- Distension of ureters and urinary bladder.
- Hard enlarged kidneys.
- Presence of calculi/ stone in kidney, ureter, bladder or urethra (Figs. 18.12 & 18.14).

There are various types of calculi, which differ in size, shape and composition. Some of them are as under:

Oxalate calculi are hard, light yellow, covered with sharp spines, found in urinary bladder and formed by calcium oxalate. They cause damage in urinary bladder leading to haemorrhage.

Uric acid calculi are composed of ammonium and sodium urates and uric acids, are yellow to brown in colour, formed in acidic urine, are spherical and irregular in shape and are not radioopaque.

Phosphate calculi are white or grey in colour, chalky in consistency, soft, friable and can be crushed with mild pressure. They are mostly multiple in the form of sand-like granules. They are composed of magnesium ammonium phosphate and occur as a result of bacterial infection.

Xanthine calculi are brownish red, concentrically laminated, fragile and irregular in shape. They rarely occur in animals.

Cystine calculi are small, soft with shiny and greasy in appearance, yellow in colour which becomes darker on exposure to air. Insoluble amino acid cystine precipitates in bladder to form calculi. Such calculi may cause obstruction of urethra with cystinuria.

Microscopic features
- Presence of crystals/stone in lumen of tubules.
- Degeneration and necrosis of tubular epithelium.
- Haemorrhage.
- Proliferation of fibrous tissue.

PATHOLOGY OF URETER
URETERITIS

Ureteritis is the inflammation of ureter characterized by enlargement, thickening of wall due to accumulation of urates, or calculi, pyonephrosis and pyelonephritis (Fig. 18.15).

Etiology
- Tuberculosis.
- Calculi.
- Hydronephrosis.
- Pyelonephritis.
- Pyonephrosis.

Macroscopic features
- Deposits of whitish/yellowish urates in ureter in poultry.
- Obstructions of ureter due to calculi leads to its enlargement and formation of diverticulum.

Microscopic features
- Thickening of the wall due to congestion and infiltration of inflammatory cells.
- Extensive fibrosis with infiltration of mononuclear cells in chronic cases.

PATHOLOGY OF URINARY BLADDER
CYSTITIS

Cystitis is the inflammation of urinary bladder characterized by congestion and fibrinous, purulent or haemorrhagic exudate (Fig. 18.16).

Etiology
- Urinary calculi.
- Tuberculosis.
- Blockage in urethra.
- Bracken fern poisoning.

Macroscopic features
- Congestion, haemorrhage.
- Enlargement of urinary bladder.
- Thickening of the wall.
- Presence of small nodules on wall.

Microscopic features
- Congestion, haemorrhage.
- Thickening of wall due to infiltration of neutrophils and macrophages.
- Granuloma in tuberculosis.
- Fibrosis
- Presence of neoplasm.

PATHOLOGY OF URETHRA
URETHRITIS

Inflammation of urethra is known as urethritis, which occurs as a result of catheter injury or calculi. It is characterized by congestion, obstruction, hydronephrosis and strictures (Fig. 18.17).

Etiology
- Calculi.
- Catheter injury.
- *Trichomonas foetus* infection.
- Picorna virus infection.

Macroscopic features
- Transient inflammation, congestion and haemorrhage.
- Strictures (male), diverticulum (female).

- Obstruction due to calculi, presence of calculi.

Microscopic features
- Thickening due to inflammatory exudate.

MODEL QUESTIONS

Q. 1.   *Fill in the blanks with suitable word(s).*
1. Increased amount of urine leading to..........urination is known as ....which is caused by ...., ...and .... to remove the ....at a faster rate.
2. Uremia is presence of ....like ...., ...and ....in blood.
3. Presence of ketones bodies in urine has been observed in.........., ..., ...and ....
4. .... are fungal toxins which may cause interstitial nephritis.
5. Environmental pollutants such as ....may induce the formation of ....in body leading to ....in animals characterized by proteinuria.
6. Pyelonephritis is caused by ...., ..., ..., ...and ....; of which ....is the main etiological agent causing disease in cattle.
7. Nephrosclerosis is ....of kidney characterized by ...., ...and ....and mostly occurs as a sequaelae to ...., ...and ....

Q.2.   *Write true or false against each statement and correct the false statement.*
1. ....Glycosuria occurs in enterotoxaemia in sheep.
2. ....Arteriolosclerosis may lead to pyelonephritis.
3. ....In cattle, *Corynebacterium ovis* causes pyelonephritis.
4. ....Oxalate calculi are hard and composed of diammonium and sodium oxalates.
5. ....Urolithiasis is presence of foreign body in kidneys.
6. ....In poultry, ureteritis is common feature of visceral gout.
7. ....Urinary calculi may cause urethritis in bullocks.
8. ....Low blood pressure may cause polyuria
9. ....Epithelial cresent is feature of interstitial nephritis.
10. ....Hypovitaminosis A may predispose the animal for calculi formation in urinary tract.

Q. 3.   *Define the following*
1. Hematuria
2. Pyuria
3. Cystitis
4. Anuria
5. Hemoglobinuria
6. Polyuria
7. Ketonuria
8. Oligouria
9. Epithelial crescents
10. Bracken fern toxicity

Q. 4.   *Write short notes on.*
1. Uremia
2. Glomerulonephritis
3. Pyelonephritis
4. Nephrosclerosis
5. Urolithiasis
6. Cystic kidney

Q. 5. *Select the most appropriate word(s) from the four options given against each statement.*

1. C_3 component of complement is found in which type of glomerulonephritis (MPGN).
    (a) Type-I   (b) Type-II   (c) Type III   (d) Type-IV

2. In cattle, pyelonephritis is caused by ....
    (a) *E. coli*   (b) *Proteus* spp. (c) *Corynebacterium renale* (d) *Actinomyces pyogenes*

3. Nephrosclerosis is .... disease of kidney
    (a) Acute   (b) Chronic   (c) Subacute   (d) Peracute

4. Hypovitaminosis ....may cause urolithiasis
    (a) A   (b) B   (c) C   (d) D

5. Ureteritis is the inflammation of ....
    (a) Uterus   (b) Uterine glands   (c) Ureter   (d) Uterine tube

6. .... amino acid forms calculi in animal which causes obstruction in urethra.
    (a) Arginine   (b) Lucine   (c) Cystine   (d) Gsolucine

7. Bracken fern causes ....
    (a) Hematuria   (b) Pyuria   (c) Hemoglobinuria   (d) Anuria

8. Urethra may become infected by ....virus.
    (a) Picorna   (b) Picobirna   (c) Birna   (d) Adeno

9. Hyperplasia of collecting tubes with their dilation causes ....cysts in kidneys.
    (a) Type-I   (b) Type-II   (c) Type-III   (d) Type-IV

10. Uremia is caused by the increased level of .... in blood.
    (a) Urea   (b) Uric acid   (c) Creatinine   (d)All of the above

19
PATHOLOGY OF GENITAL SYSTEM

- **Female Genital System**
  - **Developmental anomalies**
  - **Cystic ovaries**
  - **Oophoritis**
  - **Salpingitis**
  - **Metritis**
  - **Pyometra**
  - **Endometritis**
  - **Cervicitis**
  - **Vaginitis**
  - **Abortion**
  - **Placentitis**
  - **Mastitis**
- **Male genital system**
  - **Developmental anomalies**
  - **Orchitis**
  - **Epididymitis**
  - **Funiculitis**
  - **Seminal vesiculitis**
  - **Prostatitis**
  - **Balanoposthitis**
- **Model Questions**

FEMALE GENITAL SYSTEM

DEVELOPMENTAL ANOMALIES

Agenesis
Absence of ovary, uterus, oviduct and cervix in females. It may be unilateral or bilateral.

Hypoplasia
Complete or partial lack of germ cells in ovaries. Hypoplasia of uterus is related with agenesis of gonads. Ovaries of freemartin are also hypoplastic. Hermaphrodite animal has ovary and testicular tissue both in the gonads.

Hermaphroditism
In hermaphrodites, there is presence of organs of both sexes in same individual animal. Both ovarian and testicular tissue occur in one animal leads to sterility in animal (true hermaphrodite) while in pseudohermaphrodite the gonadal tissue of only one sex is present but there is some degree of development of opposite sex organs.

Uterus unicornis
Uterus unicornis is presence of only one horn of uterus instead of two, seen in animals with white heifer disease.

White heifer disease
White heifer disease occurs due to a single sex linked gene defect responsible for white coat colour. In such animals, there are normal ovaries, oviduct but uterus is incomplete and may lack communication with cervix. There is hypoplasia of cervix and vagina.

Uterus didelphys
Uterus didelphys is the occurrence of two cervix with two uterine bodies and single or double vagina. It occurs due to failure of mullerian ducts to fuse at their distal end. Sometimes failure of fusion may affect only cervix and there are two cervix which termed as *Cervix bifida*.

CYSTIC OVARIES
Cystic ovaries are defined as an ovary, which contains one or more clear cysts ranging from one to several centimeters in size (Fig. 19.1).

Etiology
- Hormonal imbalance

Macroscopic features
- Presence of cysts in ovaries.
- Hormonal imbalance of animal leads to sterility, continuous estrus, nymphomania due to follicular cyst.
- Lutein cysts may cause pyometra leading to pseudopregnancy.

Microscopic features
- Follicular cyst.
- Ova absent several layers of granulosa or a single layer of epithelium.
- Many follicular cysts are present.
- Lutein cyst covered by fat containing granulosa cells.

OOPHORITIS
Oophoritis is the inflammation of ovary caused by trauma, infection and characterized by granulomatous or lymphocytic inflammation of ovary (Figs. 19.2 to 19.4).

Etiology
- *Mycobacterium tuberculosis*.
- Herpes virus.

Macroscopic features
- Hard, nodular lesions in ovary, encapsulated with fibrous tissue.

Microscopic features
- Granuloma of tuberculosis through hematogenous infection.
- Infiltration of lymphocytes leading to lymphofollicular reaction in follicles.
- Atrophy or absence of ova.

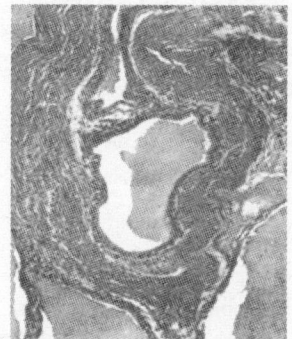

Fig. 19.1 Photomicrograph showing
cystic ovary (ARS/USDA)

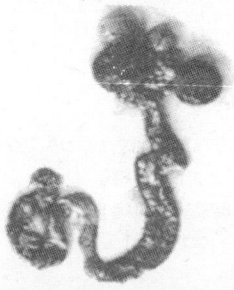

Fig. 19.2 Photograph showing oophoritis
and salpingtis

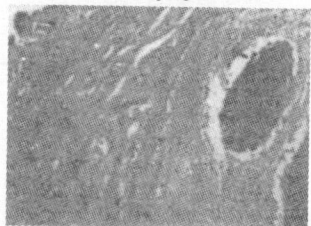

Fig. 19.3 Photomicrograph showing oophoritis

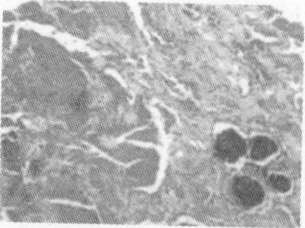

Fig. 19.4. Photomicrograph showing oophoritis

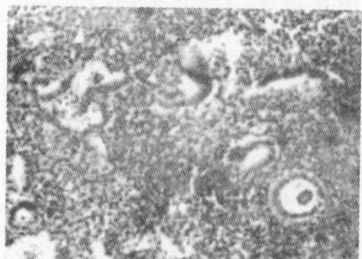

Fig. 19.5 Photomicrograph showing metritis

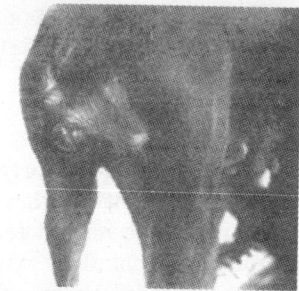

Fig. 19.6. Photograph showing prolapse of vagina

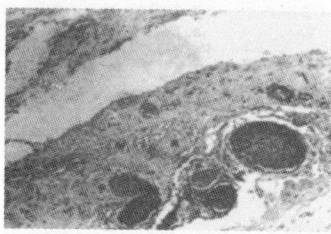

Fig. 19.7.Photomicrograph showing oedema and
congestion in placenta (Placentitis) due to brucellosis

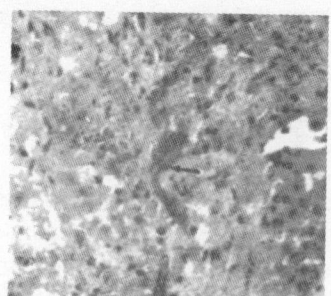

Fig. 19.8. Photomicrograph showing fungal
placentitis (ARS/USDA)

SALPINGITIS

Salpingitis is the inflammation of oviduct or fallopian tube characterized by congestion, catarrhal or purulent exudate leading to distended lumen (Fig. 19.2).

Etiology
- Mycoplasma.
- Streptococci.
- Tuberculosis (*Mycobacterium tuberculosis*).
- Trichomoniasis (*Trichomonas foetus*).

Macroscopic features
- Congestion, abscess formation
- Distension of oviduct lumen due to accumulation of serous exudate which is known as **Hydrosalpinx**.
- Accumulation of pus in oviduct is termed as **Pyosalpinx**.
- Fibrosis, hardness.
- Occlusion of lumen due to inflammatory exudate resulting in sterility.
- Inflammatory exudate is toxic to ova as well as sperms leading to sterility.

Microscopic features
- Congestion.
- Suppurative inflammation.
- Infiltration of neutrophils, macrophages and lymphocytes.
- Proliferation of fibrous tissue.
- Debris of desquamated cells.

METRITIS

Metritis is the inflammation of uterus characterized by suppurative exudate, haemorrhage and necrosis of uterus (Fig. 19.5).

Etiology
- *Actinomyces pyogenes.*
- *E. coli.*
- Staphylococci.
- Streptococci.
- *Trichomonas foetus.*
- *Campylobacter foetus.*

Macroscopic features
- Congestion, catarrhal or purulent exudate.
- Haemorrhage.
- Enlargement, oedema.
- Oozing out of pus from uterus on pressure.

Microscopic features
- Seropurulent exudate in uterine wall.
- Oedema.
- Infiltration of macrophages and lymphocytes.
- Desquamation of lining epithelium.

PYOMETRA

Pyometra is an acute or chronic suppurative inflammation of uterus resulting in accumulation of pus in the uterus.

Etiology
- Occurs under the influence of progesterone.
- *E. coli.*
- *Actinomyces pyogenes.*
- *Proteus* spp.
- *Staphylococcus aureus.*
- *Trichomonas foetus.*

Macroscopic features
- Discharge of thin cream like pus from vulva soiling the tail and perineal region.
- Pus discharge is more on sitting position of animal.
- Enlargement of abdomen due to distension of uterus.
- Uterus looking like a pregnant uterus as a result of accumulation of pus. This condition is also known as **Pseudocyesis** or **pseudopregnancy**.
- Rention of lutein cyst.

Microscopic features
- Congestion, infiltration of neutrophils, lymphocytes and plasma cells.
- Necrosis of mucosal epithelium of uterus.
- Proliferation of endometrial epithelium.
- Oedema, glandular hyperplasia.

ENDOMETRITIS

Endometritis is the inflammation of endometrium, the mucosa of uterus. It may be catarrhal or purulent and may occur after metritis.

Etiology

- *Trichomonas foetus.*
- *Campylobacter foetus.*
- Staphylococci.
- Streptococci.
- Organism enters in uterus as a result of coitus, artificial insemination or as iatrogenic infection.
- Strong chemicals/medicines administered in uterus.

Macroscopic features

- Catarrhal discharge from uterus containing desquamated cells.
- Sterility due to toxic environment of uterus to sperms.
- Congestion.

Microscopic features

- Congestion.
- Moderate infiltration of lymphocytes, plasma cells and neutrophils in mucosa.

CERVICITIS

Cervicitis is the inflammation of cervix as a result of either descending infection from uterus or ascending infection from vagina and characterized by catarrhal inflammation.

Etiology

- Etiological agents are similar as in endometritis.

Macroscopic features

- Congestion.
- Enlargement of cervix.

Microscopic features

- Catarrhal inflammation of cervical mucosa.
- Hyperplasia of mucous glands with tall mucin containing epithelial cells.
- Presence of mucin in lumen.

VAGINITIS

Vaginitis is the inflammation of vagina characterized by congestion, granularity as a result of elevations in mucosa. This is also known as **infectious pustular vulvovaginitis** in cattle caused by herpes virus.

Etiology

- *Mycoplasma bovigenitalium.*
- Bovine herpes virus-1 (BHV-1).
- Picorna virus.
- *Trichomonas foetus.*

Macroscopic features

- Granular elevation in vaginal mucosa.
- Congestion.
- Prolapse due to limitation (Fig. 19.6).

Microscopic features

- Accumulation of lymphocytes in sub-epithelial region.
- Congestion.

ABORTION

Abortion is expulsion of dead embryo or foetus before attaining normal gestation. There are two other terms related to abortion i.e. stillbirth and premature birth. **Stillbirth** is defined as expulsion of dead foetus on its full maturity while **premature birth** is birth of a live foetus before attaining full gestation period.

Etiology

- Brucellosis (*Brucella abortus, B. meletensis, B. ovis*).
- *Campylobacter foetus.*
- *Salmonella abortus-equi* – mares.
- Equine herpes virus – mares.
- Bovine herpes virus-1 – cattle.
- *Chlamydia psittasci.*
- *Trichomonas foetus.*
- *Listeria monocytogenes* (*Listeria ivanovii*).
- *Leptospria* spp.
- *Mycobacterium tuberculosis.*
- *Toxoplasma gondii.*

- *Mycoplasma mycoides.*
- Fungi – *Aspergillus* spp., *Coccidioides* spp. *Absidia* spp.
- Toxins / poisons.

Macroscopic features
- Expulsion of dead foetus in early stage (3-4 month) of gestation (Trichomoniasis).
- Abortion in middle of gestation (Campylobacteriosis).
- Late abortions (7-9 months) occur due to Brucellosis, BHV-1 infection.
- Liver of foetus has necrotic foci, congestion.
- Stomach contents used for confirmation of etiology.
- In some cases of abortion, there is retention of placenta (*e.g.* Brucellosis).
- Placenta becomes oedematous and necrotic (Placentitis).
- If the foetus dues and is not expelled outside the body due to non-opening of cervix, the dead foetus remains in uterus under sterile conditions. Such foetus undergoes autolysis and is liquified. Liquid material is absorbed in uterus through lymph or blood but bones/skin etc. remain in uterine horn sometimes causing irritation or damage to endometrium. Such foetus becomes shrunken with wrinkled skin and dried as mummy and is known as *"Mummified foetus"*.

Microscopic features
- Necrotic hepatitis with lymphofollicular reaction in foetus (Brucellosis, BHV-1 infection).
- Granulomatous lesions (tuberculosis, fungal infection), lymphofollicular reaction (mycoplasma, chlamydia).
- Demonstration/isolation of causative organisms in foetal stomach contents.
- Liver of foetus icteric (leptospirosis).
- Endometritis in dam.
- Bronchopneumonia in foetus *e.g.* brucellosis.

RETAINED PLACENTA/PLACENTITIS
Retention of placenta occurs after abortion or parturition as a result of inflammation characterized by swelling, oedema or fibrosis which prevent the separation of chorion from endometrium (Figs. 19.7 & 19.8).

Etiology
- Lack of progesterone.
- Infection *e.g.* Brucellosis, Trichomoniasis.

Macroscopic features
- Retained placenta undergoes autolysis, putrefaction.
- Toxaemia in dam.
- Endometritis, pyometra.

Microscopic features
- Placenta is oedematous and congested.
- Infiltration of neutrophils, mononuclear cells.
- Proliferation of fibroblasts.

MASTITIS
Mastitis is the inflammation of mammary gland characterized by oedema, haemorrhage and fibrosis of udder. Mastitis is always infectious and is a disease of lactating glands. There is no hematogenous infection and infections enter through teat canal to cause mastitis (Figs. 19.9 to 19.12).

Etiology
- Bacteria *e.g. Streptococcus agalactiae, Streptococcus dysgalactiae, Staphylococcus aureus, Actinomyces pyogenes, Pseudomonas aeruginosa, Brucella abortus, Mycobacterium tuberculosis, E. coli, Pasteurella multocida* and many more.
- Virus *e.g.* FMD virus, pox virus, BHV-1.
- Mycoplasma *e.g. Mycoplasma mycoides.*
- Fungi *e.g. Candida ablicans, Trichosporon* spp. *Nocardia asteroids, Cryptococcus neoformans.*

Macroscopic features
- Oedema of udder.

231

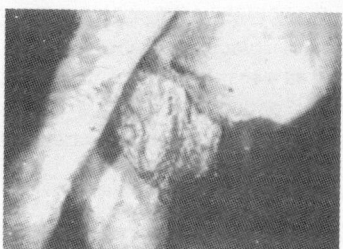

Fig. 19.9. Photograph showing mastitis due to
fusarium toxicosis

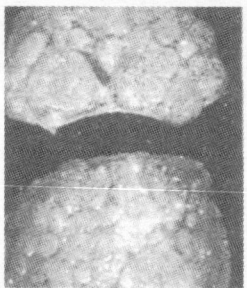

Fig. 19.10. Photograph showing chronic
granulomatous mastitis (ARS/USDA)

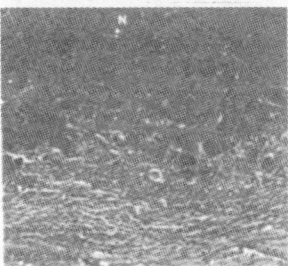

Fig. 19.11. Photomicrograph showing chronic
granulomatous mastitis (ARS/USDA)

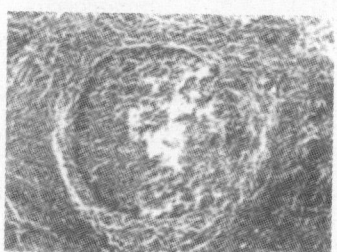

Fig. 19.12 Photomicrograph showing mycoplasmal
mastitis

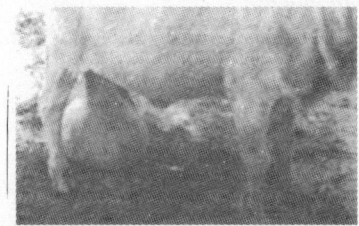

Fig. 19.13. Photograph showing orchitis in a ram

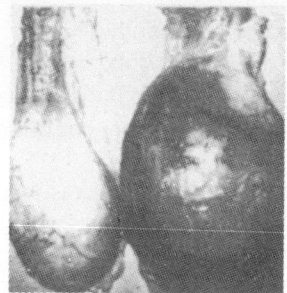

Fig. 19.14. Photograph of testicles showing
(A) normal (b) Acute orchitis.

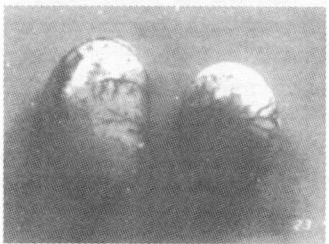

Fig. 19.15. Photograph of testicles of poultry
showing orchitis due to slamonellosis

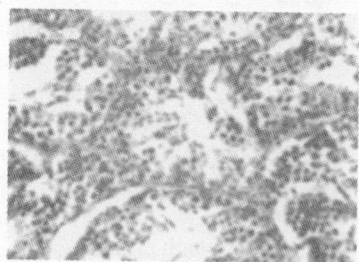

Fig. 19.16. Photomicrograph showing orchitis

- Flakes (coagulated milk proteins) in milk.
- Blood mixed milk.
- Watery dirty grey or dark colour milk in animals. In dry period it is caused by *Actinomyces pyogenes* and is known as *"summer mastitis"*.
- Terminal atrophy or shrunken quarter.
- Gangrene formation.

Microscopic features
- Congestion, haemorrhage.
- Infiltration of neutrophils, macrophages, lymphocytes.
- Necrosis of alveolar epithelium, hyperplasia of epithelial lining.
- Proliferation of fibrous tissue.
- Increase in WBC count in milk (more than 100/ml milk).

MALE GENITAL SYSTEM
DEVELOPMENTAL ANOMALIES

Testicular hypoplasia
Testicular hypoplasia occurs in animals with chromosomal abnormality such as XXY chromosomes or Klinefelter's syndrome. Hypoplasia is also seen in hermaphrodites and in animals with cryptorchidism.

Spermatocele
There is failure of development of mesonephric tubules and it does not connect with vas deferens resulting in blind tubules filled with spermatozoa. Rupture of tubules may lead to spermatic granuloma.

Cryptorchidism
The testicles fail to descend in scrotum through inguinal canal after birth and remains in abdominal cavity. This permanent retention of testicles in abdominal cavity causes their hypoplasia leading to lack of spermatogenesis. Such testes are more prone to development of neoplastic growth.

Phimosis
Phimosis is the failure of extension of penis from its sheath.

Paraphimosis
Paraphimosis is the failure of withdrawal of extended penis.

Hypospadias
In hypospadias, there is urethral opening in ventral side of the penis.

Epispadias
There is urethral opening on the dorsal side of the penis.

Phallocampsis
Phallocampsis is the deviation of penis, which may be spiral (*Cork screw penis*) or ventral deviation (*rainbow penis*).

ORCHITIS
Orchitis is the inflammation of testes characterized by oedema, necrosis and infiltration of neutrophils, macrophages, lymphocytes and proliferation of fibrous tissue leading to atrophy in chronic cases (Figs. 19.13 to 19.16).

Etiology
- *Brucella* spp.
- *Campylobactor* spp.
- *Salmonella* spp.
- *Trichomonas* spp.
- *Corynebacterium pseudotuberculosis.*
- *Actinomycess pyogenes.*
- *Pseudomanas aeruginosa.*
- *Actinomyces bovis.*

Macroscopic feature
- Enlargement of testes, oedema.
- Accumulation of serus fluid in scrotal sac/tunica vaginalis is called as *hydrocele*.
- Enlargement of scrotum.
- Congestion.
- Atrophy and hardening in chronic cases.

Microscopic features

- Congestion.
- Infiltration of neutrophils and mononuclear cells.
- Necrosis of germinal cells.
- Proliferation of fibrous tissue and infilteration of mononuclear cells.
- Granulomatous lesions in case of actinomycosis and tuberculosis.
- Aspermatogenesis.

EPIDIDYMITIS

Epididymitis is the inflammation of epididymis characterized by catarrhal or suppurative exudate with necrosis of lining epithelium.

Etiology

- *Brucella ovis* in sheep.
- Other organisms that cause orchitis which is preceded by epididymitis.

Macroscopic features

- Enlargement of epididymis.
- Oedema of scrotum.
- Accumulation of mucus and/or purulent exudate in epididymis.
- Accumulation of serus exudate in scrotum.

Microscopic features

- Necrosis of lining epithelium of epididymis.
- Infiltration of neutrophils, macrophages and lymphocytes.
- Oedema.
- Formation of granuloma in chronic cases.

FUNICULITIS

Funiculitis is inflammation of scirrhous cord characterized by enlargement of scrotum due to chronic abscess.

Etiology/Occurrence

- Botryomycosis.
- Actinomycosis.
- Castration.
- Unsanitary conditions.

Macroscopic features

- Enlargement of scrotum.
- Hard swelling/ chronic abscess.

Microscopic features

- Chronic hyperplastic/proliferative changes.
- Fibroplasia.
- Infiltration of macrophages, lymphocytes, neutrophils around sulphur granules forming rosette.

SEMINAL VESICULITIS

Seminal vesiculitis is the inflammation of seminal vesicle characterized by metaplasia of the columnar epithelial lining to cornfied stratified squamous epithelium.

Etiology

- *Pseudomonas aeruginosa.*
- *Chlamydia psittasci.*
- *Mycoplasma bovigenitalium.*
- *Actinomyces pyogenes.*
- *Corynebacterium renale.*
- *Brucella abortus.*
- *E. coli.*

Macroscopic features

- Melanosis in bulbourethral glands.
- Enlargement/hardness of seminal vesicle.

Microscopic features

- Metaplasia of columnar epithelium into severely cornified stratified squamous epithelium.
- Proliferation of melanoblasts/melanocytes.

PROSTATITIS

Prostatitis is the inflammation of prostate gland by formation of painful abscess, atrophy, hyperplasia of epithelial cells, proliferation of fibroblasts and formation of cysts. It occurs in dogs.

Etiology

- Hormonal imbalance.
- Pyogenic staphylococci, streptococci.

Macroscopic features

- Presence of abscess encapsulated by fibrous tissue.
- Enlargement of prostate causing obstruction of urethra.
- Obstruction in rectal passage.
- Hematuria.

Microscopic features

- Infiltration of neutrophils and liquefied necrosis.
- Chronic inflammation is characterized by hyperplasia of glandular epithelium, fibroblasts and smooth muscle fibres.
- Cystic glandular hyperplasia.
- Infiltration of lymphocytes.

BALANOPOSTHITIS

Balanoposthitis is the inflammation of prepuce and glans penis characterized by phimosis or paraphimosis and pain during copulation. Balanitis is inflammation of glans penis and posthitis is inflammation of prepuce.

Etiology

- *Trichomonas foetus.*
- BHV-1 virus.
- Vesicular exanthema virus.
- *Mycoplasma* spp.
- *Pseudomonas aeruginosa.*
- *Actinomyces pyogenes.*
- *Corynebacterium renale.*

Macroscopic features

- Phimosis and paraphimosis due to pain, adhesions.
- Congestion.

Microscopic features

- Fibrinopurulent exudate.
- Lymphocytic infilteration, congestion.

MODEL QUESTIONS

Q. 1. *Fill in the blanks with suitable word(s).*

1. Cystic ovary occurs due to...........imbalance and is characterized either by...........cyst manifested by............., ... and...........or..........cyst that leads to .... confused with ....
2. Pyometra is .... inflammation of uterus characterized by accumulation of .... in uterus under the influence of .... hormone secreted by..................
3. Endometritis is mostly characterized by .... inflammation.
4. Early abortions in cattle are caused by .... while late abortions are caused by ...., ... and ....
5. Fungal infection causes .... inflammation of placenta that leads to abortion and .... formation in foetal river.
6. Infectious vulvovaginitis is caused by .... which is transmissible to male counter part through coitus and characterized by .... and jointly this disease is known as.................

Q. 2. *Write true or false against each statement. Correct the false statement.*

1. ....Mastitis is caused by chemical poisons.
2. ....Acute placentitis leads to abortion.
3. ....Hypoplasia of cervix and vagina is seen in uterus unicornis.
4. ....Pseudocyesis is seen during endometritis.
5. ....Brucellosis causes early abortion in cows.
6. ....Salpingitis may cause death of sperms and zygote.
7. ....Balanitis may cause vaginitis through coitus.
8. ....Hematogenous infection of *Pasteurella multocida* infection causes mastitis.
9. ....Retention of placenta occurs in trichomoniasis.

10. ....Rainbow penis is seen as a developmental defect characterized by spiral shape of the penis.

Q. 3.   *Define the following*

1. Uterus unicornis
2. Vulvovaginitis
3. Hydrosalpinx
4. Stillbirth
5. Pseudohermaphrodite
6. Pseudocyesis
7. Placentitis
8. Premature birth
9. Cervix bifida
10. Spermatocele
11. Pyosalpinx
12. Phimosis
13. Epispadias
14. Cervicitis
15. Mummified foetus
16. Hypospadias
17. Uterus didelphys
18. Shrunken udder
19. Pseudopregnancy
20. Phallocampsis
21. Paraphimosis
22. Funiculitis
23. Balanitis
24. Posthitis
25. Corkscrew penis

Q. 4.   *Write short notes on*

1. Cystic ovary
2. Pyometra
3. Endometritis
4. Late abortions
5. Summer mastitis
6. Cryptorchidism
7. Orchitis
8. Prostatitis
9. Mastitis
10. Epididymitis

Q. 5.   *Select most appropriate word(s) from the four options given against each statement.*

1. Cryptorchidism may lead to .... of testicles.
   (a) Hypoplasia   (b) Aspermatogenesis   (c) Neoplasia   (d)All of the above
2. Ventral deviation of penis is known as ....
   (a) Corkscrew penis   (b) Phallocampsis   (c) Rainbow penis   (d) None
3. Hydrocele is accumulation of serus fluid in ....
   (a) Oviduct   (b) Testes   (c) Mammary gland   (d) Tunica vaginalis
4. Funiculitis is the inflammation of ....
   (a) Scirrhous cord   (b) Seminal vesicle   (c) Glans penis   (d) Prepuce
5. Phimosis is caused by ....
   (a) Balanitis   (b) Posthitis   (c) Balanoposthitis   (d)All of the above
6. Presence of follicular cysts in ovary may lead to ....
   (a) Sterility   (b) Nymphomania   (c) Continuous oestrus   (d)All of the above
7. Inflammation of oviduct leads to sterility due to .... nature of the exudate to sperms.
   (a) Toxic   (b) Obstructive   (c) Penetrative   (d) None
8. Mastitis is mostly caused by ....
   (a) Trauma   (b) Hematogenous infection (c) Toxins/poisons   (d) Infection
9. Summer mastitis is caused by ....
   (a) Staphylococci   (b) *Actinomyces pyogenes* (c) Streptococci   (d) *Candida albicans*
10. Parturition of a dead foetus on its full development and gestation is termed as ....
    (a) Abortion   (b) Stillbirth   (c) Premature birth   (d) Normal birth

20

PATHOLOGY OF NERVOUS SYSTEM

- **Encephalitis**

- **Encephalomalacia**

- **Spongiform Encephalopathy**

- **Meningitis**

- **Neuritis**

- **Model Questions**

Nervous system is composed of brain, spinal cord, and peripheral nerves. The neuron is a basic functional unit of nervous system. Necrosis of neurons in brain is known as *encephalomalacia* while necrosis of neurons in spinal cord is termed as *myelomalacia*. If the necrosis occurs in grey matter it is known as *polioencephalomalacia* while necrosis of neurons in white matter is called as *leukoencephalomalacia*. There are three types of scavenger cells in nervous system known as *microglial*, *oligodendroglial* and *astrocytes*. Microglial cells surround the necrotic neurons and are known as *satellite cells* and the process is called as *satellitosis*. As the neuron dies, it is engulfed by microglial cell and this process is termed as *neuronophagia*. The necrosis of nerve fibres starts from myelin sheath and this change is called *demyelination* or *Wallerian degeneration*.

The brain and spinal cord is covered by meninges. The inflammation of meninges is termed as *meningitis*. *Meningoencephalitis*. The term is used for inflammation of both meninges and brain. Inflammation of duramater is known as *pachymeningitis* and of piamater is termed as *leptomeningitis*. *Hydrocephalus* means accumulation of clear fluid in ventricles and in sub arachnoid space due to obstruction in drainage. Hydrocephalus occurs in neonatal calves due to influenza and parainfluenza virus and is termed as *congenital hydrocephalus*.

Some nutritional deficiency like vitamin A, folic acid, vitamin B_{12}, niacin and zinc may also lead to hydrocephalus. Cerebeller hypoplasia has been observed due to bovine virus diarrhoea, hog cholera and feline panleukopenia virus. Some other congenital malformations are as under.

Anencephaly means absence of brain.

Microencephaly means small size of brain. *Cranioschisis* is failure of cranium to fuse which results in hernia of meninges known as *meningocele*. Hernia of meninges and brain is known as *meningoencephalocele*.

ENCEPHALITIS

Encephalitis is the inflammation of brain characterized by purulent/lymphocytic or proliferative changes. Encephalomyelitis is the inflammation of brain as well as spinal cord (Figs. 20.1 to 20.11).

Etiology
- Bacteria
  - *Listeria monocytogenes (L. ivanovii)* main cause
  - *Haemophius* spp.
  - *Pasturella* spp.
- Virus.
- Mycoplasma.
- Strychnine poisoning.

Macroscopic features
- Congestion.
- Haemorrhage.
- Small, tiny abscess.
- Necrosis also known as encephalomalacia.
- Involvement of spinal cord leads to encephalomyelitis and of meninges and is termed as meningoencephalitis.

Microscopic features
- Tiny or micro abscess in cerebrum.
- Infiltration by neutrophils and lymphocytes.
- Perivascular cuffing in Virchow Robin space by lymphocytes.
- Necrosis of neurons.
- Satellitosis, neuronophagia.
- Pleocytosis- Increase in number of white blood cells in cerebrospinal fluid.

ENCEPHALOMALACIA

Encephalomalacia is the necrosis of nervous tissue in brain characterized by loss of normal architecture and soft friable liquefied mass (Figs. 20.12 & 20.13).

Etiology
- Deficiency of copper, thiamine, vitamin E.
- Poisons: Bracken fern, lead, mercury, salt poisoning, enterotoxaemia, mycotoxins.

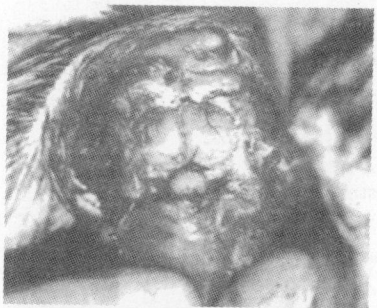

Fig. 20.1. Photograph of brain showing congestion in poultry

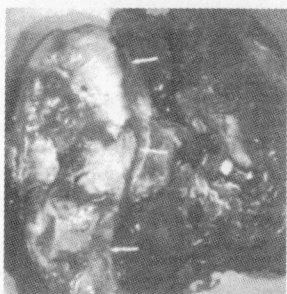

Fig. 20.2. Photograph showing abscess in brain (ARS/USDA)

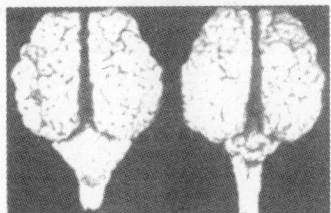

Fig. 20.3. Photograph of cerebeller hypoplasia

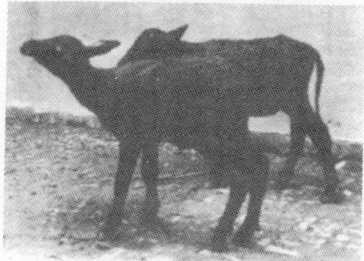

Fig. 20.4. Photograph showing staggering gait in buffalo calf due to strychnine poisoning

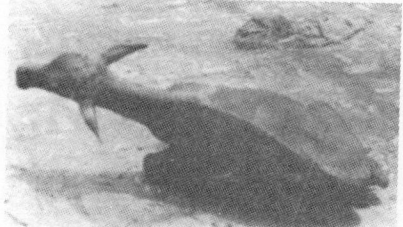

Fig. 20.5. Photograph showing spasms in neck due to strychnine poisoning

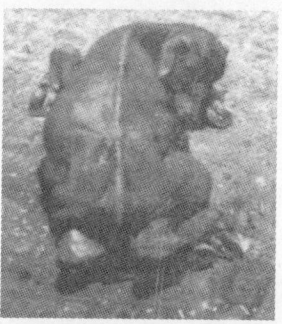

Fig. 20.6. Photograph showing torticollis in buffalo calf due to strychnine poisoning

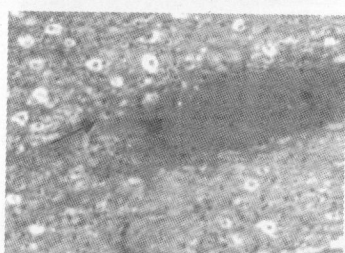

Fig. 20.7. Photomicrograph showing perivascular cuffing in brain.

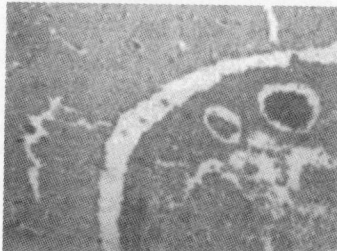

Fig. 20.8. Photomicrograph showing menigoencephalitis

Macroscopic features
- Encephalomalacia - necrosis in brain.
- Myelomalacia - necrosis in spinal cord.
- Poliomalacia - necrosis in brain gray matter.
- Leukomalacia - necrosis in brain white matter.
- Soft, friable liquefied mass in brain.
- Congestion.

Microscopic features
- Liquefactive necrosis.
- Surrounded by neurological cells/scavenger cells.
- Proliferation of small new capillaries

SPONGIFORM ENCEPHALOPATHY

Spongiform encephalopathy is characterized by the presence of vacuoles in grey and/or white matter.

Etiology
- Prion proteins.
- Scrapie in sheep.
- BSE in cattle.

Macroscopic features
- No characteristic gross lesion.
- Oedema of brain or hydrocephalus.
- Congestion.

Microscopic features
- Vacuolation in white and grey matter.
- Vacuoles are usually in neurons, glial cells and in myelin.
- Vacuoles are more extensive in medulla, pons and mid brain and give brain "spongy form".

MENINGITIS

Meningitis is the inflammation of meninges, usually occurs along with encephalitis or encephalomyelitis and is characterized by congestion and infiltration of neutrophils and mononuclear cells. Pachymeningitis is inflammation of dura mater while leptomenigitis involves the pia mater.

Etiology
- Virus *e.g.* swine fever.
- Trauma.
- Bacteria *e.g.* Pasturella, Listeria.
- Toxoplasma.
- Leptospira.

Macroscopic features
- Congestion.
- Thickening of meninges.
- Petechial haemorrhage.

Microscopic features
- Congestion.
- Infiltration of neutrophils and lymphocytes.
- Fibrosis.

NEURITIS

Neuritis is the inflammation of nerves along with degenerative changes characterized by oedema, infiltration of inflammatory cells (Fig. 20.14 to 20.16).

Etiology
- Toxins.
- Trauma.
- Virus *e.g.* Marek's disease MD.
- Lead and Mercury.
- Bacteria *e.g.* Strangles.
- Deficiency of vitamin E.

Macroscopic features
- Wallerian degeneration.
- Infiltration of neutrophils and lymphocytes.
- More destruction at distal end of the neuron.

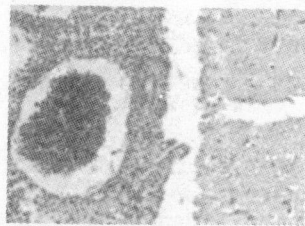

Fig. 20.9. Photomicrograph showing congestion and infiltration of inflammatory cells in brain

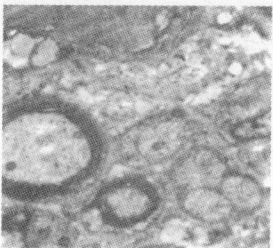

Fig. 20.10. Electronmicrophotograph of brain showing increase in endoneural space and Wallerian degeneration in nerve fiber.

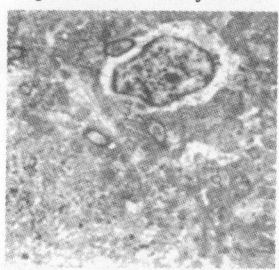

Fig. 20.11. Electronmicrophotograph of brain showing phagocytosis of degenerated nerve cell by phagocytic cell (Neuronophagia)

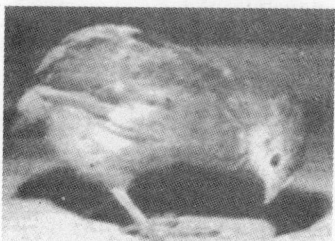

Fig. 20.12. Photograph showing encephalomalacia in a chick

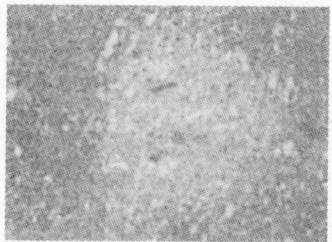

Fig. 20.13. Photomicrograph showing encephalomalacia

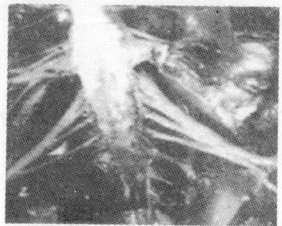

Fig. 20.14. Photograph showing neuritis due to Marek's disease

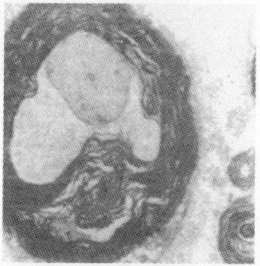

Fig. 20.15. Electronmicrophotograph of sciatic nerve showing degeneration of myelinated fibres with swelling and fragmentation

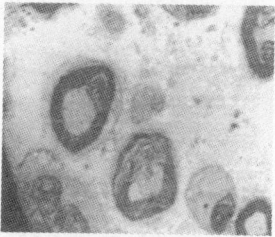

Fig. 20.16. Electttronmicrophotograph of sciatic nerve showing advanced Wallerian degeneration and increased endoneural space.

MODEL QUESTIONS

Q. 1. *Fill in the blanks with suitable word(s).*
1. Necrosis of neurons in brain is known as .... while that of spinal cord in termed as ....
2. Encephalitis is the .... of brain caused mainly by .... and characterized by ...., ..., ..., ... and ....
3. Necrosis of nerve cells in grey and white matter is known as .... and ...., respectively. The necrosed neurons are surrounded by .... cells and the process is termed as .... while they are eaten away by these cells and the process is known as................
4. Vacuoles in ...., ... and .... and which are more prominent in .... , ...and...............and give the brain .... are only diagnostic lesions of BSE in cattle.
5. The inflammation of pia mater is .... and of dura mater is ....

Q. 2. *Write true or false against each statement and correct the false statement.*
1. ....Meningoencephalomyelitis is the inflammation of brain and meninges.
2. ....Vitamin B$_{12}$ deficiency may cause cerebral hydrocephalus.
3. ....Neuronophagia is necrosis of nerve fibres.
4. ....Inflammation of dura mmter is known as patchymeningitis
5. ....Polioencephalomalacia is inflammation of white matter of brain.
6. ....Spongiform encephalopathy is caused by a virus.
7. ....Vacuoles in neurons in brain are main diagnostic lesion which helps in diagnosis of BSE.
8. ....Leptospira may cause meningitis and myelitis.
9. ....Neuritis can be observed in Marek's disease.
10. ....Mycotoxins may cause encephalomalacia in calves.

Q. 3. *Define the following*
1. Myelomalacia
2. Satellitosis
3. Neuronophagia
4. Pleocytosis
5. Cranioschisis
6. Microencephaly
7. Anencephaly
8. Meningoencephomyelitis
9. Cerebellar hypoplasia
10. Leptomeningitis
11. Leukomalacia
12. Wallerian degeneration
13. Poliomalacia
14. Pachymeningitis
15. Perivascular cuffing

Q. 4. *Write short notes on*
1. Bovine spongiform encephalopathy
2. Encephalomalacia
3. Encephalitis
4. Meningitis
5. Hydrocephalus

Q. 5. *Select the most appropriate word(s) from the four options given against each statement.*

1. Neuritis is observed in ....
   (a) Mucosal disease (b) Infectious bursal disease (c) Marek's disease (d) ILT
2. Necrosis of brain in known as ....
   (a) Encephalomalacia (b) Polioencephalomalacia (c) Myelomalacia (d) None of the above
3. Removal of dead neurons through microglial cells in known as ....
   (a) Satellitosis (b) Neuronophagia (c) Perivascular cuffing (d) None
4. Increase in number of white blood cells in cerbrospinal fluid in termed as ....
   (a) Encephalitis (b) Satellitosis (c) Pleocytosis (d) Leucoencephalomalacia
5. Spongiform encephalopathy is caused by ....
   (a) Virus (b) Viroids (c) Prions (d) Deficiency of vit B_{12}
6. Inflammation of dura mater is known as ....
   (a) Leptomeningitis (b) Pachymeningitis (c) Meningitis (d) Meningoencephalitis
7. Congenitally small size brain is termed as ....
   (a) Anencephaly (b) Hydrocephalus (c) Microencephaly (d) Cranioschisis
8. Phagocytic cells of brain are ....cell(s)
   (a) Astrocytes (b) Microglial (c) Oligodendroglial (d) All of the above
9. Increase in CSF in sub arachnoid space is known as ....
   (a) Pleocytosis (b) Hydrocephalus (c) Microencephaly (d) Hypoplasia
10. Hernia of meninges through cranioschisis is known as ....
    (a) Hydrocele (b) Meningocele (c) Meningoencephalocele (d) None

21
PATHOLOGY OF ENDOCRINE SYSTEM, EYES AND EAR

- **Pathology of Endocrine System**
  - Pathology of Hypothalamus
  - Pathology of Pituitary
  - Pathology of Thyroid
  - Pathology of Parathyroid
  - Pathology of Adrenal glands
  - Pathology of Pancreas
  - Pathology of Pineal gland
- **Pathology of Eyes**
  - Keratoconjunctivitis
  - Cataract
- **Pathology of Ear**
  - Otitis externa
  - Otitis media
  - Otitis interna
- **Model Questions**

PATHOLOGY OF ENDOCRINE SYSTEM
PATHOLOGY OF HYPOTHALAMUS

The lesions in hypothalamus may cause diabetes insipedus characterized by polydipsia and polyuria with low specific gravity of urine. It occurs due to deficiency of antidiuretic hormone vasopressin.

Etiology/ Occurrence

- Lesions in hypothalamus and/or pituitary.
- Adenoma and adenocarcinoma of pituitary.
- Necrosis of hypothalamic nuclei due to larval migration.

PATHOLOGY OF PITUITARY GLAND
HYPERPITUITARISM

Hyperpituitarism is increased secretion of hormone(s) from pituitary gland such as excessive secretion of somatotropic hormone which may cause gigantism characterized by increased length of long bones, heavy and thick bones leading to large hands, feet, skull bones (*acromegaly*). Hyperpituitarism also increases adrenal cortical stimulating hormone leading to hyperplasia of adrenal cortex. Pituitary adenoma or adeno-carcinoma is responsible for hyperpituitarism.

HYPOPITUITARISM

Hypopituitarism is decrease in pituitary hormone secretions due to atrophy, aplasia or hypoplasia of pituitary. Systemic diseases such as meningitis of bacterial or viral origin may also cause lesions in pituitary *e.g.* infectious canine hepatitis, hog cholera. It is characterized by dwarfism, genital hypoplasia and prolonged gestation period.

PATHOLOGY OF THYROID
HYPERTHYROIDISM

Hyperthyroidism is increased activity of thyroid gland leading to increased production of thyroxin characterized by tachycardia, increased basal metabolic rate, bulging of eyeballs and early maturity. It occurs due to presence of tumor in thyroid. Other signs include polydipsia, polyuria, and loss of weight, weakness, fatigue and hyperthermia.

HYPOTHYROIDISM

Hypothyroidism is reduced activity of thyroid gland characterized by decreased basal metabolic rate, obesity, retardation of growth and sexual development leading to cretinism. In adult, it is characterized by myxomatous mucoid degeneration in subcutaneous region giving floppy and oedematous appearance. Hypothyroidism is caused by aplasia or hypoplasia of thyroid gland.

Goiter

Goiter is enlargement of thyroid gland, which may be accompanied by hypo- or hyperthyroidism. The enlargement of thyroid is due to hyperplasia, inflammation, or proliferation of connective tissue. The hyperplasia of gland is characterized by increased height and number to epithelial cells in acini of gland. It may be caused by deficiency of iodine, thiouracil toxicity and by use of goiterogenic substances such as soybean and cabbage. The goiter has been classified into 6 forms described as under:

Hyperplastic goiter

Due to iodine deficiency, there is hyperplasia of thyroid gland with reduction in thyroxin production. It occurs due to increased level of thyrotropic hormone from pituitary gland.

Familial goiter

There is hyperplasia of thyroid gland with reduced thyroxin secretion caused by defective or absence of enzymes responsible for thyroxin synthesis. It is not related with iodine deficiency but has congenital basis of occurrence

Colloid goiter

Colloid goiter is enlargement and distention of acini filled with colloid and flat epithelium caused by deficiency of iodine.

Adenomatous goiter

This is characterized by nodular enlargement of thyroid gland, with one or many hard nodules of variable size and characteristic adenoma of gland.

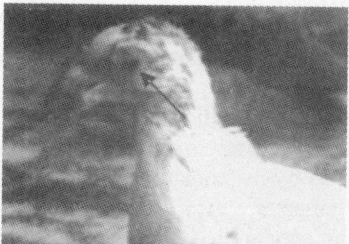

Fig.21.1. Photograph showing conjunctivitis in pigeon due to poxvirus infection

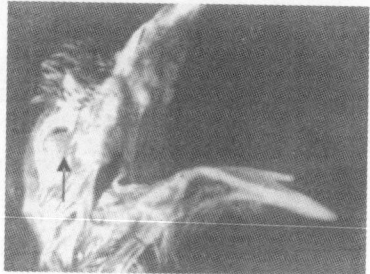

Fig.21.2. Photograph showing conjunctivitis in pigeon due to poxvirus infection

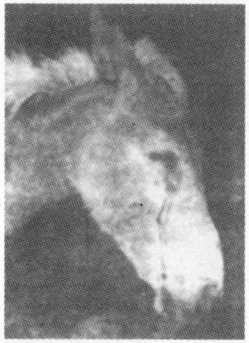

Fig.21.3. Photograph showing mucopurulant discharge from eyes due to mallein test in horse

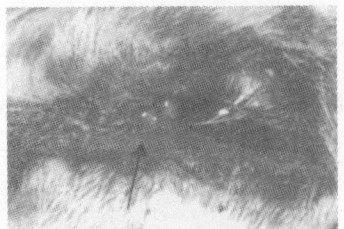

Fig.21.4. Photograph showing mucopurulant exudate in eye

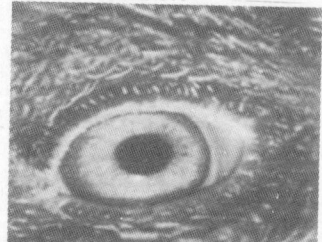

Fig.21.5. Photograph showing iridocyclitis

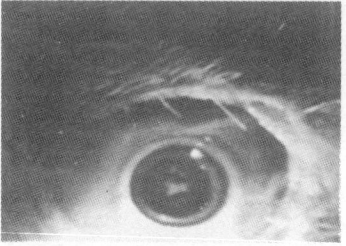

Fig.21.6. Photograph showing cataract

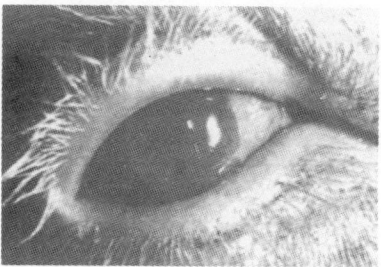

Fig.21.7. Photograph showing corneal opacity

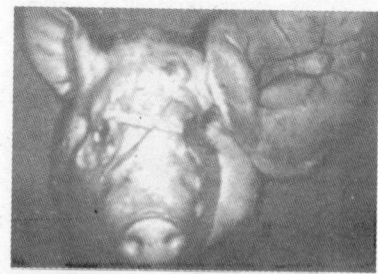

Fig.21.8. Photograph showing otitis externa in pig.

Toxic goiter

Toxic goiter is characterized by exophthalmus due to hyperthyroidism, enlargement of thyroid due to hyperplasia, and occurs as a hypersecretion of thyrotropic hormone from pituitary.

Equine goiter

Equine goiter is caused by excessive iodine levels in feed and occurs in new born foals with weakness from a goiterous mare. These foals have enlarged thyroid gland.

LYMPHOCYTIC THYRODITIS

Lymphocytic thyroditis is characterized by infiltration of lymphocytes in gland causing destruction and is caused by autoimmune mechanism. The infiltration of lymphocytes is so severe that it gives lymphofollicular appearance.

PATHOLOGY OF PARATHYROID GLAND HYPOPARATHYROIDISM

Hypoparathyroidism is decreased activity of parathyroid gland characterized by decreased concentration of blood calcium and tonic spasms of muscles. It occurs due to infection, neoplasms, low calcium diets and hypersecretion of thyrocalcitonin.

HYPERPARATHYROIDISM

Hyperparathyroidism is the increased activity of parathyroid gland characterized by weakness, polydipsia, polyuria, hypercalcemia nephrocalcinosis, demineralization of bones, metastatic calcification in soft tissues and fibrous osteodystrophy. It may occur in adenoma or adenocarcinoma of parathyroid and hyperplasia of gland. Hyperparathyroidism is also associated with renal disease and chronic hypocalcemia and produces more parathormone hormone.

PATHOLOGY OF ADENAL GLANDS HYPOADRENOCORTICISM

Hypoadrenocorticism is decreased activity of adrenal cortex characterized by atrophy, necrosis and decreased hormones leading to low blood pressure, decreased blood volume, hypoglycemia, gastrointestinal malfunction and hyperpigmentation

in skin. It may occur in tuberculosis, histoplasmosis, amyloidosis, neoplasms and drug toxicity.

HYPERADRENOCORTICISM

Hyperadrenocorticism is increased activity of adrenal cortex characterized by hyperplasia and neoplasia of the gland leading to alopecia, muscle weakness, pendulous abdomen, obesity, polyuria, polydipsia, lymphopenia, eosinophilia, neutrophila and excessive secretion of 17- ketogenic steroids.

PATHOLOGY OF PANCREAS

Pancreatic islets or islets of Langerhans' are responsible for production of insulin, deficiency of which may cause hyperglycemia or diabetes mellitus. It is characterized by polyuria, glycosuria, hyperglycemia, polydipsia, loss of secretory granules in β-cells of pancreatic islets. It is caused by inflammation of pancreas causing excocrine pancreatitis. This condition may lead to arteriosclerosis in blood vessels of animals.

PATHOLOGY OF PINEAL GLAND

The pineal gland is responsible for secretion of melatonin hormone which inhibits gonadotropic hormone synthesis and release by pituitary and thus plays an important role in seasonal estrus/reproductive capacity of animals. Degeneration and necrosis of gland may cause its decreased function but it is not well reported. Adenoma of gland may be associated with increased sexual libido and activity.

PATHOLOGY OF EYE

Blepheritis is the inflammation of eyelids while the term *conjunctivitis* is used to describe the inflammatory condition of conjunctiva and *keratitis* for cornea. In ward turning of eyelid is known as *entropion* which may result in keratitis or conjunctivitis. Conjunctivitis is also caused by double row of eye lashes (*disctichiasis*).

DEVELOPMENTAL ANOMALIES

Aphakia is the absence of lens.
Microphakia is the small size of lens.

Hypoplasia of optic nerve is underdeveloped optic nerve with absence of optic nerve layer and ganglion cell layer of retina.

Agenesis of optic nerve is absence of optic nerve.

Coloboma is the congenital defect in the continuity of one of the tunics of the eye *i.e.* iris.

Congenital anophthalmos is the absence of the eye which may occur due to vitamin A deficiency in dam.

Congenital microphathalmos is the decreased size of eyes and may occur due to maternal vitamin A deficiency

Congenital opacity of cornea occurs in cattle and dogs due to effect of inherited recessive gene trait.

Hemeralopia is day blindness which may occur in dogs due to single autosomal recessive gene.

KERATOCONJUNCTIVITIS

Keratoconjunctivitis is the inflammation of cornea and conjunctiva characterized by congestion of eyes, blindness, opacity and corneal oedema (Figs 21.1 to 21.7).

Etiology
- Penetrating foreign objects *e.g.* Awns of wheat.
- *Moraxella bovis.*
- *Mycoplasma* spp.
- BHV-1, poxvirus.
- *Rickettsia conjunctivae.*
- *Chlamydia* spp.
- *Thelazia* spp.
- Allergy.

Macroscopic features
- Congestion of conjunctiva leading to redness "pink eye".
- Oedema, pain
- Increased lacrimation (decreased lacrimation also causes conjunctivitis).
- Corneal opacity.

CATARACT

Cataract is opacity of lens and is classified as under:

Subcapsular cataract is the opacity of lens due to abnormal proliferation of lens epithelium in anterior end as a result of injury.

Posterior polar cataract is opacity of lens due to abnormal growth of lens epithelium at posterior face of lens

Cortical cataract is opacity of lens due to disorganization of the lens fibres.

Nuclear cataract is the increased density of fibres of lens at the centre and occurs in old animals.

Morgagnian cataract is the liquefaction of cortical substance and has not been observed in animals.

Congenital cataract is seen in neonatal animals and occurs due to failure of closure of primary lens vesicle at the periphery of lens vesicle and is associated with chediak - Higashi Syndrome.

RETINITIS

Retinitis is the inflammation of retina caused by trauma, iritis, iridocyclitis and choroiditis. When it is associated with inflammation of choroids, it is known as chorioretinitis. It may lead to detachment of retina. *Iritis* is inflammation of iris. *Iridocyclitis* is the inflammation of iris and uvea. *Choroiditis* is inflammation of choroid plexus.

The *chorioretinitis* is characterized by glaucoma occurs in canine distemper, feline panleukopenia, toxoplasmosis, tuberculosis, coccidioidomycosis, deficiency of vitamin A and bracken fern poisoning.

GLAUCOMA

Glaucoma is the intraoccular hypertension due to occlusion of the filtration angle and is caused by trauma, iridocyclitis, intraoccular haemorrhage and neoplasm. It may be unilateral or bilateral. It is characterized by enlargement of eye ball, opaque cornea and increase aqueous humor.

PATHOLOGY OF EAR
OTITIS EXTERNA

Otitis externa is inflammation of external ear caused by *Actinomyces bovis*, parasites and fungus and characterized by granulomatous inflammation (Fig. 21.8).

Etiology
- *Actinomyces bovis*.
- *Psoroptes communis* – mite.
- *Otobius megnini* – tick.
- Fungi – (otomycosis).
- Grass of wheat awns.

Macroscopic features
- Swelling and congestion leading to obstruction of ear canal.
- Excessive production of thick, tenacious and brownish wax.
- Granulomatous lesions filling the external auditory meatus

Microscopic features
- Granulomatous lesions of actinomycosis in subcutaneous region around the cartilage.

OTITIS MEDIA

Otitis media is inflammation of middle ear including tympanic cavity and eustachian tube.

Etiology
- Infections from otitis externa or nasopharynx.
- Mites.
- Awns of wheat.
- *Pasteurella* spp.

Macroscopic features
- Occlusion of eustachian tube.
- Purulent inflammation.

Microscopic features
- Suppurative inflammation.

OTITIS INTERNA

Otitis interna is the inflammation of inner ear including membranous and osseous labyrinth. This is also known as *labyrinthitis*.

Etiology
- Infection from otitis media.
- *Mycoplasma* spp.
- Mumps .
- Measles.

Macroscopic features
- Disturbance in equilibrium.
- Deafness.

Microscopic features
- Suppurative inflammation.

MODEL QUESTIONS

Q. 1. *Fill in the blanks with suitable word(s).*
1. Pathological lesions in hypothalamus may cause....................characterized by................... and ....with low specific gravity of....................
2. Hyperpituitarism is excessive secretion of...........hormone which may cause............ characterized by..................., ...leading to large..................., ...and..................
3. Goiter is...................of thyroid gland accompanied by...................or..................
4. Hypoparthyroidism is characterized by...................and...................and caused by..................., ..., ...and...................secretion of thyrocalcitonin.
5. Hypoadrenalism may occur in..................,.................,.................,.................. and..................

Q. 2. *Write true or false against each statement. Correct the false statement.*
1. ....Hypoadrenocorticism may cause lymphopenia.
2. ....Disctichiasis is protrusion of eyelid.
3. ....*Moraxella canis* causes pink eye.
4. ....Diabetes mellitus is related with insulin deficiency.

5. ....Hemeralopia is night blindness
6. ....Aphakia is absence of eyelid.
7. ....BHV-1virus is responsible for keratoconjunctivitis.
8. ....Iridocyclitis is inflammation of iris and lens.
9. ....Bracken fern poisoning may cause chorioretinitis
10. ....Cretinism is related with hypothyroidism.

Q. 3.   *Define the following*

1. Aphakia
2. Disctichiasis
3. Labyrinthitis
4. Glaucoma
5. Conjunctivitis
6. Microphakia
7. Retinitis
8. Lymphocytic thyroditis
9. Iritis
10. Keratitis
11. Hypothyroidism
12. Iridocyclitis
13. Coloboma
14. Gigantism
15. Hemeralopia

Q. 4.   *Write short notes on*

1. Goiter
2. Cataract
3. Pink eye
4. Otitis externa
5. Hyperparathyroidism

Q. 5.   *Select the most appropriate word(s) from the four options given against each statement.*

1. Metastatic calcification occurs in...................
   (a) Hyperthyroidism   (b) Hyperparathyroidism   (c) Hypothyroidism   (d) Hypoparathyroidism
2. Goiter is related with...................
   (a) Hypothyroidism   (b) Hyperthyroidism   (c) Both a & b   (d) None
3. Otitis media is the inflammation of middle ear including............
   (a) Tympanic cavity   (b) Eustachian tube   (c) Both a & b   (d) None
4. Disturbance in equilibrium occurs in animals with disease of ....
   (a) External ear   (b) Eyes   (c) Middle ear   (d) Inner ear
5. Glaucoma is caused by...................
   (a) Neoplasm   (b) Trauma   (c) Haemorrhage   (d) All of above
6. *Thelazia* spp worms may cause...................
   (a) Keratoconjunctivitis   (b) Microphakia   (c) Aphakia   (d) Coloboma
7. Cleft in iris is known as...................
   (a) Iritis   (b) Microphakia   (c) Aphakia   (d) Coloboma
8. Equine goiter is caused by...................
   (a) Iodine deficiency   (b) Iodine excess   (c) Cabbage   (d) Radiation
9. Exophthalmos is a feature of................... goiter
   (a) Colloid   (b) Adenomatous   (c) Toxic   (d) Familial
10. Acromegaly is caused by...................
    (a) Hyperpituitarism   (b) Hypopituitarism   (c) Hypothyroidism   (d) Hyperthyroidism

22

APPENDICES

I. Techniques of post-mortem examination

II. Steps in post-mortem examination

III. Writing of post-mortem report

IV. Collection, preservation and dispatch of specimens for laboratory diagnosis

V. Histopathological techniques

VI. Post-mortem examination of veterolegal cases

VII. Collection, preservation and dispatch of material to forensic laboratory

VIII. Examination of blood, urine and faeces

IX. Self assessment

TECHNIQUES OF POST-MORTEM EXAMINATION (NECROPSY)

Necropsy is examination of animal after death. It helps in diagnosis of diseases and their control. It is said that "Necropsy is a message of wisdom from dead to living". Necropsy include systemic examination of dead animal, recording of pathological lesions and their interpretation to make diagnosis of disease. Sometimes it is difficult to arrive at any conclusion merely based on gross examination of dead animal. Then one should seek the help of laboratory examinations from other branches of pathology such as Histopathology, Microbiology, Immunology and Toxicology for confirmation.

Necropsy examination is an integral part of disease investigation. Therefore, veterinarians must have the knowledge of the techniques of post-mortem examination, recording of lesions, collection of proper material for laboratory and most importantly their correlation to arrive at conclusive diagnosis. The technique of post-mortem examination is as under:

POST-MORTEM EXAMINATION OF LARGE ANIMAL

- Place animal on left side (ruminants) (Fig. 22.1).
- Place horse on right side and dog on vertebral column (Figs. 22.2 & 22.3).
- Make midventral incision with knife from chin to anus.
- Surround the prepuce, scrotum/mammary gland.
- Remove skin dorsoventrally. Remove skin at face, neck, thorax and abdomen.
- Cut the muscles and fascia in between scapula and body; remove fore legs.
- Raise hind legs, cut the coxofemoral ligament.
- Examine s/c tissue, muscles, superficial lymphnodes — prescapular, prefemoral supramammary, etc.

- Open abdominal cavity by cutting muscles and peritoneum.

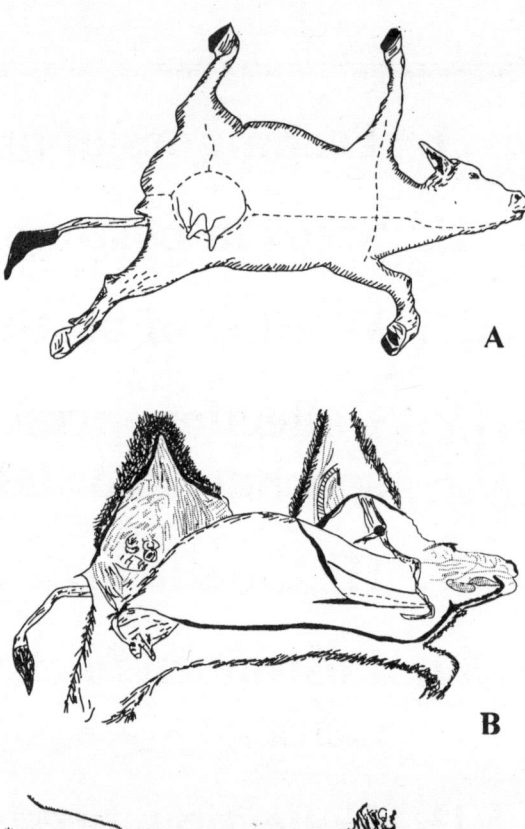

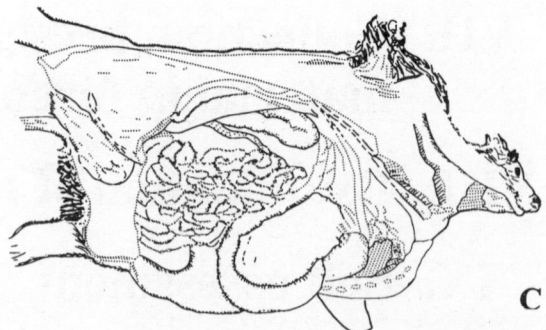

Fig. 22.1. Diagram showing post-mortem examination of ruminant (A) position of cow and the marking for incision (B) after removal of skin and (C) after exposure of abdominal cavity

- Open thoracic cavity by cutting xiphoid cartilage at sternum; lift ribs and press them to break at joints with vertebral column.
- Examine the visceral organs in both cavities:

Thorax : Heart, Lungs, Trachea, Oesophagus, Mediastinal lymphnodes, Diaphragm

Abdominal cavity :

Ruminants : Rumen, Reticulum, Omasum, Abomasum

Other animals : Stomach

In all animals : Liver, Pancreas, Intestines, Mesenteric lymphnodes, Spleen, Kidneys, Ureter

Pelvic cavity : Urinary bladder, uterus

POST-MORTEM EXAMINATION
(POULTRY, Figs. 22.4 to 22.21)

- Dip the dead bird in antiseptic solution or in water to avoid feather contamination.
- Keep the bird on post-mortem table at vertebral column and look for any lesion or parasite on skin.
- Examine the eyes, face and vent.
- Remove skin through a cut with knife and with the help of fingers. Expose thymus, trachea, oesophagus in neck.
- Break the coxofemoral joint by lifting the legs. Examine the chest and thigh muscles.
- Cut on lateral side of chest muscles. Lift the chest muscle dorsally and break bones at joints with thorax. Cut bones at both sides and remove muscles, bones to expose thorax, abdomen.
- Examine different organs.
- Cut proventriculus and pull the organs of digestive tract out. Separate liver, spleen, intestines, caecum, proventriculus, gizzard, etc.
- Expose bursa just beneath the cloaca.
- Cut beak at joint, examine mouth cavity and expose oesophagus and trachea.
- Remove skin of head and make a square cut on skull to expose brain.

- Take a forceps and place in between thigh muscles, remove fascia and expose the sciatic nerve.
- Separate each organ, examine them for the presence of lesion.

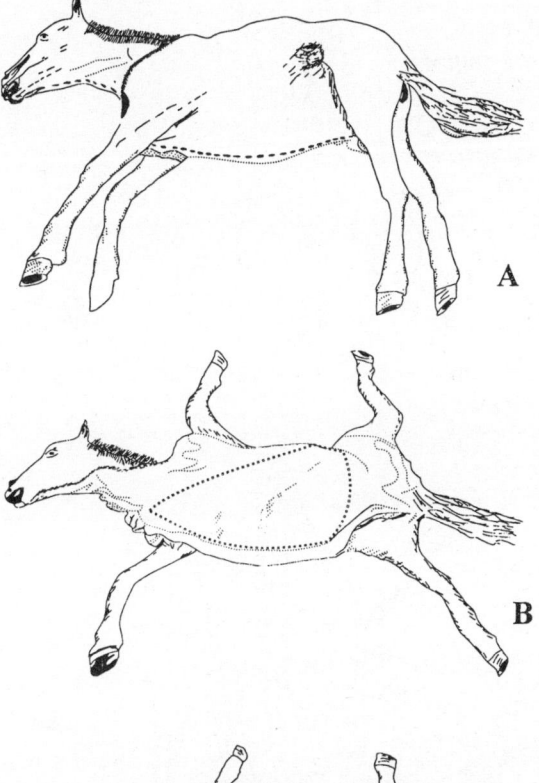

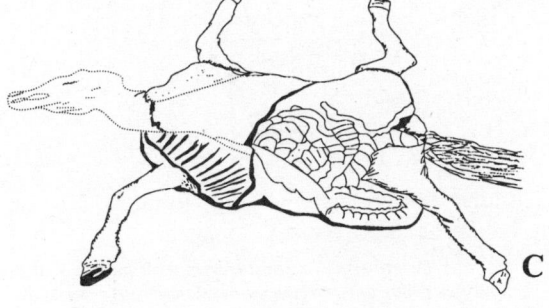

Fig. 22.2. Diagram showing post-mortem examination of horse (A) position of horse and marking for incision (B) after removal of skin and (C) after exposure of abdominal cavity

253

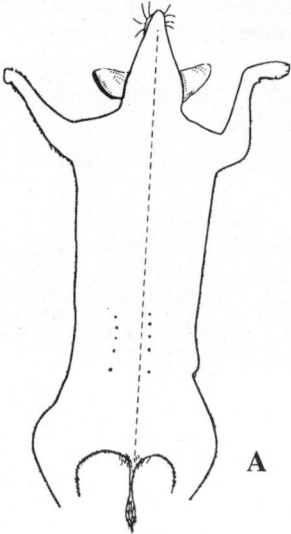

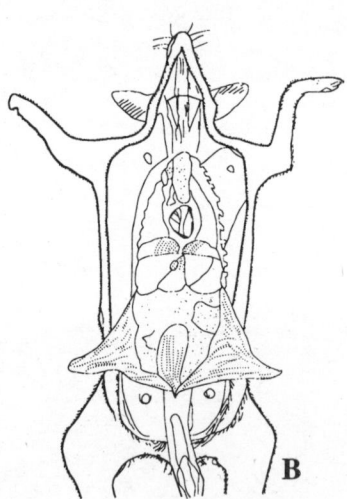

Fig. 22.3. Diagram showing post-mortem examination of dog (A) position of dog and marking for incision (B) after exposure of thoracic and abdominal cavity

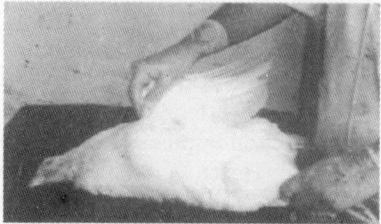

Fig. 22.4. Photograph showing position of bird on post-mortem table

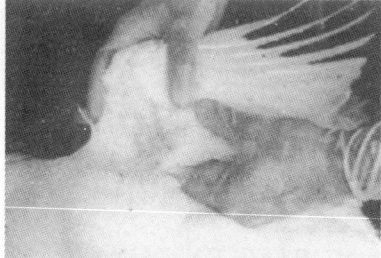

Fig. 22.5. Photograph showing external examination for presence of lice, mites & ticks

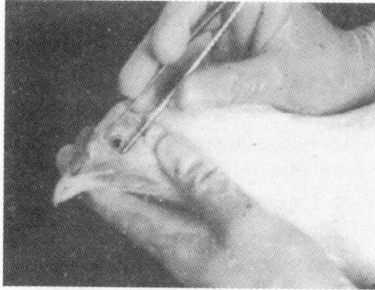

Fig. 22.6. Photograph showing external examination of eyes

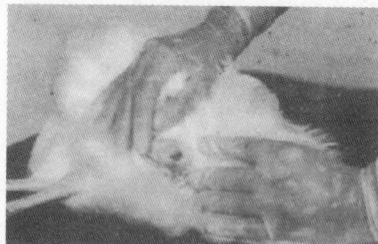

Fig. 22.7. Photograph showing examination of vent

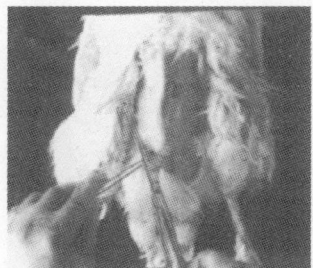

Fig. 22.8. Photograph showing removal of skin

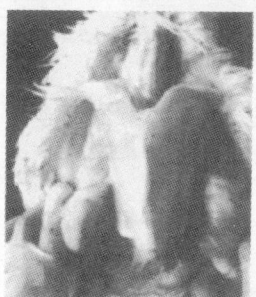

*Fig. 22.9. Photograph showing breaking
of coxofemoral joint*

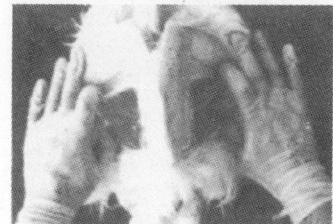

*Fig. 22.10. Photograph showing exposure of
muscles for examination*

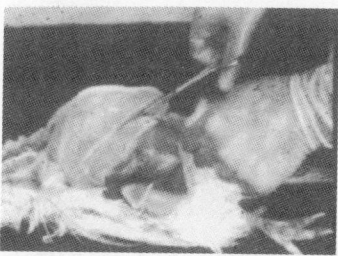

*Fig. 22.11. Photograph showing removal of breast
muscles*

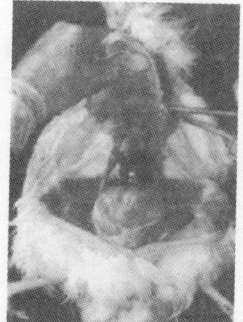

*Fig. 22.12. Photograph showing cutting of
neck bones*

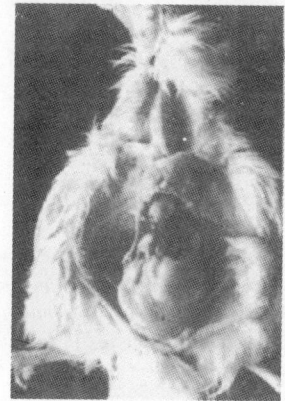

*Fig. 22.13. Photograph showing exposure
of internal organs*

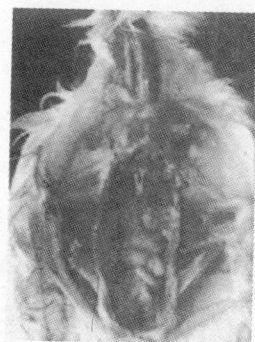

*Fig. 22.14. Photograph showing kidneys, ovary,
oviduct after removal of digestive system and heart*

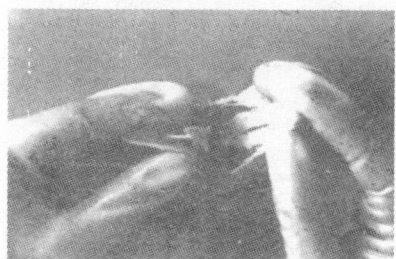

Fig. 22.15. Photograph showing examination
of mouth cavity

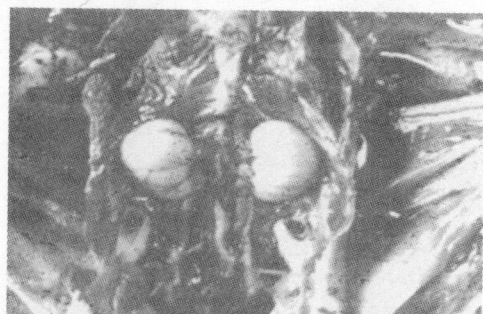

Fig. 22.19. Photograph showing examination of
testes

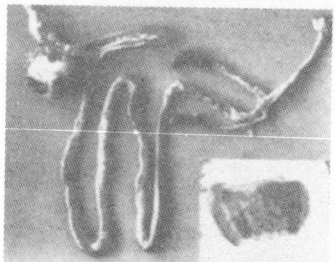

Fig. 22.16. Photograph showing examination of
intestines including caeca and proventriculus

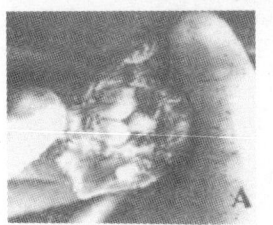 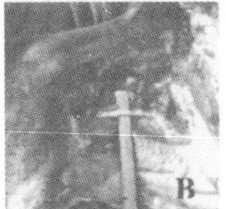

Fig. 22.20. Photograph showing examination of nervous
system (A) brain (B) sciatic nerve

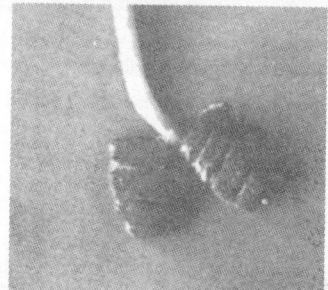

Fig. 22.17. Photograph showing examination of
trachea, bronchi and lungs.

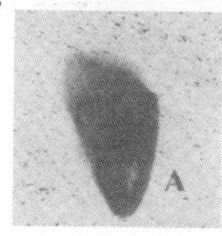 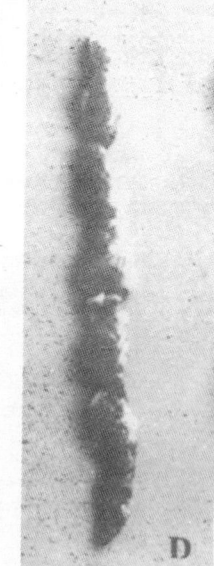

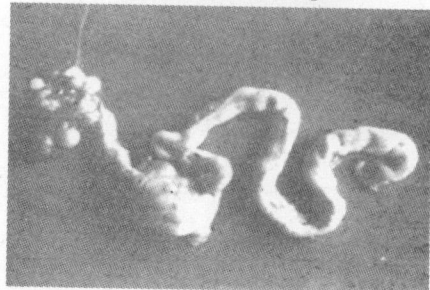

Fig. 22.18. Photograph showing examination of
female genital tract.

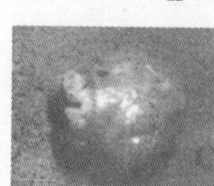

Fig. 22.21. Photograph showing (A) Heart, (B)Spleen
(C) Bursa of Fabricious and (D) Thymus

STEPS IN POST-MORTEM EXAMINATION

Post-mortem examination should be conducted only after receiving a formal request from the owner of animal having details of anamnesis and date and time of death. Without a formal written request, one should not do post-mortem examination of animal. The post-mortem record includes the animal's identification, illness, therapeutic and preventive measures adopted and date and time of death. This information is provided by the owner or person requesting autopsy, which helps in post-mortem examination and recording of lesions to make a conclusive diagnosis.

Various steps in post-mortem examination are as under:

1. External examination

Animal should be examined externally before opening the body for the presence of lesions on body surface. Eyes, ear, anus, vulva, mouth, nares etc. should be specifically examined for the presence of blood and any other lesion. If the blood is coming out from natural orifices, it should be examined for the presence of anthrax bacilli and such carcasses must not be opened for post-mortem examination. Following points should be taken into consideration while conducting external examination.

- Trauma, wound, fracture, cuts, etc.
- Fungal infection *e.g.* ringworm.
- Parasitic infestation *e.g.* mange, lice, ticks.
- Side of animal lying down on earth..
- Discharges from openings.
- Burn, ulcers, erosions etc.

2. Subcutaneous tissue and musculature

Examine the subcutaneous tissue and musculature after removal of skin for the presence of lesions such as:

- Congestion, haemorrhage, oedema, nodule, anemia, icterus.
- Fat deposits.
- Necrosis on muscles, hardening, calcification.

3. Abdominal and thoracic cavity

Just after opening the carcass, one should observe the presence of any lesion in abdominal and thoracic cavity and following points must be kept in mind.

- Accumulation of fluid (serus, serosanguinous, blood, pus etc.).
- Fibrinous or fibrous adhesions.
- Parasites.
- Abscess, tumor etc.

4. Respiratory system
Organs/tissues to be examined

External nares, nasal passage, larynx, trachea, bronchi, lungs, air sacs (poultry) mediastinal lymphnodes.

Lesions to be observed

- Discharge from external nares.
- Growth (granuloma/polyp) in nasal passage if there is blood mixed nasal discharge.
- *Trachea and Bronchi* — Congestion, haemorrhage, presence of caseous exudate, frothy exudate etc.
- *Lungs* — Congestion, consolidation, nodules, presence of exudate on cut surfaces, oedema, atelectasis, emphysema, haemorrhage, necrosis.
- *Mediastinal lymphnodes* — Oedema, hardening, calcification, congestion, haemorrhage.

5. Cardiovascular system
Organs/tissues to be examined

Heart, aorta, arteries, veins and lymphatics.

Lesions to be observed

- Fluid, blood, pus etc. in pericardial sac.
- Adhesions, fibrin, fibrosis.
- Congestion, haemorrhage, necrotic foci.
- Hardening of blood vessel, obstruction, thrombi.
- Presence of parasites.

- Post-mortem clot/thrombi.

6. Digestive system

Organs/tissues to be examined

Mouth cavity, oesophagus, crop, proventriculus, gizzard (poultry), rumen reticulum, omasum, abomasum (ruminants), stomach, intestine (duodenum, jejunum, ileum, caecum, colon, rectum), cloaca, vent (poultry), anus, liver, pancreas, gall bladder, mesenteric lymphnodes etc.

Lesions to be observed

- Erosions, ulcers, vesicles.
- Congestion, haemorrhage, oedema.
- Necrosis.
- Icterus.
- Abscess/pus.
- Perforation, needles or hard objects in reticulum.
- Intussusception, torsion, volvulus.
- Parasites.
- Atrophy, hardening, nodules.
- Contents, catarrhal, blood mixed, digested/undigested feed material, thickening of wall of intestines.
- Cut surface of liver for parasites, lesions in bile duct.

7. Cardiovascular system

Organs/tissues to be examined

- Kidneys, ureter, urinary bladder, urethra

Lesions to be observed

- Congestion, haemorrhage, infarction, oedema.
- Necrosis, hardening, nodules.
- Deposition of salts, calculi.
- Obstruction.

8. Genital system

Organs/tissues (female)

- Ovaries, oviduct, uterus, cervix, vagina.

Male

- Testicles, Epididymis, penis, prepuce.

Lesions to be observed

- Cysts in ovary.
- Congestion, haemorrhage, oedema.
- Foetus in uterus, pus, fluid.
- Necrosis, overgrowth, nodules.
- Atrophy, adhesions, granularity.

9. Immune system

Organs/tissues to be examined

- Spleen, lymphnodes, bursa and thymus (poultry), bone marrow.
- Peyer's patches, GALT, RALT.

Lesions to be observed

- Size, shape, atrophy, hardening.
- Oedema, congestion, haemorrhage.

10. Nervous system

Organs/tissues to be examined

- Brain, spinal cord, nerves, meninges.

Lesions to be observed

- Congestion, haemorrhage, hematoma.
- Oedema, swelling.
- Abscess.
- Hypoplasia.

11. Miscellaneous observation

- Adhesions in pleural/peritoneal cavity.
- Any other left over information pertinent to post-mortem examination/diagnosis.

12. Post-mortem diagnosis

- Diagnosis should be made on the basis of above findings about any system or organ. The most involved organ based diagnosis should be written with suggestion of etiological factors or etiology based diagnosis.

WRITING OF POST-MORTEM REPORT

Post-mortem report consists of two parts, post-mortem record and post-mortem examination as given in the format on next page. The first part *i.e.* post-mortem record contains information related to animal and is supplied by the owner or person requesting post-mortem examination. Actually, it is a part of request form of the case for post-mortem examination. This is necessary for the identification of animal. It should be filled in before conducting post-mortem examination. The proper record will be helpful in establishing accurate diagnosis based on post-mortem examination.

POST-MORTEM RECORD

1. **Species:** Here one should write the species of animal such as bovine, porcine, equine, poultry, etc.

2. **Date:** Date of the post-mortem examination.

3. **Case number:** The serial number of your post-mortem book. It shows cumulatively how many animals are examined by you in necropsy.

4. **Breed:** Mention the breed of animal, if known or supplied, in the request form, such as Murrah buffalo, Jersey cattle, etc.

5. **Age/Date of birth:** Age of animal or its date of birth. In case the exact age is not known then mention young, adult or chick, grower, adult in case of poultry.

6. **Sex:** Sex of animal (male or female).

7. **Identification number/mark:** It must be filled with utmost care; the number (tattoo number or brand number) should be the same as on animal. If the identification number is not available/illegible then write the characteristic mark of animal.

8. **Owner:** Here, the name of owner with complete address must be filled clearly. The address should be complete enough so that the report can reach the owner through post also.

9. **Referred by:** In this column, the name of Veterinary Officer/any other officer who has referred the case for post-mortem examination should be written. Sometimes owner himself/herself is interested in post-mortem examination of animal; in such cases the name of owner should be written.

10. **History of the case:** This includes the clinical illness of animal, duration of illness, epidemiological data, tentative diagnosis, therapeutic and preventive measures adopted. This is very important and information of this column has an important role in making the diagnosis.

11. **Reported date and time of death:** It should have the exact date and time of death of animal. Sometimes, it is difficult to note the exact time then one can write morning, noon, evening, midnight etc. to approximate the timing of death of animal. In some large farms, it is very difficult to record information with regard to each individual animal/bird so here one can write "previous night" as time of death.

12. **Date and time of post-mortem examination:** Pathologist conducting post-mortem examination should write here the exact time and date of the post-mortem examination.

The above information is very important to arrive at any conclusive diagnosis. The correct information enhances the specificity of post-mortem diagnosis. Some points might appear to be insignificant but one should not overlook them and write as correct information as he/she can gather from the owner's request letter/form.

POST-MORTEM REPORT

POST-MORTEM RECORD

1. Species: 2. Date: 3. Case No.:

4. Breed: 5. Age/Date of birth: 6. Sex:

7. Identification No.:

8. Owner's name with address: 9. Referred by:

10. History of the case: 11. Reported date & time of death:

12. Date and time of post-mortem examination:

POST-MORTEM EXAMINATION

1. External appearance :

2. Subcutaneous tissue and musculature :

3. General observations after opening the carcass :

4. Respiratory system :

5. Cardiovascular system :

6. Digestive system :

7. Urinary system :

8. Genital system :

9. Immune system :

10. Nervous system :

11. Miscellaneous observations :

12. Post-mortem diagnosis

Signature of officer conducting post-mortem

Date:
Place:

POST-MORTEM EXAMINATION

It includes the observations made by the pathologist conducting post-mortem examination. This part of report should be filled in as soon as possible after the post-mortem examination. It is advisable to record some points on a small paper or diary during post-mortem examination and fill them in report after the necropsy/autopsy.

1. **External appearance:** Record the lesions observed in intact animal before opening it. One should place on record the side of animal lying down, lesions on skin, external parasites, trauma etc.

2. **Subcutaneous tissue and musculature:** The observations made after removal of skin, on subcutaneous tissue and muscle should be included in this column.

3. **General observations after opening the carcass:** It contains the general information or lesions present in abdominal and thoracic cavity such as accumulation of fluid, pus, blood, clot of blood, post-mortem changes such as pseudomelanosis, etc.

4. **Respiratory system:** Record the lesions observed in respiratory system right from external nares, nasal passage, trachea, bronchi and lungs along with mediastinal lymphnodes.

5. **Cardiovascular system:** Record the lesions present in heart, aorta, arteries, veins and lymphatics.

6. **Digestive system:** Record the lesions observed in digestive tract from mouth cavity, oesophagus, crop, proventriculus, gizzard (poultry), rumen, reticulum, omasum abomasum (ruminants), stomach, intestines, rectum, anus, cloaca, vent (poultry), liver, pancreas, gall bladder etc.

7. **Urinary system:** Place on record the lesions present on kidneys, ureter and urethra.

8. **Genital system:** Record the lesions present in ovaries, uterus, oviduct, cervix and vagina in females and testes, penis etc. in males. Be careful in recording lesions in this column as it should match with the sex of animal written in post-mortem record section.

9. **Immune system:** Record the lesions present in spleen, bursa, thymus, lymphnodes, respiratory associated lymphoid tissue (RALT), gut associated lymphoid tissue (GALT) etc. Careful recording of lesions in these organs will be helpful in diagnosis.

10. **Nervous system:** Place on record the lesions present in brain, spinal cord and nerves. Most of the pathologists overlook this system and often do not taken pain to examine the brain. It should not be done and every effort should be made to examine and place on record the lesions present in this system.

11. **Miscellaneous observations:** Here one can record any missing observation which has not been covered above.

12. **Post-mortem diagnosis:** This is very important. Based on the history and lesions present in different systems, pathologist, by using his experience and conscience, concludes the diagnosis. He/she may also write suggestions along with diagnosis or some points to suggest the diagnosis and/or contain the disease in other animals.

13. **Signature of officer conducting post-mortem:** Each and every report must be signed by the officer doing post-mortem examination. Without signature of competent officer, it has no validity.

14. **Place and date:** The person signing the post-mortem report must also write date and place of post-mortem examination.

COLLECTION, PRESERVATION AND DISPATCH OF SPECIMENS FOR LABORATORY DIAGNOSIS

Tissue samples are collected from dead or live animals for laboratory examination to confirm the tentative diagnosis.

Purpose
- Diagnosis of disease or for identification of new disease.
- Confirmation of tentative diagnosis.
- Prognosis.
- To observe the effect of treatment and give directions for future therapy.

Precautions
- Collect the tissues as early as possible after death of animal.
- Representative tissue/sample should be collected.
- Sharp knife should be used for cutting tissue.
- Collect the tissues directly in fixative.
- Size of tissue should not be more than 1 cm for histopathology in 10% formalin.
- Hollow organs should be taken on paper to avoid shrinkage.
- Hard organs like liver, kidneys etc. should be collected along with capsule.

COLLECTION OF SPECIMENS FOR BACTERIOLOGICAL EXAMINATION
- Collect the tissues under sterile condition.
- Sterilize knife/ scalpel/ spatula on flame or in boiling water.
- Surface sterilized by hot spatula.
- Cut with knife and collect sample from inner tissue.
- Body fluids/blood should be collected in sterilized syringe or in Pasteur pipette.

- Specimens should be collected directly in media (liquid media-nutrient broth, peptone water, tetrathionate broth or even in normal saline solution/phosphate buffer saline).
- Seal, pack and transport the collected material to laboratory in ice/under refrigeration conditions.

BACTERIAL DISEASES
Abscesses
- Swab in sterile conditions/pus in vials.
- Collect material from margin of abscess.

Actinobacillosis/ Actinomycosis
- Tissues from affected parts in 10% formalin.
- Pus in sterile test tube/from edge of lesion.
- Slides from pus for sulphur granules.

Anthrax
- Blood smear from tip of the ear.
- Blood for cultural examination.
- Muzzle piece for biological test.
- Mark the specimen as *"Anthrax suspect"*.

Black Quarter/Black leg
- Smear from swelling.
- Affected muscle piece in ice.

Brucellosis
- Serum after 3 weeks of miscarriage.
- Foetal stomach tied off.
- Swabs from uterine discharge.
- 5 to 10 ml milk in ice.

Glanders
- Smear from discharge.

- Lung, liver and spleen in 10% formalin.
- Serum.

Johne's disease
- Bowel washings in sterile bottle.
- Smear from rectal mucosa.
- Mesenteric lymphnode in 10% formol saline.

Leptospirosis
- Serum 21 days after miscarriage.
- Milk/urine in vials (1 drop of formalin in 20 ml).
- Liver, kidney tissue in 10% formalin.

Listeriosis
- Half brain in ice.
- Half brain in 10% formalin.

Mastitis
- 10 ml milk in sterile vial in ice.

Pasteurellosis
- Heart blood.
- Lung, spleen and mediastinal lymphnodes in ice.
- Affected tissues in 10% formalin.

Salmonellosis
- Liver, spleen, kidney and intestine tied off in ice.

Strangles
- Smear, swab of pus in ice.

Erysipelas
- Blood.
- Spleen, kidney, liver in ice.

Vibriosis/Campylobacteriosis
- Foetal stomach tied off.
- Vaginal mucosa in ice.

- In pig, intestine and liver in 10% formalin.

Colibacillosis
- Heart blood in sterile vial.
- Tissues from intestine and lymphnodes in 10% formol saline.

Tuberculosis
- Lungs, mediastinal and bronchial lymphnodes in ice and in 10% formalin.

COLLECTION OF SPECIMENS FOR VIROLOGICAL EXAMINATION
- Collect tissue under sterilized condition.
- Body fluids/blood in sterilized syringe or in Pasteur pipette.
- Tissues in buffered glycerin.
  - PBS pH 7.2- 50%
  - Glycerin- 50%
- Avoid samples in glycerin from sensitive viruses *e.g.* Rinderpest, canine distemper.
- Seal and mark the specimen bottle and transport to laboratory.

VIRAL DISEASES
Foot and mouth disease
- Tongue epithelium, vesicular fluid, saliva, pancreas in 50% buffered glycerine.
- Serum.

Hog cholera/ swine fever
- Serum under refrigeration.
- Spleen, liver, kidney in 50% glycerin/ice.
- Tissues from intestine, mesenteric lymphnode and half of the brain stem in 10% formol saline.

Infectious Canine Hepatitis
- Several pieces of liver, gall bladder and kidney in 10% formol saline.

Pox
- Scabs in ice and in 10% formol saline.

Rabies

- Intact head should be soaked in 1% carbolic acid.
- Fracture the skull with hammer.
- Remove skin and bones.
- Half brain in 10% formalin.
- Half brain in 50% neutral glycerin.
- Tissues from cerebellum and hippocampus in Zenkers fluid for 20 hrs, wash in tape water for 24 hr and keep in 80% ethyl alcohol for Negribodies.

Ranikhet disease

- Liver, spleen in 50% neutral glycerin.
- Proventriculus in 10% formalin.
- Brain in ice.

Rotaviral enteritis

- Faecal sample.
- Interstinal tissue in 10% formol saline.

Gumboro disease

- Bursa of Fabricious, kidney, muscles in 10% formol saline.
- Bursa, kidney in 50% buffered glycerine.

SYSTEMIC DISEASES

Diarrhoea/Enteritis

- Faecal sample in sterile vial.
- Serum.
- Tissues of intestine, mesenteric lymphnodes in 10% formol saline.

Miscarriage/Metritis

- Foetal stomach content tide off or in sterile vials.
- Serum of dam after 21 days of miscarriage.
- Vaginal discharges in sterile conditions.
- Tissues of placenta, foetal liver, stomach, kidney in 10% formol saline.

Pneumonia

- Nasal discharge/nasal swabs.
- Lung tissue/pieces in sterile vials.
- Lung tissue and mediastinal lymphnode in 10% formol saline.

Dermatitis

- Skin scrapings in 10% KOH.
- Skin tissue in 10% formol saline.

Encephalitis

- Cerebrospinal fluid in heparinised vials.
- Brain tissue in 10% formol saline.
- Brain tissue in 50% glycerol.

Nephritis

- Urine sample in sterile vial.
- Kidney tissue in 10% formol saline.

COLLECTION OF SPECIMENS FOR TOXICOLOGICAL EXAMINATION

- Stomach/intestinal contents.
- Liver, kidneys, heart blood.
- Urine.
- In clean glass jars.
- In ice/refrigeration without any preservative.
- Seal, label, transport to laboratory.
- In veterolegal cases all specimens must be collected in presence of police.
- Type of poison suspected along with detailed history, signs, lesions/treatment etc. should be written on letter with specimens.

TOXICOSIS/POISONING

Heavy metal poisoning

- Hg, Pb, Bi, Ag.
- Liver, kidney, stomach content in ice in separate containers.

Alkaloids

- Liver, stomach contents and brain tissue in ice.

Nitrate

- Fodder.
- Stomach contents, blood in ice.

Strychnine poisoning

- Stomach contents, intestinal contents, urine, liver, kidney in ice.

Hydrocyanic acid

- Plants.
- Stomach contents, blood, liver.
- Preserved in 1% solution of mercuric chloride.

Pesticides

- Fatty tissue, liver, stomach contents, blood in ice.
- Subcutaneous, omental, mesenteric fat.

COLLECTION OF SPECIMENS FOR IMMUNOLOGICAL EXAMINATION

- Heart blood in syringe/ Pasteur pipette.
- CSF/Synovial fluid /peritonial fluid.
- Tissues in formol sublimate or in buffered formalin.
- Blood/serum/others should be sent to laboratory under refrigeration conditions.

- Add one drop of 1:10000 merthiolate in 5 ml serum as preservative.

DISPATCH OF MATERIAL

Following points must be kept in mind while dispatching the material to laboratory for diagnosis.

1. Describe the clinical signs, lesions, tentative diagnosis and treatment given to animal in your letter. Also mention the type of test you want with your tentative diagnosis.
2. Write correct address on letter as well as on the parcel preferably with pin code, if the material is sent through post.
3. Mark the parcel 'Biological Material', 'Handle with care', 'Glass material', 'Fragile' etc. in order to avoid damage in parcel. Also mark the side to be kept on upper side with arrows.
4. Seal the container so that it does not leak in transit.
5. Try to send the material soon after its collection from animal.
6. Keep one copy of cover letter inside the parcel and send another copy by hand or post in a separate cover.
7. Keep adequate material like thermocol etc. in the parcel which will save the material from outside pressures/jerks.
8. Use dry ice, if available, otherwise use ice in sealed containers.

HISTOPATHOLOGICAL TECHNIQUES

Histopathology is the branch of pathology which concerns with the demonstration of minute structural alterations in tissues as a result of disease. Most of histopathological techniques simulate those of applied for study the normal histological structures. For the demonstration of minute histological changes, the tissue must be processed in such a manner that it will provide maximum information. The histopathological diagnosis is an overlooked area specially in Veterinary Sciences. Many times it has been observed that the procedures are not properly followed or the qualified person trained for histopathology is not available, which in turn affects the interpretation and/or diagnosis. Histopathological procedures are described for the benefit of readers which will help them in diagnostic laboratory.

Scope
Though the histopathological techniques are labour intensive, cumbersome and time consuming, particularly when there are automation equipments are not available; their use in diagnosis of diseases is unequivocal. Some of the areas where histopathological diagnosis is helpful are described as follows:

- This is useful in establishing the pathogenesis and pathology of any disease caused by bacteria, virus, chlamydia, rickettsia, mycoplasma, parasite, toxin, poisons etc.

- There are certain diseases in which histopathological examination of tissues is the only alternative to diagnose the disease. *e.g.* Bovine spongiform encephalopathy. The agent of this disease has a very long incubation period and very difficult to isolate and there is no immune response and inflammation in animal. Therefore, histopathology remains the only alternative for confirmatory diagnosis.

- In some cases, the tissues from dead animals are the only available material for laboratory diagnosis. This may occur either due to lack of

time or due to negligence for not collecting the material for serological tests or isolation studies. Sometimes the transportation of material from remote areas destroys the other material and the tissues fixed in formalin only remains for making diagnosis. In all such cases the histopathological examination has its pivotal role.

- The histopathological procedures produce permanent slides, which can be stored for a longer period and one cannot manipulate the findings; therefore, it is considered the best reliable technique.

- The histopathological techniques are useful in carrying out retrospective studies. The unstained slides and blocks can be stored for indefinite period; which can be examined even after many years for further studies.

- The presence of causative agents can also be demonstrated in tissue sections using routine histopathological techniques or special stainings, In the Gram's staining, procedures are used for demonstration of bacteria while viral presence is demonstrated using hematoxylin and eoxin or other staining techniques like Macchiavello's stain or Mann's methylene blue eosin method. The Negri bodies are demonstrated by Seller's stain in case of rabies in animals. In such cases, the isolation of causative agent or their serological examination not required; since the presence of causal agent in infected tissues gives a confirmatory diagnosis.

- The detection of chemicals in tissues like enzymes, lipids etc. is included in histochemical examination; which not only describes the structural changes but also gives an idea about the functional status of the organ.

Histopathological procedures
The microscopic examination of tissues or organs can be achieved by their smears or using vital

staining or by sectioning; the latter method being more commonly used in histopathological laboratories.

Smears

The microscopic examination using smears of any organ/tissue/cells is very rapid method which gives the results within hours. A drop of blood is placed on clean glass slide and with the help of another slide, the smear is prepared (Fig. 22.22). In this the tissue pieces from organs are cut using a sharp knife and the cut surface is mildly touched with clean glass slides with some gentle pressure. Which gives an impression on the slide (Figs. 22.23 & 22.24). This is also known as impression smear; generally 2-5 smears are prepared on a slide. If the collected tissue material is too less then it is pressed between two slides and the impressions thus obtained on both the slides are used for study. The wet smears are fixed with methanol and can be stored or transported to laboratory for examination. The impression smears of hippocampus, cerebellum and cerebrum of brain are very useful for demonstration of Negri bodies in rabid animals for diagnosis of rabies. The impression smears are stained with seller's stain for a few seconds, washed and air dried and examined under oil immersion microscope for the presence of inclusion bodies also known as Negri bodies. These inclusions are characterized by intracytoplasmic, eosinophillic appearance with basophilic granules and round to oval in shape with a clear hallo.

In case of pox infection in animals, the impression smears are prepared from scabe or pustule for demonstration of intracytoplasmic inclusions. Sometimes the viral inoculum is inoculated on chorioallantoic membrane (CAM) of embryonated eggs; the impression smears of CAM may yield the viral inclusions. In certain bacterial diseases like haemorrhagic septiemia and enterotoxaemia, it becomes very difficult to demonstrate the organism in blood or in tissues. For confirmatory diagnosis, the material is inoculated in laboratory animals like mice, guinea pigs etc. The impression smears are then prepared from liver, spleen and other relevant organs of laboratory animals for demonstration of the organism.

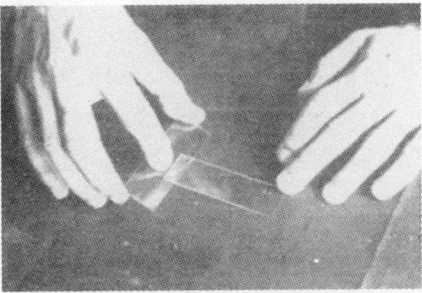

Fig. 22.22. Photograph showing preparation of blood smear

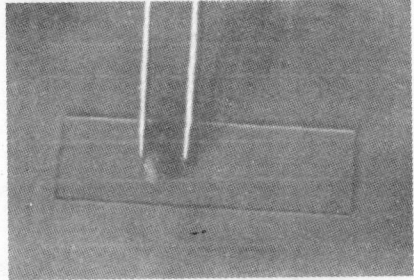

Fig. 22.23. Photograph showing preparation of impression smear

Fig. 22.24. Photograph of impression smear

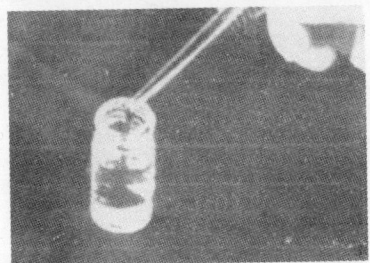

Fig. 22.25. Photograph showing collection of tissue in fixative

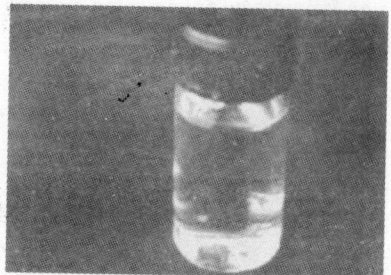

Fig. 22.26. Photograph showing collection of tissue in fixative

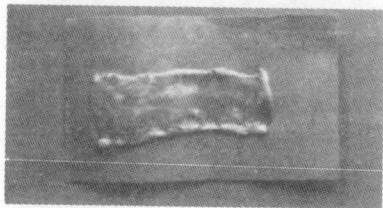

Fig. 22.27. Photograph showing the collection of intestine on a piece of paper for fixation.

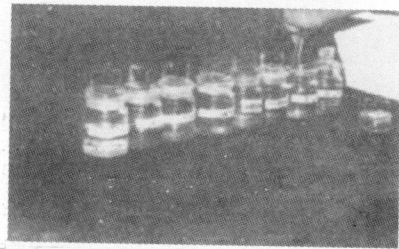

Fig. 22.28. Photograph showing the dehydration of blocks in ascending series of ethanol

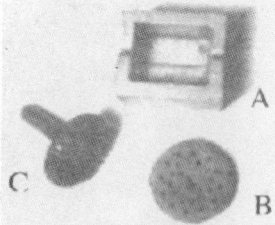

Fig. 22.29. Photograph showing (A) Mould (B) Tissue capsule and (C) Block holder.

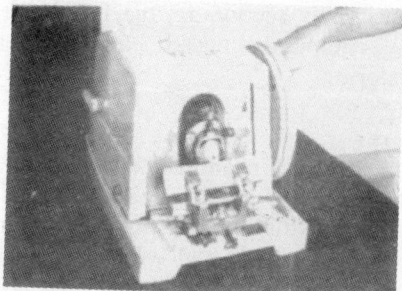

Fig. 22.30. Photograph showing section cutting on microtome

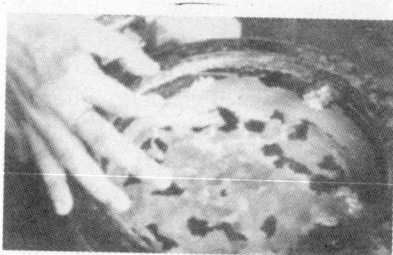

Fig. 22.31. Photograph showing lifting of tissue section from floatation bath

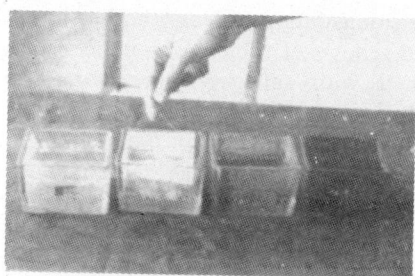

Fig. 22.32. Photograph showing staining of tissue sections

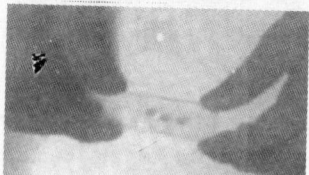

Fig. 22.33. Photograph showing mounting of slides with DPX

Vital Staining

Vital staining procedures are not much in use directly in the diagnosis. However, for detection of phagocytic cells in body the vital stains are used. In the living animals when vital staining procedures are used for localization of phagocytic cells, these are known as *intravital*. *In vitro* use of vital stains is called as *spravital staining* which is being done for the live and dead lymphocyte count in leucocyte migration inhibition test (LMIT), lymphocyte stimulation test (LST), macrophage migration inhibition test (MMIT) and macrophage function tests (MFT).

Routine Histopathological Techniques of sectioning

The tissue pieces from morbid animals should be collected properly and fixed in a suitable fixative. Then these are processed and sections of 4-5 microns are cut and taken on slides. These sections are stained and mounted to make the permanent preparations of slides. The different steps required for making the tissue slides are described briefly as follows.

1. Collection of tissue

The collection of tissues is an important step, which is many times not given proper attention. The whole diagnostic process depends upon the collection of tissue pieces. A representative tissue should have been collected carefully and should have the normal as well as abnormal (lesion) part. The tissues must be collected by qualified person after a thorough examination of each organ/system. Sometimes it has been observed that the collection of tissues is done by attendants or very casually by the qualified persons and proper attention is not paid. It should be kept in mind that a representative tissue sample will only give the correct diagnosis which cannot be corrected/altered afterwards. At the time of tissue collection following points must be kept in mind which will be beneficial for making a correct diagnosis.

- The tissue pieces from morbid animal should be collected as early as possible after the death of animal. Once the autolytic changes starts in the dead body; it will not give true picture of microscopic lesions due to autolysis.

- At the time of tissue collection, it should be kept in mind that the representative tissue piece should include a part of lesion and a part of normal tissue, which facilitates the identification of organ/tissue at the time of microscopic examination.

- The tissue pieces should be cut with sharp knife and using only one stroke. Blunt edged knife may require many attempts for cutting, which destroys the normal architecture of tissues.

- Tissue pieces for histopathological examination should be collected from all the organs. Sometimes it has been noticed that the tissue sample is taken from those parts of body which show gross lesions; merely absence of gross lesion does not mean that there will not be microscopic alteration. In many disease conditions only microscopic changes occur which do not exhibit grossly. Such selective collection of tissues gives a biased interpretation, so it is better to have tissues from all the organs for proper interpretation and unbiased conclusions of histopathological studies.

- Tissues should be collected directly in the fixative and not in any other pot or water (Figs. 22.25 & 22.26). Sometimes it has been observed that at the time of post-mortem examination, the tissue samples are collected in petridishes or in bottles and brought to the laboratory, then fixative is added. This seems to be a wrong practice. The tissue bottles filled with 2/3 fixative must be available at the time of necropsy and tissue pieces should be collected directly in the fixative.

- The size of tissue piece should not be more than 5 mm; it facilitates the homogenous and smooth fixation. Large size tissues do not get fixed properly and in the middle, the tissue gets autolysed.

- The tissue pieces from hollow organs like intestines, oviduct etc should be cut

269

transversely and placed on a hard paper, then it should be cut longitudinally in such a way that the serosal layer sticks to paper and mucosal layer gets free. Thereafter, it should be placed in fixative along with paper. This allows a good fixation and avoids the shrinkage and folding of tissue (Fig. 22.27).

- At the time of post-mortem examination, it has been noticed that the faecal matter is removed from the intestines by pressing/squeezing them or after opening the lumen by sharp objects like knife, slides etc., which causes damage in the mucosal layer. The representative tissue should not be collected from such damaged portions.

- The tissues from encapsulated organs should be collected along with capsule or covering. like brain should be collected along with meninges; kidneys and liver should be collected with their capsules. The coverings of such organs also yield useful information on histopathological examination.

2. Fixation

The fixation of tissues is required for preventing the post-mortem changes like autolysis and putrefaction by saprophytes, preservation of cellular constituents in life-like manner and for hardening of tissues by way of conversion of semisolids to solid material. For a proper histopathological preparation and their interpretation, the role of fixative is very crucial. Any faulty fixation cannot be remedied at any later stage. An ideal fixative should be one that fixes the tissues quickly and does not interfere with the refractive index of the tissue components.

The choice of fixative depends on the type of investigation required, the formol saline (10% formaldehyde in 0.85% sodium chloride solution) is considered best fixative for routine histopathological studies. The buffered formalin has certain advantages over formol saline and now a days it is recommended for routine use in histopathological laboratories. The buffered formalin can also be used for immunopathological studies. Buffered formalin is widely used and preferred because of its tolerance; tissues can be left for longer period without excessive hardening or damage and sectioned easily. Since it has neutral pH, the formalin pigment is also not formed in the tissues. However, for immunopathological studies like immunoperoxidase staining techniques, the fixative of choice is formol sublimate. But in its absence buffered formalin may also be used. The time required for proper fixation is 6-12 hrs for 5 mm thick block of tissue.

3. Washing

After 6-12 hours fixation the tissue pieces are taken out from fixative and cut into 2-3 small pieces of 2-3 mm size blocks. These blocks are then kept in tissue capsules (Fig. 22.29 B) or in a gauge tide off with the help of thread. The identification marks written by copying pencil are also kept along with tissues. These capsules/gauge containing tissues should be kept in running tap water overnight for at least 12 hours.

4. Dehydration

In routine practice, the dehydration is done in ascending series of graded ethanol. The tissue blocks are kept in 50% ethanol and then in 70%, 80%, 90%, 95% absolute ethanol I and absolute ethanol II for one hour each. These ethanol graded series should be kept in tight glass stoppered bottle or in screw cap jars to prevent evaporation. In the last bottle of ethanol II sometimes the copper sulfate is layered in the bottom, covered with filter paper, which increases the life of ethanol as it absorbs the water from alcohol. But care should be taken, as soon as the copper sulfate turns bluish due to absorption of water, the ethanol should be changed (Fig. 22.28).

To increase the process of dehydration, the tissue blocks should be agitated either mechanically in an automatic tissue processor or by shaking the container periodically. The volume of alcohol should be at least 50 times more than the tissue placed for dehydration.

5. Clearing

Usually the clearing of tissue blocks is done in xylene. Like ethanol, xylene should also be kept in

270

tightly stoppered bottle to prevent evaporation. After dehydration the tissue blocks should be kept in ethanol and xylene (1:1) mixture for one hour, then the blocks should be transferred to xylene I and xylene II for one hour each. If xylene is not available then benzene may be used for 3 hours as its action of clearing is slower than xylene. On complete clearing, the tissue becomes transparent. It should then be transferred in paraffin wax for impregnation.

6. Impregnation

For the impregnation of tissue blocks, paraffin wax is used either in paraffin embedding bath or in oven fixed at 60-62°C temperature. Both the oven and embedding bath are electrically operated with thermostat to adjust the desired temperature. At the time of transfer of tissue blocks from xylene II, the paraffin wax must be kept at 60-62°C in liquid form for impregnation. Three changes are given in paraffin wax; each of one hour duration. The paraffin wax should be free from dust or other gross impurities; which can be removed by filteration through muslin cloth.

7. Casting of blocks

After 3 hours' impregnation of tissue blocks in paraffin wax, the blocks are formed in moulds using molten wax. The tissues are placed in moulds (Fig. 22.29A) in such a way that desired surface remains downward, on the base of mould. The sections are cut from this surface, so care must be taken to keep the tissue in a proper manner and should be cut into sections homogenously. The mould is then filled with molten paraffin wax and then the blocks are cooled either at room temperature or in cold water. Various types of moulds, like 'L' shaped or ring shaped, can be used. If the moulds are not available, the blocks can be prepared in glass petridishes or in empty slide boxes. But care should be taken to lubricate the surface of such petridishes and other moulds with liquid paraffin or glycerine which facilitates the easy removal of blocks after cooling and hardening of paraffin wax.

8. Trimming

The blocks are removed from the moulds and are cut so as to give one tissue per block and the wax is trimmed by knife or by rubbing on a hot plate in order to remove the extra wax on either side of tissue. The tissue is exposed, which helps in determining the side on which the section is to be cut. The identification of tissue should by fixed on one side of the block by touching the block with the small paper kept on it with hot forcep or knife, bearing the number. Then the blocks are fixed on block holder (Fig. 22.29C). Care should be taken that the number of marking of block is kept on upper side at the time of trimming of the block on microtome to remove the extra wax and expose the whole surface of tissue. The trimming of blocks is done at 10-15µ and a separate knife should be used for trimming and section cutting.

9. Section cutting

Before the sectioning, the tissue blocks are cooled on ice or by keeping them in refrigerator. The tissue floatation bath should be cleaned and filled with water having a temperature of about 60-70°C. The blocks along with block holders are fixed in the microtome (Fig. 22.30) in such a way that the marking number is on upper side, giving a similar position to the blocks as it was during trimming. Usually the sections are cut at 4-6µ thickness on rotary microtome using a plain edge knife. The knife should be sharp enough to cut the desired thickness sections in the form of a ribbon while not causing damage to the tissue. By using a brush and forceps, the ribbon of tissue sections are placed in tissue floatation bath (Fig. 22.31). The tissue sections will spread here due to melting of paraffin wax and will take the shape similar to the tissue of that block. One can make out the selection here; the best looking 1-5 sections can be lifted on a sticky glass slide, which should be kept in a tray at an angle so that the water is removed. The glass slides are made sticky by applying on clean glass slides a sticky material consisting of egg white and glycerine in 1:1 (V/V) ratio. The sticky material

271

Flow Chart Showing Processing of Tissue for Histopathology

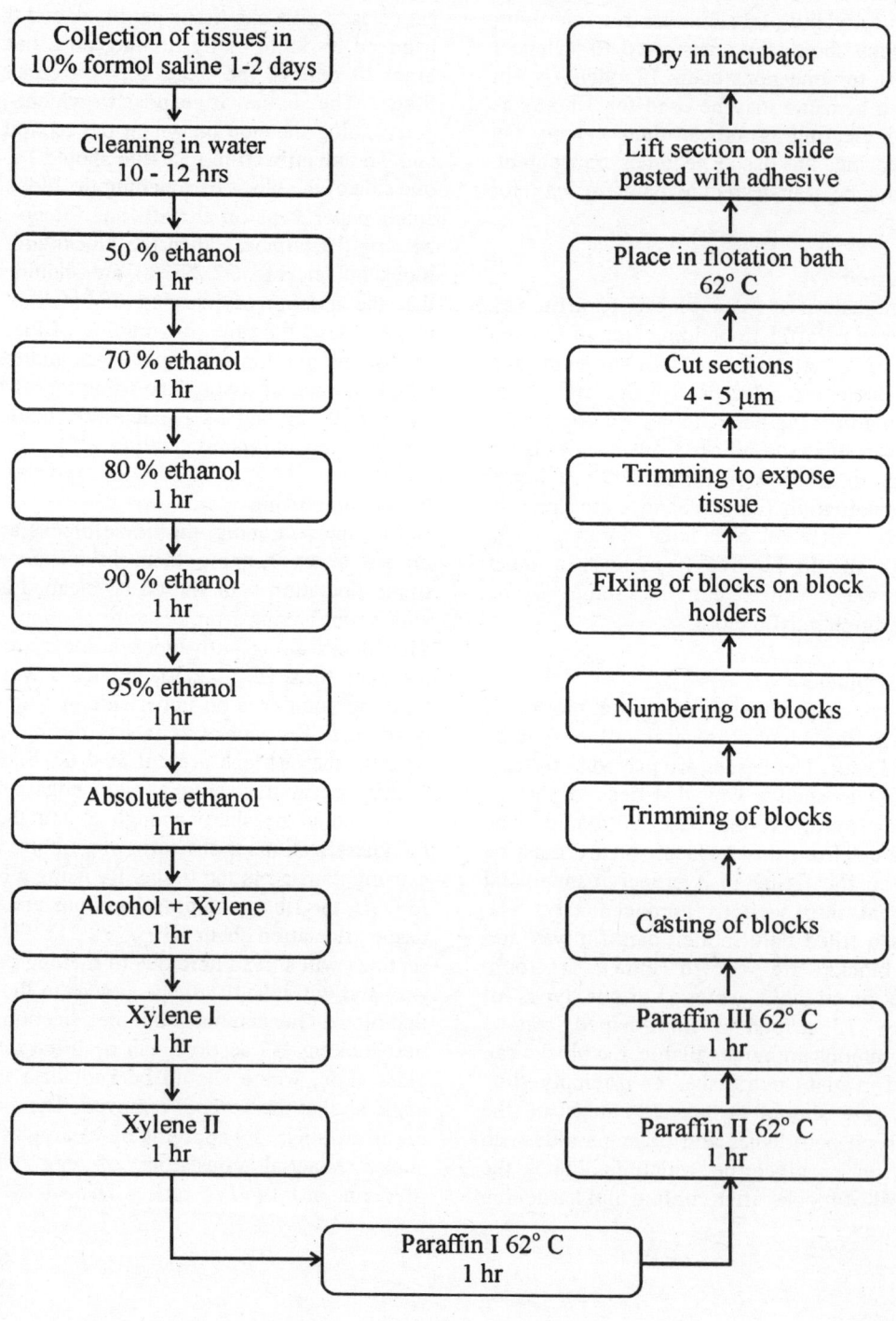

facilitates the sticking of sections on slides, so that they are not damaged or removed during further processing of staining. Generally, 4-5 slides are made from each block and air dried in incubator or at room temperature. The following precautions should be taken at the time of section cutting:

i. Adjust the microtome gauge at right place, generally it is adjusted at 4-5μ for routine histopathological examinations.

ii. Knife should be properly fixed with the help of screws at an angle of about 45 degree. Ensure that all the fittings are tightly fixed.

iii. The knife should be sharp enough to cut sections free from *nicks*. If the nicks are present on sections, the position of knife should be changed or the knife should be properly stropped.

iv. The temperature of tissue floatation bath should neither be low nor should it be higher than the prescribed limit. In low temperature, the tissue will not spread properly and its compressions and creased will not be removed, while at high temperature the paraffin wax of tissue will melt quickly making the tissue fragments and destroying the original shape of section.

v. Lift the tissue sections on slide at an angle (45°) of slide so that the air bubbles does not appear in between the slide and section.

vi. Use little sticky material on slide, if it is more then drying process will take more time.

vii. If the ribbon of sections is large then it should be cut at the junction of two sections with a sharp knife or blade and small pieces made of it.

viii. During summer, when temperature is above 40°C, the tissue sections should be cut either in a room or laboratory having air-conditioner or desert cooler. If such facilities are not available then make moisture in the environment by sprinkling water on ground. It is necessary because at high environmental temperature, the tissue sections stick to the knife and the ribbon is not properly formed.

ix. Drive the microtome smoothly at a regular speed; jerks should not be given.

x. For marking the slides, use the diamond pencil. The marking should be made at the time of section cutting itself.

10. Staining
(A) Routine procedure
After drying the slides are kept in slide cabinets. One slide of each block is selected for staining using the following procedures (Fig. 22.32):

(a) *Removal of paraffin*
The slides are slightly warmed either in incubator or by the flame of a spirit lamp and placed in jar having xylene. Replace the xylene after 10-15 min with fresh xylene for another 10-15 min. This removes the paraffin from the tissue sections.

(b) *Rehydration*
After removal of paraffin, the slides are kept in descending series of alcohol. For this first they should be kept in absolute ethanol and xylene (1:1) mixture for 5 min; then in absolute ethanol, 95%, 90%, 80%, 70%, 50% ethanol for 5-6 min in each dilution. After that the slides are taken in water.

(c) *Cleaning of slides*
With the help of muslin cloth, clean the slides at both the sides. Leave only 1 or 2 section on a slide and remove the extra sections and/or paraffin wax. Wash the slides in running tape water.

(d) *Staining in hematoxylin*
Place the slides in Harris hematoxylin or Meyer's hematoxylin for 10-15 min. Shake the slides 2-3 times for proper staining. Remove the hematoxylin solution and wash the slides in running tap water, then dip in acid alcohol for few seconds, which helps in differentiation. Wash in tap water and place the slides in ammonia water for few seconds for blueing and place in running tap water in order to remove the ammonia.

(e) *Staining in eosin*
Place the slides in 2% aqueous eosin or alcoholic eosin for 2-5 min. After staining in eosin, quickly proceed for dehydration.

Flow Chart Showing Staining Procedure

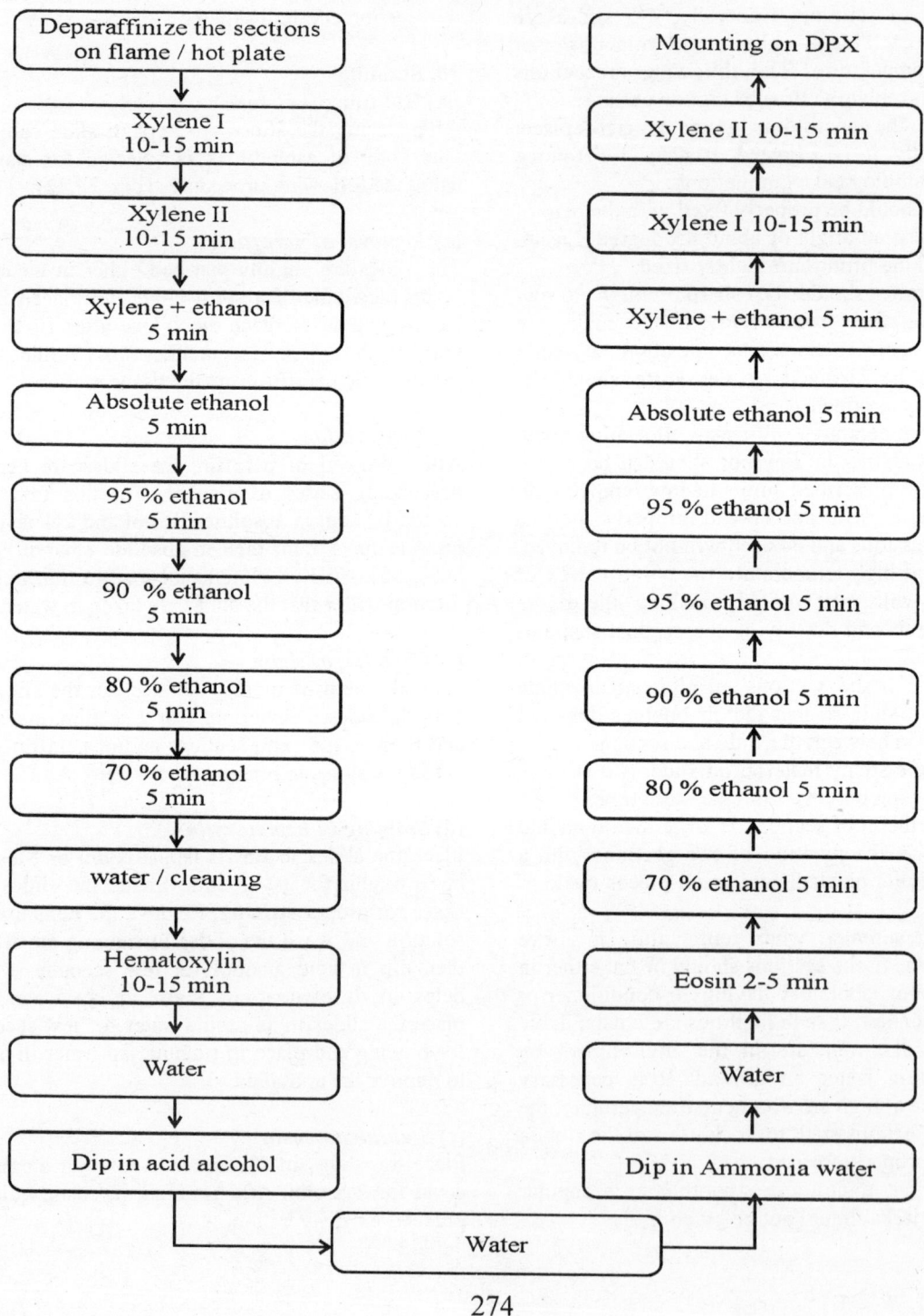

Deparaffinize the sections on flame / hot plate	Mounting on DPX
Xylene I 10-15 min	Xylene II 10-15 min
Xylene II 10-15 min	Xylene I 10-15 min
Xylene + ethanol 5 min	Xylene + ethanol 5 min
Absolute ethanol 5 min	Absolute ethanol 5 min
95 % ethanol 5 min	95 % ethanol 5 min
90 % ethanol 5 min	95 % ethanol 5 min
80 % ethanol 5 min	90 % ethanol 5 min
70 % ethanol 5 min	80 % ethanol 5 min
water / cleaning	70 % ethanol 5 min
Hematoxylin 10-15 min	Eosin 2-5 min
Water	Water
Dip in acid alcohol	Dip in Ammonia water

Water

274

(f) Dehydration

The slides are placed in 70%, 80%, 90% 95% absolute ethanol for dehydration for at least 5 min in each solution; then they are placed in absolute ethanol: xylene mixture (1:1) for 5 min.

(g) Clearing

Clear the sections in xylene and give 2 changes at least for 10-15 min each. The clearing in xylene II can be extended for even upto one hour.

(h) Mounting

Mount the slides with coverslip using Canada balsam or DPX mountant. For this the cover slips of desired size and shape are kept on filter paper and one or two drop of mountant is placed on coverslip. Takeout the slides from xylene and place on coverslip in such a way that the section touches with mountant, press gently and lift the slide (Fig. 22.33). Remove air bubble, if any, by pressing the coverslip with fine forcep and keep the slides in horizontal position in a tray for drying.

(i) Cleaning and labelling

After drying, clean the slides with muslin cloth and xylene. Remove the extra mountant using a blade. Label the slide with a piece of paper and stick it on one corner of slide using gum or other adhesive. At the time of examination, the histopathologist should put the name of organ, main changes in sections/disease condition with other remarks on this label for future identification of the slide.

(j) Examination

On hematoxylin and eosin staining, the nuclei of the cells take blue stain while the cytoplasm is pink or red. Examine the tissue section using 10 x objective and, if required, in high power or oil immersion. Precautions and important tips which should be considered at the time of staining:

i. Check the sections for staining after blueing in ammonia water for hematoxylin stain and after dehydration for eosin stain. If under stained then repeat the process and in case of overstaining, the sections can be differentiated for some more time in acid alcohol to remove the excess hematoxylin and in ethanol for removing the excess eosin.

ii. Clean the slides thoroughly in water and remove all patches/spots of paraffin; which gives a good look to slides.

iii. If on clearing in xylene, cloudyness appears then repeat the dehydration process in absolute ethanol for 10-15 min. The cloudyness appears due to presence of water in the sections which reacts with xylene.

iv. At the time of mounting, ensure that the tissue section does not get dried. To eliminate the chance of drying, proceed fast. Ensure the proper mounting of section on slides. Sometimes the opposite side of the section is mounted and the section becomes dry. To ensure proper mounting, one should feel/touch the diamond pencil marking present on the same surface and then mount the sections. This can also be checked by touching the slide on reverse side for the presence/absence of tissue sections.

v. Labelling with paper should be done on same side on which the section is present; which will be helpful at the time of examination.

(B) Special procedures

In histopathological techniques, one can demonstrate bacteria, fungus, chlamydia, rickettsia or viral inclusions in the tissue sections by using special staining procedures. These special staining techniques, however, require special expertise but can be used in diagnostic laboratory as routine methods. Some important special staining techniques are described as under:

I. Staining for acid fast bacilli

The acid fast bacilli are demonstrated in tuberculosis or Johne's disease in animals. The tissues are collected in formol saline or buffered formalin and processed in same manner as for routine histopathological techniques. For special staining of acid fast bacilli following procedures are followed:

1. Deparaffinize the sections and hydrate in descending series of ethanol as described earlier.
2. Clean the slides in water and give a wash in distilled water for 5 min.
3. Place the slides in carbol fuchsin solution and keep the chamber of slides in a water bath at 56°C for 1 hr.
4. Thereafter, remove the slides from water bath and keep at room temperature for a few min, wash in running tap water. Dip in acid alcohol for differentiation till the colour of tissue becomes pale pink.
5. Wash in running tap water.
6. Place the slides in methylene blue working solution for a few seconds, wash in tap water till the colour of sections becomes pale blue.
7. Dehydrate in ascending series of ethanol, clear in xylene and mount in DPx as described earlier in histopathological procedures. Examine the slides under oil immersion. The acid fast bacilli will be of bright red colour with a light blue back ground.
8. **Precautions**
(a) Care should be taken that at 56°C for 1 hr, the stain does not get dry so it is always advisable to keep it in a covered jar in water bath to prevent drying.
(b) Differentiation with acid alcohol is a very crucial step and should be controlled carefully; it depends on experience of a histopathologist to stain the slides properly.

II. Demonstration of Gram-positive/Gram negative bacteria in tissue sections
i. Deparaffinize and hydrate the sections in water, clean them.
ii. Stain the slides with crystal violet for 2 min.
iii. Wash in distilled water.
iv. Keep the slides in Gram's iodine solution for 5 min.
v. Wash in distilled water.
vi. Differentiate in cellosolve (Ethylene glycol monomethyl ether) until blue colour no longer comes out from sections.
vii. Wash in distilled water.

viii. Place in basic fuchsin for 5 min and wash in distilled water.
ix. Place the slides in differentiating solution for 5 min., wash in distilled water and blot dry.
x. Dip the slides in tetrazine for a few seconds.
xi. Place the slides in cellosolve, 3 changes of 6 dip in each.
xii. Clear in xylene I and II for 15 min each.
xiii. Mount in DPX
xiv. Examine the slides under oil immersion. The Gram-positive bacteria will be of blue colour while Gram-negative will take a red colour against a yellow background.

III. Demonstration of spirochaetes
1. During post-mortem examination, cut about 1 mm thick slice of tissues from several sites of an organ and fix them in 10% buffered formalin for 24hrs, wash in running tap water overnight and place in 95% alcohol for 24hr.
2. Transfer the tissues in distilled water and keep till the tissues sink to bottom.
3. Stain in silver nitrate at 37°C in dark for 3-5 days and change the solution daily.
4. Wash in distilled water and place the tissues in reducing solution for 1-3 days.
5. Rinse in distilled water and dehydrate in ascending series of ethanol.
6. Clear in cedar wood oil for 2 hrs.
7. Impregnation/embedding is done in paraffin wax as in case of routine histopathology, cut sections at 4-5μ, dry and deparaffinise in xylene (3 changes of 5 min each)
8. Clean the slides, remove artifacts and spots of paraffin wax
9. Mount 1-2 sections per slide with DPX
10. Examination is done under microscope; the spirochaete will be of black colour with yellow to light brown background.

IV. Demonstration of fungi
1. Collect the tissues in formol saline or buffered formalin and process the samples in a same way as in routine histopathology and cut the section at 4-5μ, deparaffinize and hydrate to water.

2. Place the slides in 4% chromic acid for 1 hr.
3. Wash in running tap water and keep the slides in 1% sodium bisulfite solution for 3-5 min.
4. Wash in running tape water and then in distilled water.
5. Stain with methanamine-silver nitrate working solution at 60^0C in water bath till sections become yellowish brown.
6. Wash in distilled water and place in gold chloride solution for 5 min.
7. Wash in distilled water and place in sodium thiosulfate solution for 5 min and wash in running tap water.
8. Stain with light green for 1 min, wash in water; dehydrate in ascending series of ethanol, clear in xylene and mount in DPX.
9. Examine the sections under microscope, the fungi will take a black colour, mycelia and hyphae will be of rose coloured with a pale green back ground.

V. Demonstration of rickettsia

1. Tissues are fixed in formol saline or buffered formalin and processed in same manner, sections of 4-5μ thick are cut, dried, deparaffinized and hydrated in water.
2. Place in methylene blue solution for overnight and decolourize in 95% ethanol for a few seconds or till blue colour is lost.
3. Wash in distilled water and place the slides in basic fuchsin solution for 30 min.
4. Decolourize in citric acid solution for 1-2 sec.
5. Differentiate in absolute ethanol for a few min, clear in xylene and mount in DPX.

Examine the slides, the rickettsia will be of bright red colour and nucleus of the cell will take blue colour.

POST-MORTEM EXAMINATION OF VETEROLEGAL CASES

The post-mortem examination of veterolegal cases is performed as described in previous sections. However, following points must be kept in mind during post-mortem examination and while preparing the report.

1. For veterolegal cases, post-mortem request should be signed by a police officer not below the rank of inspector or by magistrate; without this no post-mortem examination should be done.

2. Always collect maximum information on history, date and time of death of animal and treatment given. Use self knowledge and experience to determine the time of death such as rigor morits, autolysis, putrefaction, pseudomelanosis etc.

3. Animal identification, including species, breed, age and number or mark, must be clearly established before starting post-mortem examination. It is specially necessary in case of insured animals as well as in religion-related disputes..

4. All the lesions present on skin surface should be clearly defined as laceration, wound, trauma, incision, erosion, vesicle, ulcer, and if there is suspected sharp edge wound or bullet injury its depth and width (diameter), as the case may be, should also be stated. Also mention the side on which the animal is lying down (ventral portion touching earth).

5. In case of dispute whether it was still birth or the calf was born alive, a piece of lung should be placed in water. The lung piece will sink in water in case of atelectasis neonatum while it will float if the calf was born alive.

6. If the case is suspected for toxic condition/poisoning, try to mention the type of poison in your report. This will help the police authorities to establish/confirm the type of toxin/poison in forensic laboratory.

7. The post-mortem examination of wild animals should be conducted as a special case. One should conduct the post-mortem examination only when DFO or higher officer makes request for post-mortem examination. It should be noted on the report that all the viscera, including skin, bones, teeth, etc. have been returned to the person who requested for the necropsy and no item has been left behind.

8. Fill the post-mortem report clearly with neat handwriting and in clear language and avoid ambiguity in presentation. Avoid writing general sentences. Be specific in your findings and conclusions. Sign the report with date and keep a copy of it with you for record and future evidence in the court of law.

9. Post-mortem examination should be conducted in daylight. In darkness, where the pathologist is not able to recognize the lesions, the post-mortem examination should not be conducted.

10. At the time of post-mortem examination outsiders should not be allowed in. To avoid them, and wild birds and animals, post-mortem examination should be done in closed premises.

COLLECTION, PRESERVATION AND DISPATCH OF MATERIAL TO FORENSIC LABORATORY

The collection, preservation and dispatch of different tissues/organs, fluids and viscera should be done as described in section 4 of appendix. However, in veterolegal cases, these materials should be sent to forensic laboratory under sealed packings.

- In suspected cases of toxic condition or poisoning, the stomach and intestinal contents should be sent after proper ligation at both the ends and in ice to prevent putrefaction. Besides, samples of blood, liver, spleen and kidneys should be sent in separate container.

- All the materials should be collected in leak proof glass or plastic bottles.

- Tissues for histopathological examination must be collected in 10% formalin or formol saline, this can be sent to laboratory under normal temperature.

- The materials suspected for toxicity should be sent in ice without adding any preservative.

- The bottles or containers should be sealed and labelled properly indicating the name of owner, identification of animal (number, name, mark etc.), type of tissue collected and preservative used. The examination requested and disease or poisoning suspected should also be written.

- A copy with details of post-mortem report containing above information should be sent separately under separate cover.

- The address of the forensic laboratory should be clearly written.

- All the containers should be packed with cloth and sealed with sealing wax and should preferably be sent through person in order to avoid any breakage in transit.

- One copy of the forwarding letter should be kept in file for future reference, one copy should accompany the material and one copy should be sent by post. The forwarding letter bearing number and date should have the information about materials sent, type of preservative used, type of examination requested and identification of animals, including other details of owner.

EXAMINATION OF BLOOD, URINE AND FAECES

BLOOD EXAMINATION
TOTAL ERYTHROCYTE COUNT

- Clean New Bauer's counting chamber/ hemocytometer counter and place clean coverslip on ruled areas.
- Suck fresh or anticoagulant mixed blood in RBC diluting pipette (red ball in bulb) upto 0.5 mark and fill the pipette with RBC diluting fluid upto 101 mark.
- Hold pipette in horizontal position and remove rubber tube. Mix the contents by rotating the pipette in between palms.
- Discard first few drops from pipette and then place a drop near the edge of cover slip to fill the space between cover slip and counting chamber.
- Keep counting chamber 1-2 min for settling of the cells.
- Count the cells under high power of the light microscope.
- Cells are counted in 5 medium squares of the central large square or 80 tertiary squares.
- Cells on top of square or left side are included in count.
- Calculate RBC per μl of blood by multiplying 10,000 to the total number of cells counted in 80 tertiary squares. It can be converted into ml by further multiplying by 1000 and in litre by 10,00,000.

TOTAL LEUCOCYTE COUNT

- Clean the New Bauer's chamber/ hemocytometer. Put the cover slip on the area demarcated for counting.
- Suck fresh/anticoagulant mixed blood in WBC diluting pipette (white ball in bulb) upto 0.5 mark and fill the pipette with WBC diluting fluid upto 11 mark.

- Hold the pipette in horizontal position and remove rubber tube. Mix the contents by rotating the pipette in between palms.
- Discard first few drops from pipette and then place a drop near the edge of cover slip to fill the space between cover slip and chamber.
- Keep counting chamber 1-2 min for settling of the cells.
- Count the cells under low power in four large/ primary corner squares of the ruled area.
- Cells on top of square and left side are included in count.
- Calculate WBC per μl of blood by multiplying the total number of cells counted in 4 primary squares by 50. It can be converted into ml by multiplying by 1000 and in litre by 10,00,000.

PACKED CELL VOLUME (HEMATOCRIT VALUE)

- Clean and dry the wintrobe tube.
- With the help of a long needle (6") and syringe fill the blood in wintrobe tube upto mark 100.
- Take precaution to prevent air bubble from entering the tube.
- Centrifuge the wintrobe tube at 3000 rpm for 30 min.
- Record the reading of packed cell volume in percent *i.e.* mass of erythrocytes settling down in tube.

ERYTHROCYTE SEDIMENTATION RATE

- Clean and dry Westergren pipette.
- Suck anticoagulant mixed blood in Westergren pipette upto mark 'O' and fix it in stand in vertical position.
- Leave this for one hour in room temperature.
- Record the reading on pipette, it is the mm fall of erythrocytes per hour.

HEMOGLOBIN

- It is measured by using Hellige- Sahli hemoglobinometer.
- Clean and dry the graduated tube of the hemoglobinometer.
- Take 5 drops of N/10 hydrochloric acid in tube.
- Suck the anticoagulant mixed blood in pipette upto 20 marks.
- Place the pipette in tube containing N/10 HCl and transfer the blood into acid.
- Suck acid in pipette and leave in tube.
- Keep the tube for 5 min in dark.
- Add distilled water in the tube drop-by-drop using dropper, mix with stirring rod and match the colour with standard. Add water till the colour matches with standard.
- Read the scale on tube; it is the value of hemoglobin gram per 100 ml of blood.

DIFFERENTIAL LEUCOCYTE COUNT (DLC)

- Prepare a thin blood smear on clean glass slide. Place a drop of blood on one end of slide and spread as smear with the help of another slide using its edge at 45° angle.
- Dry the smear in air and mark identification number in the thick portion of smear.
- Fix the smear in methanol for at least 5 min and dry in air.
- Stain the smear with Giemsa stain diluted to 1:10 in distilled water for 30 min or with Leishman's stain without fixing the smear.
- Wash the slide, dry in air and examine under oil immersion microscope. Count at least 200 cells by battlement/zigzag method. Cells counted are lymphocytes, neutrophils, monocytes, eosinophils and basophils. (Figs. 9.12 - 9.16) Cell count is presented in percent.

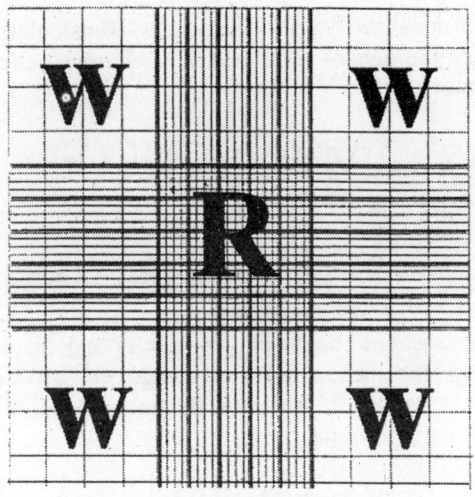

Fig. 22.34 Neubauer s chamber
(W=Counting area for leucocytes;
R= Counting area for erythrocytes)

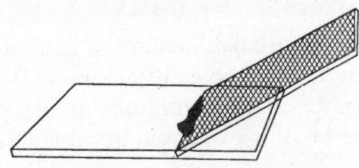

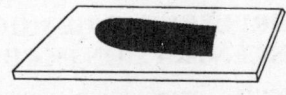

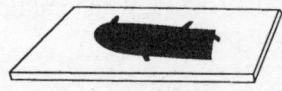

Fig. 22.35 Smear preparation for differential leucocyte count

ABSOLUTE LYMPHOCYTE COUNT (ALC)

The absolute lymphocyte count is calculated by using the data of DLC and TLC through following formula:

$$\frac{ALC}{(10^3/\mu l)} = \frac{\% \text{ Lymphocyte x TLC } (10^3/\mu l)}{100}$$

ABSOLUTE NEUTROPHIL COUNT (ANC)

The absolute neutrophil count is calculated by using the neutrophil percentage of differential leucocyte count and total leucocyte count using following formula:

$$\frac{ANC}{(10^3/\mu l)} = \frac{\% \text{ Neutrophils x TLC } (10^3/\mu l)}{100}$$

MEAN CORPUSCULAR VOLUME (MCV)

Mean corpuscular volume is determined by dividing the packed cell volume (PCV) by the total erythrocyte count in millions/μl and multiplied by 10. The MCV is expressed in cubic microns.

$$\frac{MCV}{(\text{Cubic } \mu)} = \frac{PCV}{TEC} \text{ x } 10$$

MEAN CORPUSCULAR HEMOGLOBIN CONCENTRATION (MCHC)

Mean corpuscular hemoglobin concentration is calculated by dividing the hemoglobin in grams per 100 ml of blood by the PCV and multiplied by 100. It is expressed in percent.

$$\frac{MCHC}{(\%)} = \frac{Hb}{PCV} \text{ x } 100$$

MEAN CORPUSCULAR HEMOGLOBIN (MCH)

Mean corpuscular hemoglobin is calculated by dividing hemoglobin in grams per 100 ml by TEC in millions per μl of blood and multiplying by 10.

$$\frac{MCH}{(10^{-12} \text{ g})} = \frac{Hb}{TEC} \text{ x } 10$$

ALTERATIONS IN HEMATOLOGICAL AND BIOCHEMICAL ATTRIBUTES IN VARIOUS DISEASE CONDITIONS OF ANIMALS

A. Hematological profile

1. Erythrocytosis
Brucellosis, Campylobacteriosis, Leptospirosis, Rinderpest, Haemorrhagic septicemia.

2. Erythropenia
Leukemia, Haemorrhage, Aflatoxicosis, Theileriosis, Babesiosis, Anaplasmosis.

3. Leucocytosis
Pyogenic infections, Rabies, Tuberculosis, Strangles, Leptospirosis, Theileriosis Babesiosis, Anaplasmosis, Haemorrhagic septicemia.

4. Leucopenia
Canine distemper, Infectious canine hepatitis, Swine fever, Brucellosis, Tuberculosis, Infectious bovine rhinotracheitis.

5. Neutrophilia
Acute inflammation, Pyogenic infections, Pyometra.

6. Neutrophiliamth (shift to left)
Leptospirosis, Metritis, Traumatic reticulopericarditis (TRP), Canine distemper, Glanders.

7. Neutropenia
Pasteurellosis, Infectious canine hepatitis.

8. Lymphocytosis
Leukemia, after vaccination, viral infections.

9. Lymphopenia
Canine distemper, Infectious canine hepatitis, Infectious bovine rhinotracheitis, Foot and Mouth Disease.

10. Eosinophilia
Allergy, Parasitic diseases.

11. Hypohemoglobinemia
Anemia, Theileriosis, Strangles, Anaplasmosis, Degnala disease, Fascioliosis.

12. Increased ESR
Carcinoma, Nephritis, Chronic granulomatous infection, Tuberculosis, Canine distemper, Trypanosomiasis.

13. Increased Hematocrit Value/PCV
Dehydration.

14. Decreased hematocrit Value/PCV
Anemia, Theileriosis, Strangles, Anaplasmosis, Blue tongue.

B. Biochemical attributes
1. Hyperglycemia
Diabetes mellitus, Chronic nephritis.

2. Hypoglycemia
Hepatic insufficiency, Ketosis.

3. Hyperproteinemia
Shock, Dehydration, Plasmacytoma, Infectious diseases.

4. Hypoproteinemia
Burn Diarrhoea, Renal dysfunction, Hepatic disorders, Tuberculosis.

5. Hyperglobulinema
Dehydration, Leukemia, bacterial, viral and parasitic infections.

6. Hypogammaglobulinemia
Anemia, Haemorrhage, Immunodeficiency.

7. Hypercalcemia
Hyperparathyroidism, bone cancer, Nephrolithiasis.

8. Hypocalcemia
Hypoparathyroidism, Ricketts, Osteomalacia, Ketosis.

9. Hyperphosphatemia
Renal failure, Hypoparathyroidism, Healing of fracture.

10. Hypophosphatemia
Chronic diarrhoea, Pica, Rheumatism-like syndrome, Hemoglobinuria. Hyperparathyroidism.

11. Increased levels of blood urea nitrogen
Renal impairment, nephritis, Urinary obstruction.

12. Decreased levels of BUN
Acute hepatic insufficiency, nephrosis, Chronic wasting diseases

13. Increased level of creatinin
Severe nephritis, urinary obstruction, severe toxic nephrosis.

14. Hypermagnesemia
Chronic infection, Oxalate poisoning.

15. Hypomagnesemia
Grass tetany, Lactation tetany, Wheat pasture poisoning.

16. Increased levels of SGOT
Hepatic necrosis, Myocardial infarction, Muscular degeneration/necrosis in dog and cat, Azoturia.

17. Increased levels of SGPT
Hepatic necrosis, Infectious canine hepatitis.

18. Increased levels of alkaline phosphatase
Obstructive jaundice, hepatitis, Hyperparathyroidism.

19. Decreased level of alkaline phosphatase
Chronic nephritis.

20. Increased level of acid phosphatase
Prostate carcinoma, Leukemia.

21. Increased level of lactic dehydrogenase
Malignant lymphoma.

22. Increased level of serum isocitric dehydrogenase
Hemolytic anemia in horses.

23. Increased level of ornithine carbamyl transferase
Liver disorders in dogs.

URINE EXAMINATION
PHYSICAL EXAMINATION

1. Colour:
- Note the colour of urine as
  - Watery/colourless
  - Amber colour
  - Red
  - Brown
  - Yellow/Yellowish green
  - Black
  - Pale

2. Odour
- Record the smell of the urine
  - Uremic
  - Sweetish/ Fruity
  - Fetid

3. Turbidity
- Look for the presence of suspended material in urine
  - Clear
  - Turbid +, ++, +++, +++
  - Cloudy

4. Foaming
- Shake the urine in a test tube
  - No/slight foams
  - Yellow/Green foams
  - Red/brown foams

5. Specific Gravity
- This is measured by urinometer
  - Urine is filled in cylinder and urinometer is left in the urine.
  - Record the specific gravity in urinometer.

CHEMICAL EXAMINATION

1. Reaction
- Reaction is determined by using pH strips or pH meter.
- For this take a pH strip and dip in urine.
- Read the change in colour on scale given with pH strips.

2. Glucose
- Take 0.5 ml urine in a clean and dry test tube.
- Mix 5.0 ml Benedict's reagent in the urine and keep it in boiling water bath/flame for 5 min.
- Remove the tube and cool it on test tube stand.
- Record the changes of colour in tube as follows:
  - Blue (-) : No glucose
  - Blue to green (+): Mild glucose
  - Yellow with heavy sediment (++): Moderate glucose
  - Orange with heavy sediment (+++): Highly positive for glucose

3. Protein
- Take 2 ml of urine in a clean and dry test tube.
- Place 2 ml Robert's reagent over urine.
- If protein is present in urine, then a white ring will appear at the interjunction of two fluids. It is graded as follows:
  - No ring (-): Negative
  - Mild ring (+): Mild positive
  - A wide ring (++): Moderate positive
  - Heavy ring (+++): Positive
  - Very heavy ring (++++): Highly positive

Ketone bodies

1. Acetone

- Take 1.0 gm mixed powder of sodium nitropruside and ammonium sulfate (Sod. Nitropruside 1 part, Amm. Sulfate 100 parts) in a test tube.
- Add 5 ml urine in the salts and mix them properly.
- To this slowly overlay 20% ammonium hydroxide solution.
- Record the colour at the interjunction of two fluids.
- If it is red to purple then it is acetone positive.

2. Acetoacetic acid

- Take 10 ml urine in a clean and dry test tube.
- Add 5 drops of Lugol's iodine and 3 ml chloroform, mix them and allow to stand.
- Record the colour of urine
  Colour less   : Positive
  Red/ violet colour : Negative

3. Beta hydroxybutyric acid

- Take 20 ml urine in a small beaker and add 20 ml distilled water and a few drops of acetic acid.
- Boil the contents over flame till it remains 10 ml, add distilled water to make it 20 ml and place in two test tubes, 10 ml in each.
- In one test tube add 1 ml H_2O_2 and warm it for 1 min, cool it.
- Add 1 ml glacial acetic acid, 1 ml freshly prepared sodium nitropruside solution in both tubes, mix thoroughly.
- To this overlay strong ammonia water and allow to stand for 3-4 hrs.
- Record the change in colour in H_2O_2 added tube if it is purple colour ring then it is positive.

Bile salts

- Take 4-5 ml urine in a test tube and shake it. If persistent foams are present then it is positive for bile salts.
- Add sulphur granules over surface of urine. In case of positive, sulphur granules will sink in urine.

Blood

- Take 2 ml urine in test tube I.
- Take 1 ml saturated solution of Benzidine in test tube II. Add 1 ml 3% H_2O_2 and mix well.
- Mix the contents of tubes I and II.
- Record the development of colour. In positive case a green to blue colour will appear.

Hemoglobin/Myoglobin

- Take 5 ml urine in a test tube.
- Add 2.8 gm ammonium sulfate.
- Shake well and allow to stand for a few min.
- If urine becomes clear/ watery in colour. Then it is positive for hemoglobin. If colour remains same as before the test then it is positive for myoglobin.

Microscopic examination

- Take 5-10 ml urine in a centrifuge tube and centrifuge it at 1000 rpm for 10 min.
- Discard supernatant and place a drop of sediment on clean, dry glass slide.
- Cover it with a cover slip and examine it under microscope for the followings:
  o Epithelial cells
  o Leucocyte
  o Erythrocytes
  o Microorganisms
  o Casts

FAECAL EXAMINATION
GROSS EXAMINATION

- Collect faeces in clean and dry petridish or in small sample bottle.

- With clean spatula and glass rod spread the faeces and note the following:
  - Colour
  - Consistency
  - Odour
  - Presence of blood
  - Presence of parasite/segments of parasite

MICROSCOPIC EXAMINATION
Direct smear method

- Place a drop of distilled water on clean and dry glass slide.
- Add small amount of faeces in distilled water on slide.
- Mix with glass rod/tooth pick/ matchstick.
- Place a cover slip on it.
- Examine under microscope for the presence of parasitic ova.

Qualitative concentration method (Simple floatation method)

- Take about 1.0 gm faeces and mix it in small amount of distilled water.
- Filter it through sieve/muslin cloth.
- Filterate is mixed with 4-5 ml of saturated salt solution.

- Place the mixture in a tube or cylinder and fill it upto the top.
- A clean coverslip or glass slide is placed on the mouth of tube/cylinder.
- Keep it for 30 to 60 min at room temperature.
- Remove the coverslip or slide and examine it under microscope for parasitic ova.

Qualitative concentration method (Centrifugation floatation method)

- Take about 1.0 gm faeces and mix it in small amount of distilled water.
- Mixture is filtered through fine sieve/muslin cloth.
- Mix the filterate with saturated salt solution (1:3) in a centrifuge tube.
- Centrifuge it at 1500 rpm for 5 min.
- Take a drop of superficial contents on a clean glass slide and examine under microscope.
- Sediment is examined for eggs of liver flukes.

Appendix-IX
SELF ASSESSMENT

1. INTRODUCTION

Q. 1.   (1) 8% (2) 3% (3) 37.5% (4) 16 days (5) (a) Clinical Pathology (b) Post-mortem Pathology (c) Chemical Pathology (d) Histopathology (e) Humoral Pathology (f) Clinical Pathology.

Q. 3.   (1) Renatus Vegetius (2) Cornelius Celsus, Redness, Swelling, Heat, Pain, Loss of function, Claudius Galen. (3). Comparative Pathology (4) Immune mechanisms, immunodeficiency, Autoimmunity, Hypersensitivity. (5) Subjective, objective (6) Pathogenesis, entry/action, recovery, death (7) Biopsy.

Q. 5.   (1) b , (2) a, (3) b, (4) d, (5) b, (6) a, (7) d, (8) d, (9) a, (10) b

2. ETIOLOGY

Q. 1.   (1) Immunosuppression, Neutrophils (2) Dividing, ovary, testicles/ sperm, lymphocytes, Intestine/ Bone marrow (3) DNA, RNA, nucleic acid (4) Tuberculosis, Paratuberculosis, Leprosy, (5) Iatrogenic (6) Phospholipase A_2, hyaluronidase, phosphodiesterase, peptidase, hemolytic anemia, shock (7) Paddy straw, Degnala (8) Aflatoxin, ochratoxin. (9) Insecticides, weedicides, fungicides, rodenticides insecticide (10) Lead, cadmium, mercury (11) Skeletal muscle, myocardium, brain (12) young (13) Deprivation, Fatty degeneration of liver, anemia, skin diseases (14) Acetoatcetate, hydroxybutyrate, acetone, (15) Testicles, ovary, thymus, lymphoid tissue (16) lysin, tryptophane (17) Linolenic acid, linoleic acid, arachdonic acid (18) Conjunctivitis, keratitis (19) E (20) Biotin, choline, manganese.

Q. 2.   (1) T,   (2) F,   (3) F,   (4) F,   (5) T,   (6) F,   (7) T,   (8) T,   (9) F,   (10) T,   (11) F,   (12) T,   (13) F,   (14) F,   (15) T,   (16) F,   (17) T,   (18) T,   (19) F,   (20) T.

Q. 5.   (1) a,   (2) b,   (3) c,   (4) c,   (5) d,   (6) d,   (7) c,   (8) c,   (9) a ,   (10) d,   (11) d,   (12) b   (13) c,   (14) d,   (15) c,   (16) a,   (17) b,   (18) d,   (19) d ,   (20) b.

3.   GENETIC DISORDERS, DEVELOPMENTAL ANOMALIES AND MONSTERS

Q. 1.   (1) Length, location of centromere, Karyotyping (2) Translocation, reciprocal, non-reciprocal (3) cranium, abrachia (4) Atresia, atresia ani (5) Chelioschisis, harelip (6) Cleft, cleft palate (7) Dextrocardia, right side (8) Single ovum, incomplete (9) Pyopagus (10) Renarcuatus, horseshoe kidneys.

Q. 2.   (1) F,   (2) F,   (3) F,   (4) T,   (5) T,   (6) T,   (7) F,   (8) F,   (9) T,   (10) F.

Q. 5.   (1) a,   (2) b,   (3) c,   (4) d,   (5) c,   (6) a,   (7) d,   (8) c,   (9) b,   (10) c. (11) c,   (12) a (13) d, (14) c,   (15) c,   (16) a,   (17) d,   (18) c,   (19) b,   (20) a .

4.   DISTURBANCES IN GROWTH

Q. 1.   (1) Abnormal, improperly, development (2) Reduced, full size (3) Decreased (4) More (5) Hyperplasia (6) Hypertrophy, myometrium (7) Change (8) Embryonic, differentiated (9) Anaplasia (10) Metaplasia.

Q. 2.   (1) T,   (2) F,   (3) T,   (4) F,   (5) T,   (6) F,   (7) F,   (8) F,   (9) T,   (10) T.

Q. 5.   (1) c,   (2) c,   (3) a,   (4) d,   (5) a,   (6) a,   (7) d,   (8) c,   (9) a,   (10) d.

5.   DISTURBANCES IN CIRCULATION

Q. 1.   (1) Congestion/ hyperemia (2) Hematuria, hemoptysis, melena (3) Linear (4) Anasarca, hydrocele (5) Hydropericardium, HPS(6) Total blood volume, blood flow, hemoconcentration (7) Sludged blood, emboli, obstruction of blood vessel, ischemia, infarction (8) Metrorrhagia, hematemesis.

Q. 2.   (1) F,   (2) T,   (3) F,   (4) F,   (5) T,   (6) T,   (7) T,   (8) F,   (9) F,   (10) T.

Q. 3.   (1) a,   (2) b,   (3) d,   (4) d,   (5) b,   (6) d,   (7) d,   (8) c,   (9) d,   (10) c.

6.   DISTURBANCES IN CELL METABOLISM

Q. 1.   (1). Hydropic degeneration, stratum spinosum, food & mouth (2) pustules (3) Mildest, mild / any, first (4) Thyroid, cachexia, Starvation, parasitism, chronic wasting disease (5) Cystadenoma, cystadenocarcinoma, transparent, slimy, (6) Starch, black / brown / blue, Protein polysaccharide (7) Old scars, nutrients, homogenous, strong acidophilic (8). Keratinized epithelium, horn.

Q. 2.   (1) F,   (2) T,   (3) F,   (4) F,   (5) T,   (6) T,   (7) T,   (8) T,   (9) F,   (10) T.

Q. 3.   (1) a,   (2) c,   (3) d,   (4) b,   (5) a,   (6) c,   (7) b,   (8) d,   (9) c,   (10) a.

7.   NECROSIS, GANGRENE AND POST-MORTEM CHANGES

Q. 1.   (1) Caseative, proteins, lipids (2) Chromatin (3) Living, pyknosis, karyorrhexis, karyolysis (4) liquifactive, pyogenic (5) Pancreas, chalky white (6) Moist (7) Fusarium, dry (8) Clostridia, oedema, blackening, crepitating sound (9) Digestion, own (10) Pseudomelanosis, saprophyte, hydrogensulfide, iron.

Q. 2.   (1) F,   (2) T,   (3) F,   (4) F,   (5) T,   (6) F,   (7) F,   (8) F,   (9) T,   (10) F.

Q. 3.   (1) d,   (2) d,   (3) c,   (4) b,   (5) a,   (6) b,   (7) a,   (8) b,   (9) b,   (10) c.

8. DISTURBANCES IN CALCIFICATION AND PIGMENT METABOLISM

Q. 1. (1). Hypercalcemia, hyperparathyroidism, renal failure, Excess of vit. D, Increased calcium intake (2) Bright yellow, macrophages (3) Brown/black, skin, hairs, retina (4) Bile, hemolysis, damage to liver, obstruction in bile duct, yellow, mucous membranes (5) Glucuronic acid, bilirubin diglucuronide, urobilinogen, urobilin, stercobilin.

Q. 2. (1) T, (2) T, (3) F, (4) T, (5) T, (6) F, (7) T, (8) T, (9) F, (10) F.

Q. 3. (1) d, (2) a, (3) c, (4) b, (5) a, (6) c, (7) b, (8) d, (9) a, (10) d.

9. INFLAMMATION AND HEALING

Q. 1. (1). Redness, heat, swelling, pain, loss of function (2) Vascular changes, proliferative (3) Stomatitis, Lampas/palatitis, glossitis, Sialadenitis. (4) Vasoconstriction, vasodilation, cationic proteins, hydrogen peroxide, hydrolytic enzymes, lysozymes, proteases, cytokines (kinins, histamine, serotonin, heparin, complement are also true) (5) B-lymphocytes, N.K. Cells, T-lymphocytes, T-helper, T-cytotoxic T-suppressor cells (6) Multinucleated cells, macrophages, Langerhans, foreign body (7) Linoleic acid, C_5a, cyclo-oxygenase, lipo-oxygenase (8) 5- hydroxytryptamin, gastrointestinal tract, spleen, mast, blood vessels, vasodilatation, increased permeability. (9) Acid proteases, collagenases, elastases, plasminogen activator (10) Hormone, lymphocytes, monocytes, glycoprotein (11) Small macrophages, fibroblasts, endothelial cells, lymphocytes, granulocytes, hepatocytes, keratinocytes, basophils, neutrophils, T-cells (12) Fibrous tissue, granulation tissue/ fibroblasts.

Q. 2. (1) F, (2) T, (3) F, (4) F, (5) F, (6) T, (7) F, (8) T, (9) T, (10) T. (11)T, (12)F, (13)T, (14) F, (15)T, (16) T, (17) F, (18) T, (19) T, (20) F.

Q. 3. (1) c, (2) c, (3) b, (4) c, (5) c, (6) a, (7) c, (8) a, (9) c, (10) d, (11) a, (12) d, (13) a (14) a, (15) a, (16) c, (17) c, (18) a, (19) c, (20) c.

10. CONCRETIONS

Q. 1 (1) Calculi, fibrin, mucus, desquamated epithelial cells, bacterial clumps (2) Calcium phosphate, magnesium phosphate, aluminium phosphate, calcium oxalate (3) cholecystitis, cholangitis obstruction of bile duct, post hepatic /obstructive jaundice (4) Colon (5) Dogs, bones

Q. 2. (1) F, (2) T, (3) F, (4) F, (5) T.

Q. 3. (1) a, (2) c, (3) d, (4) b, (5) b, (6) d, (7) a, (8) b, (9) d, (10) a.

11. IMMUNITY AND IMMUNOPATHOLOGY

Q. 1. (1) Horse, pig, cat (2) Oil, wax, alum, aluminium hydroxide, increase (3) 7,900, 5, J-chain, Primary (4) Absent (5) Long, dendrites, lobulated, cytoplasmic granules (6) T-suppression, suppresses (7) 200-300 (8) IgG, IgM (9) Alteration, Immunodeficiency autoimmunity, hypersensitivity. (10) Suppression, drugs, diseases, deficiency of nutrition, neoplasm, environmental pollution, increased susceptibility to infections, vaccination failures, recurrent infections, occurrence of new diseases, neoplasms (11) Systemic lupus erythematosus, polyarteritis nodosa, glomerulonephritis, rheumatoid arthritis, opsonization, chemotaxis, phagocytosis (12) Macrophages T-helper cells, destruction, immunosuppression, lymphadenopathy, lymphocytolysis, reduction in lymphokine production (13) T-suppressor cells (14) Macrophages (15) Insecticide, weedicide, fungicide rodenticide, Immunopathology, immunosuppression, autoimmunity, hypersensitivity.

Q. 2. (1) T, (2) F, (3) F, (4) T, (5) F, (6) T, (7) T, (8) F, (9) T, (10) F, (11) F, (12) T, (13) F, (14) T, (15) F, (16) F, (17) T, (18) F, (19) T, (20) T.

Q. 3. (1) c, (2) d, (3) b, (4) c, (5) d, (6) a, (7) b, (8) d, (9) b, (10) a, (11) a, (12) c, (13) b, (14) c, (15) a, (16) b, (17) d, (18) d, (19) a, (20) a, · (21) c, (22) a, (23) b, (24) b, (25) d, (26) a, (27) b, (28) c, (29) c, (30) b.

12. PATHOLOGY OF CUTANEOUS SYSTEM

Q. 1. (1) Vesicle, stratum lucidum/ corneum, pustule (2) Erosion, excoriation, ulcer (3) Scaly, (4) Epithliogenesis imperfecta (5) Melanin, hormonal imbalance, testicles, pituitary gland.

Q. 2. (1) T, (2) F, (3) F, (4) T, (5) T, (6) T, (7) T, (8) T, (9) T, (10) T.

Q. 3. (1) b, (2) c, (3) b, (4) d, (5) a, (6) b, (7) a, (8) a, (9) c, (10) b.

13. PATHOLOGY OF MUSCULOSKELETAL SYSTEM

Q. 1. Clostridia, crepitating, gas, water/fluid (2) Monday, pain, sweating, unable to more, hardening. (3) Adult rickets, vit-D, calcium, phosphorus, softening of bones (4) Hormonal imbalance, copper deficiency/vit-c deficiency, atrophy (5) Osteopetrosis, increase (6) Bone, bone marrow, trauma, pyogenic bacteria, destruction, replacement, excessive growth of new bone (7) Callus (8) Joints, swelling.

Q. 2. (1) F, (2) T, (3) T, (4) T, (5) T, (6) T, (7) T, (8) T, (9) F, (10) F.

Q. 3. (1) b, (2) a, (3) d, (4) b, (5) a, (6) b, (7) b, (8) c, (9) b, (10) a.

14. PATHOLOGY OF CARDIOVASCULAR SYSTEM

Q. 1 (1) Lungs, left sided heart, juglar (2) Hypertrophy of myocardium, cyanosis (3) Low oxygen, dilation of heart, chronic passive congestion, sternal (4) Hardening, atherosclerosis, medial sclerosis, arteriosclerosis. (5) Hypercholesterolemia, hyperlipidemia, hypertension (6) *Corynebacterium ovis*, inflammation of lymph vessels, aggregation of lymphocytes, oedema (7) atherosclerosis, hypercholesterolemia/fatty streaks, plaques, lumen (8) Lipid, cholesterol, fatty acids, triglycerides, phospholipids.

Q. 2. (1) F, (2) T, (3) T, (4) F, (5) T, (6) T, (7) T, (8) F, (9) T, (10) F.

Q. 5. (1) d, (2) a, (3) a, (4) d, (5) d, (6) d, (7) a, (8) a, (9) b, (10) b.

15. PATHOLOGY OF RESPIRATORY SYSTEM

Q. 1 (1) Pneumonia, congestion, consolidation (2) Thickening (3) Fibrinous, hyaline membrane diposition, alveoli, bronchiole (4) Drenching, necrosis, gangrene (5) Granulomatous, tubercle, caseative, macrophages, epithelioid cells, giant cells, fibrous (6) Retrovirus, metaplasia, cuboidal, columnar, glandular (7) Moldy hay/ fungus, hypersensitivity pneumonitis, interestitial pneumonia, emphysema, hyaline membrane formation, hyperplasia, (8) Granulomatous, dust particles, sand, silica /beryllium, carbon/asbestos, anthracois, (9) Air sacculitis, *E. coli Mycoplasma gallisepticum*, avian reovirus, thickening of air sac wall, cheesy exudate (10) Tuberculous pearly disease, chylothorax.

Q. 2. (1) F, (2) F, (3) T, (4) F, (5) T, (6) F, (7) F, (8) F, (9) F, (10) T.

Q. 5. (1) b, (2) d, (3) a, (4) c, (5) b, (6) c, (7) a, (8) c, (9) d, (10) d.

16. PATHOLOGY OF DIGESTIVE SYSTEM

Q. 1 (1). *Spirocerca lupi* (2) Tympany, distended (3) Omasum, *Actinobacillus ligneiresi*, granulomatous *(4)* Braxy, congestion oedema, haemorrhage (5) Intestine, haemorrhagic, *E. coli, Bacillus anthracis, Salmonella* sp., Petechiae, echymotic (6) Chronic, proliferative, proliferation of fibrous tissue, infilteration of mononuclear cells, plasma cells, hardening (7) *Clostridium* sp. Coccidia (8) Hjarre's disease, *E. coli* (9) *Candida albicans, Turkish towel (10)* Diffused necrosis.

Q. 2. (1) T, (2) F, (3) F, (4) F, (5) F, (6) T, (7) T, (8) T, (9) F, (10) .

Q. 5. (1) a, (2) d, (3) c, (4) d, (5) d, (6) c, (7) a, (8) d, (9) c, (10) a(11) c, (12) c, (13) c, (14) b, (15) c, (16) a, (17) d, (18) d, (19) b, (20) c, (21) b, (22) c, (23) b, (24) a, (25) a.

17. PATHOLOGY OF HEMOPOIETIC AND IMMUNE SYSTEM

(1). Erythropoiesis, reduced vitality, erythropenia, leucopenia (2) Phagocytic cells, neutrophils, macrophage, chemotaxis, engulfment, killing (3) Macrocytic, normocytic, microcytic, normochromic hypochromic (4) Lysis, blood vessel, icterus, hemoglobinuria.(5) *Hemonchus contortus* (6) Iron, copper, cobalt, B$_{12}$, pyridoxine, riboflavin, folic acid, pale mucus membrane, weakness, decreased number of erythrocytes. (7) Increased, blood, infections, neoplasms.

Q. 2. (1) F, (2) F, (3) T, (4) F, (5) T, (6) F, (7) T, (8) F, (9) F, (10) T.

Q. 5. (1) d, (2) b, (3) a, (4) c, (5) d, (6) b, (7) d, (8) a, (9) d, (10) c.

18. PATHOLOGY OF URINARY SYSTEM

Q. 1. (1) Frequent, polyuria, diabetes insipedus, hormonal imbalance, polydipsia, wasteproduct (2) Harmful wasteproducts, urea, uric acid, creatinine (3) Diabetes mellitus, acetonemia, pregnancy toxaemia, starvation (4) Ochratoxins (5) Pesticides, immune complexes, glomerulonephritis (6) *Corynebacterium renale, Staphylococcus aureus, E. coli. Actinomyces pyogenes, Pseudomonas aeruginosa, corynebacterium. renale. (7) Chronic fibrosis, loss of glomeruli, loss of tubules, extensive fibrosis, glomerulonephritis, interstitial nephritis, arteriolosclerosis.*

Q. 2. (1) T, (2) F, (3) F, (4) F, (5) F, (6) T, (7) T, (8) F, (9) F, (10) T.

Q. 5. (1) b, (2) c, (3) b, (4) a, (5) c, (6) c, (7) a, (8) a, (9) a, (10) d.

19. PATHOLOGY OF GENITAL SYSTEM

Q. 1. Hormonal, follicular, sterility, continuous oestrus, nymphomania, lutein, pyometra, pseudopregnancy (2) Acute or chronic, pus, progesterone, lutein cyst /corpus luteum (3) catarrhal (4) *Trichomonas foetus, Brucella* spp, BHV-1, *Leptospira* spp (5) chronic, granuloma (6) BHV-1 virus, Epididymitis, Epi-vag.

Q. 2. (1) F, (2) T, (3) F, (4) F, (5) F, (6) T, (7) T, (8) F, (9) T, (10) F.

Q. 5. (1) d, (2) c, (3) d, (4) a, (5) d, (6) d, (7) a, (8) d, (9) b, (10) b.

20. PATHOLOGY OF NERVOUS SYSTEM

Q. 1. (1) Encephalomalacia, myelomalacia, (2) Inflammation, *Listeria monocytogenes,* congestion, haemorrhage, tiny abscess, necrosis, meningoencephalomyelitis (3) Polioencephalomalacia, leucoencephamalacia, microglial cells, satellitosis, neuronophagia, (4) Neurons, glial cells, myelin, medulla pons, mid brain, spongy form (5) Leptomeningitis, pachymeningitis.

Q. 2.   (1) F,   (2) T,   (3) F,   (4) T,   (5) F,   (6) F,   (7) T,   (8) F,   (9) T,   (10) T.

Q. 5.   (1) c,   (2) a,   (3) b,   (4) c,   (5) c,   (6) b,   (7) c,   (8) d,   (9) b,   (10) b.

21.   PATHOLOGY OF ENDOCRINE SYSTEM EYES AND EAR

Q. 1. (1). Diabetes insipedus, polydipsia polyuria, urine. (2) Somatotropic, gigantism, long bones, heavy and thick bones, hands, feet, skull bones (3) Enlargement, hypothyroidism, hyperthyroidism (4) Hypocalcemia, tonic spasms of muscles, infections, neoplasms, low calcium diet, hyper/ increased (5) Tuberculosis, histoplasmosis, amyloidosis, neoplasms, drug toxicity.

Q. 2.   (1) F (2) F,   (3) T,   (4) T,   (5) F,   (6) F,   (7) T,   (8) F,   (9) T,   (10) T.

Q. 5.   (1) b,   (2) c,   (3) c,   (4) d,   (5) d,   (6) a,   (7) d,   (8) b,   (9) c,   (10) a.

Index